WI
S22
Emm

D1628682

**Irritable Bowel Syndrome**

**DATE DUE**

# Irritable Bowel Syndrome

## Diagnosis and Clinical Management

EDITED BY

### Anton Emmanuel, MD

Senior Lecturer in Neurogastroenterology & Consultant Gastroenterologist
GI Physiology Unit
University College Hospital
London, UK

### Eamonn M.M. Quigley, MD, FRCP, FACP, FACG, FRCPI

Professor of Medicine and Human Physiology
Department of Medicine, University College Cork
Consultant Gastroenterologist, Cork University Hospital
Principal Investigator, Alimentary Pharmabiotic Centre
University College Cork
Cork, Ireland

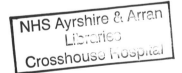
## ⊗WILEY-BLACKWELL

A John Wiley & Sons, Ltd., Publication

*Registered Office*
John Wiley & Sons, Ltd, The Atrium, Southern Gate, Chichester, West Sussex, PO19 8SQ, UK

*Editorial Offices*
9600 Garsington Road, Oxford, OX4 2DQ, UK
The Atrium, Southern Gate, Chichester, West Sussex, PO19 8SQ, UK
111 River Street, Hoboken, NJ 07030-5774, USA

For details of our global editorial offices, for customer services and for information about how to apply for permission to reuse the copyright material in this book please see our website at www.wiley.com/wiley-blackwell

*Library of Congress Cataloging-in-Publication Data*

Irritable bowel syndrome : diagnosis and clinical management / edited by Anton Emmanuel, Eamonn M.M. Quigley.
      p. ; cm.
   Includes bibliographical references and index.
   ISBN 978-1-118-53862-3 (pbk) – ISBN 978-1-118-44468-9 (obook) –
ISBN 978-1-118-44473-3 (Mobi) – ISBN 978-1-118-44474-0 (epub) – ISBN 978-1-118-44475-7 (ePDF/ebook)
   I. Emmanuel, Anton.   II. Quigley, Eamonn M. M.
   [DNLM:  1. Irritable Bowel Syndrome–diagnosis–Handbooks.   2. Irritable Bowel Syndrome–therapy–Handbooks.   WI 39]
   616.3′42–dc23

                                   2012029834

A catalogue record for this book is available from the British Library.

Wiley also publishes its books in a variety of electronic formats. Some content that appears in print may not be available in electronic books.

Cover image: iStock © David Marchal
Cover design by Andy Meaden

Set in 9.5/13pt Meridien by SPi Publisher Services, Pondicherry, India
Printed and bound in Singapore by Markono Print Media Pte Ltd

1   2013

# Contents

# List of Contributors

**Qasim Aziz, PhD, FRCP**
Director, Centre for Digestive Diseases
Blizard Institute;
The Wingate Institute of
Neurogastroenterology
Barts and the London School of Medicine and
Dentistry
Queen Mary University of London
London, UK

**Pamela Barney, MN, ARNP**
Research Nurse
Department of Biobehavioral Nursing and
Health Systems
University of Washington
Seattle, WA, USA

**Nicholas S. Coleman, DM, FRCP**
Consultant Gastroenterologist
Department of Gastroenterology
University Hospital Southampton
Southampton, UK

**Michel Dapoigny, MD, PhD**
Professor of Gastroenterology
Médecine Digestive, CHU Estaing
CHU Clermont-Ferrand, Université d'Auvergne
Inserm U 766
Clermont-Ferrand, France

**Douglas A. Drossman, MD**
Drossman Center for Education
and Practice of Biopsychosocial Care and
Center for Funpctional GI and Motility
Disorders
Adjunct Professor of Medicine and Psychiatry
University of North Carolina at Chapel Hill
Chapel Hill, NC, USA

**Hazel Everitt, MBChB, BSc, MSc, PhD**
Primary Medical Care
School of Medicine
University of Southampton
Southampton, UK

**Adam D. Farmer, PhD, MRCP**
Centre for Digestive Diseases
Blizard Institute;
Wingate Institute of Neurogastroenterology
Barts and the London School of Medicine &
Dentistry
Queen Mary University of London
London, UK

**Alexander C. Ford, MD, FRCP**
Senior Lecturer and Honorary Consultant
Gastroenterologist
Leeds Gastroenterology Institute
St. James's University Hospital
Leeds, UK

**Kok-Ann Gwee, FRCP, PhD**
Adjunct Associate Professor of Medicine
Yong Loo Lin School of Medicine
National University of Singapore;
Gastroenterologist
Gleneagles Hospital
Singapore

**Margaret M. Heitkemper, RN,
PhD, FAAN**
Professor
Department of Biobehavioral Nursing and
Health Systems
University of Washington
Seattle, WA, USA

**Monica E. Jarrett, PhD**
Professor
Department of Biobehavioral Nursing and
Health Systems
University of Washington
Seattle, WA, USA

**Gururaj J. Kolar, MD**
Division of Gastroenterology and Hepatology
Mayo Clinic College of Medicine
Rochester, MN, USA

**Ching Lam, MB BCh, MRCP**
Clinical Research Fellow, NIHR Nottingham
Digestive Diseases Biomedical Research Unit,
University of Nottingham
Nottingham, UK

**G. Richard Locke III, MD**
Professor of Medicine
Division of Gastroenterology and Hepatology
Mayo Clinic College of Medicine
Rochester, MN, USA

**Carolina Malagelada, MD**
Attending Gastroenterologist
Digestive Diseases Department
Vall d'Hebron University Hospital
Barcelona, Spain

**Juan-R. Malagelada, MD**
Associate Professor of Medicine
Autonomous University of Barcelona, Spain;
Digestive System Research Unit
University Hospital Vall d'Hebron
Vall d'Hebron University Hospital

**Stefan Müller-Lissner, MD**
Professor of Medicine
Park-Klinik Weissensee
Berlin, Germany

**Madusha Peiris, PhD**
Centre for Digestive Diseases
Blizard Institute;
Wingate Institute of Neurogastroenterology
Barts and the London School of Medicine &
Dentistry
Queen Mary University of London
London, UK

**Magnus Simrén, MD, PhD**
Professor of Gastroenterology
Department of Internal Medicine
Institute of Medicine
Sahlgrenska Academy
University of Gothenburg
Gothenburg, Sweden

**Robin Spiller, MB Bchir, MSc,
MD, FRCP**
Professor of Gastroenterology
Director, NIHR Nottingham Digestive Diseases
Biomedical Research Unit, University
of Nottingham
Nottingham, UK

**Jan Tack MD, PhD**
Translational Research Center for
Gastrointestinal Disorders (TARGID)
University of Leuven
Leuven, Belgium

**Hans Törnblom, MD, PhD**
Senior Consultant in Gastroenterology
Department of Internal Medicine
Institute of Medicine
Sahlgrenska Academy
University of Gothenburg
Gothenburg, Sweden

**Stephan R. Weinland, PhD**
Clinical Psychologist and Assistant Professor of
Medicine and Psychiatry
Division of Gastroenterology and Hepatology
UNC Center for Functional GI and Motility
Disorders
University of North Carolina at Chapel Hill
Chapel Hill, NC, USA

**Peter J. Whorwell, MD, BSc,
PhD, FRCP**
Professor of Medicine and Gastroenterology
Education and Research Centre,
Wythenshawe Hospital and University Hospital
of South Manchester
Manchester, UK

# Foreword

One of the last great medical mysteries waiting to be unravelled is MUPS, or so-called medically unexplained physical symptoms. Examples include the irritable bowel syndrome (IBS), functional (or non-ulcer) dyspepsia (FD), fibromyalgia and chronic fatigue syndrome. Disorders such as IBS and FD are remarkably common, impact on quality of life, often overlap and share a number of features in common including co-morbid anxiety or depression. Some attribute MUPS to somatoform disorder, itself a controversial entity. Yet is IBS really unexplained, or are gut biological markers emerging? Is it a psychological disorder? Is a positive diagnosis of IBS possible or is the disorder still a diagnosis of exclusion? And, most importantly, what should you do when faced with a patient with this diagnosis? What treatments really work and what should you do first? Is a pathophysiologically tailored approach now the way to go? If initial therapy for IBS fails, what's next?

It is with great pleasure that I introduce this excellent new book on IBS. Dr Emmanuel and Professor Quigley are international authorities in the field. As editors they have brought together the cream of the crop in IBS, a veritable who's who in neurogastroenterology worldwide. The editorial team and authors have developed a refreshingly readable book; it presents a practical management approach. Impressively, in a relatively brief space the book summarizes the current state-of-the-art. The text is evidence-based and contains illustrative case histories, potential pitfall boxes, key points, management algorithms and useful web links that will guide you undertake best practice.

In my opinion, IBS has evolved into a particularly exciting field and translational research has exploded in this area in recent years. You will read about new hints in terms of the aetiopathogenesis (including genes, inflammation, infections and the gut microbiome). I predict the pathophysiological advances are so major that this is likely to translate into objective diagnostic testing and possibly curative rather than suppressive therapies. The role of diet has dramatically changed and increasingly fibre is now recognized to be far from the only option. I am impressed that new dietary approaches can provide striking relief for some sufferers. You will see why the mind–body connection is so important, with neurological signalling going in both the up and down directions; this may explain the overlap of IBS with other disorders, and why psychological treatments such as cognitive behavioural therapy are so valuable.

I commend the editors and authors for crafting this new book on IBS; its creation signals an approaching maturity in the field. Despite all the inherent difficulties studying a condition based on a characteristic symptom profile, translational research in IBS represents a triumph starting to bear fruit. While IBS has a bright future as evidenced by this book, I remain doubtful that the concept of MUPS will survive long term!

*Nicholas J. Talley, MD, PhD*
*University of Newcastle, Australia*

# Preface

Patients with irritable bowel syndrome frequently report unhappiness with their care and the manner in which their disorder is approached by healthcare professionals. These clinical experiences contrast sharply with the research arena, where our understanding of the condition is increasing rapidly based on findings in both laboratory and clinical studies. There is a need and an opportunity to bridge this clinical–research divide; thus the motivation to write this book. We consider ourselves immensely fortunate to have been able to recruit enthusiastic support for this project from what is truly an 'A-team' of IBS experts who have generously contributed to this book.

The book is intended to be of direct assistance in clinical practice. Each chapter includes information, tips and techniques that will help in your next clinic with an IBS patient. The book is structured to match this aim. There are four sections, the first of which is a necessary and complete introduction to the condition. Section two focuses on assessment – the importance of making a positive diagnosis, a practical approach to quantifying the condition and the increasingly important topic of the care pathway between general practitioner and specialist. The next section comprises a range of chapters focusing on state-of-the-art advice regarding treatment of specific symptoms and treatment modalities – it offers a review of established and more recent therapies. This segues into the final section, which addresses emerging areas of therapy in IBS.

We wish to express our deep appreciation to our colleagues in Wiley-Blackwell. From the initiation of the project through to the review of proofs we have been met with outstanding speed, clarity and vision from every member of an excellent team. The quality of presentation of this book owes as much to them as the content does to the authors.

*Anton Emmanuel and Eamonn Quigley*
*London and Cork, December 2012*

# PART 1

# Overview of Irritable Bowel Syndrome

# CHAPTER 1

# Definitions and Classifications of Irritable Bowel Syndrome

*Alexander C. Ford*

Leeds Gastroenterology Institute, St. James's University Hospital, Leeds, UK

---

**Key points**

- Irritable bowel syndrome is common.
- The condition can be difficult to diagnose.
- Physicians should try to make a positive diagnosis, without need for extensive investigation.
- Existing symptom-based diagnostic criteria for the diagnosis of IBS perform modestly.
- The Rome criteria have not been extensively validated.

---

## Background

Irritable bowel syndrome (IBS) is a chronic functional gastrointestinal disorder characterized by abdominal pain or discomfort, in association with altered bowel habit. The natural history of the condition is a relapsing and remitting one [1–4], with most sufferers experiencing episodes of exacerbation of symptoms and other periods where symptoms are less troublesome, or even quiescent. The prevalence of IBS in the general population varies between 5 and 20% in cross-sectional surveys [5–7], and may be influenced by the demographics of the population under study. For example, IBS is commoner in females [8, 9] and younger individuals [7, 10, 11], although evidence for any effect of socioeconomic status is conflicting [12–14]. The prevalence of IBS appears to be comparable among Western nations and those of the developing world and the Far East [7, 10, 15, 16], although there are fewer data available from the latter regions. Prevalence is also higher in those with coexisting functional gastrointestinal diseases [17], particularly dyspepsia and gastro-oesophageal reflux disease [18, 19], and other functional disorders, such as fibromyalgia and chronic fatigue [20].

At the time of writing, there is no known structural, anatomical, or physiological abnormality that accounts for the symptoms that IBS sufferers

---

*Irritable Bowel Syndrome: Diagnosis and Clinical Management*, First Edition.
Edited by Anton Emmanuel and Eamonn M.M. Quigley.
© 2013 John Wiley & Sons, Ltd. Published 2013 by John Wiley & Sons, Ltd.

experience, and it seems unlikely that there is a single unifying explanation for them. It is more plausible that a combination of factors contributes to the abdominal pain and disturbance in bowel habit. Proposed etiological mechanisms that may be involved in the disorder include altered gastrointestinal motility [21, 22], visceral hypersensitivity [23, 24], abnormal pain processing in the central nervous system [25, 26], dysregulated intestinal immunity [27], low-grade inflammation and altered gastrointestinal permeability following enteric infection [28, 29], imbalances in intestinal flora [30] and altered psychological state [31]. Irritable bowel syndrome also aggregates in families [32] but whether this is due to genetic factors, shared upbringing, or both is unclear.

Individuals with IBS are more likely to consume healthcare resources than those without gastrointestinal symptoms [33]. Up to 80% of sufferers may consult their primary care physician as a result of symptoms [34, 35], and the condition accounts for approximately 25% of a gastroenterologist's time in the outpatient department [36]. Diagnosing IBS can be challenging for the physician, due to the potential for overlap between the symptoms that sufferers report and those of organic gastrointestinal conditions such as coeliac disease, small intestinal bacterial overgrowth, bile acid diarrhoea, exocrine pancreatic insufficiency, inflammatory bowel disease and even colorectal cancer. Several studies have examined the yield of diagnostic testing for these conditions in individuals with symptoms suggestive of IBS [37–41], but clear evidence for the routine exclusion of any of these disorders, with the exception of coeliac disease, is lacking. Attempts to identify a biomarker for the condition have, to date, been unsuccessful [42].

As a result of this uncertainty, and despite recommendations made by various medical organizations for a diagnosis of IBS to be made on clinical grounds alone [43–46], many patients with symptoms suggestive of IBS will undergo investigation, in an attempt to reassure both the patient and the physician that there is no organic explanation for the symptoms [47]. However, once a diagnosis of IBS is reached it is unlikely to be revised following further investigations of the gastrointestinal tract for the same symptoms in the future [48], and the subsequent detection of a 'missed' diagnosis of organic disease, which may have been the underlying explanation for the patient's original presentation with symptoms, is unlikely [49].

Medical treatment for IBS is considered to be unsatisfactory, with patients representing a significant financial burden to health services. The annual cost of drug therapy for IBS has been estimated at $80 million in the US [50]. Placebo response rates in treatment trials for IBS are high [51], perhaps because there is no structural abnormality that can be corrected by successful therapy, and therefore any benefit following treatment is often assessed by an improvement in global symptoms, an endpoint that may be less objective than those used in trials conducted for organic diseases.

Despite this, there is evidence that fibre, antispasmodic drugs, antidepressants and probiotics are all more effective than placebo in the short-term therapy of IBS [52–54], although no single medical treatment has been demonstrated to alter the long-term natural history of the disorder.

The definition and classification of IBS are both of paramount importance to the management of sufferers. Accurate definitions allow physicians to diagnose IBS with confidence, hence reducing the costs of managing the condition to the health service. Whether or not this approach is cost effective is uncertain [55], but it should discourage physicians from over-investigating young patients who are otherwise well and clearly meet these criteria, and in whom the diagnostic yield of such investigations is likely to be low. It may also avoid unnecessary surgery in patients with IBS. Cholecystectomy, appendectomy and hysterectomy rates in IBS patients have been shown to be two to threefold higher than those observed in controls without IBS [56]. Classification of IBS according to symptoms allows the tailoring of therapy according to the predominant symptom reported by the patient, as well as the assessment of which of the existing, as well as novel, treatments are effective in particular subgroups of patients.

## Definitions of irritable bowel syndrome

Functional bowel disorders were described in the medical literature as early as the nineteenth century, but it was not until 1950 that the term irritable bowel syndrome was first coined [57], eventually replacing spastic colon or irritable colon syndrome as the accepted nomenclature. There were descriptions of case series of patients in the 1960s that studied the clinical features of the condition as well as reporting the prognosis [58, 59], but it was not until the 1970s that attempts were made to define the condition using the symptoms reported by sufferers.

### Individual symptoms in irritable bowel syndrome

Medical students are taught that up to 90% of diagnoses are made through obtaining a thorough symptom history from the patient. Subjects with IBS often report abdominal pain or discomfort that is relieved by defaecation, altered stool form (looser or harder), altered stool frequency (more or less frequent), a sensation of bloating or visible abdominal distension, a sensation of incomplete evacuation and the passage of mucus per rectum. The presence of these symptoms suggests a diagnosis of IBS and it has often been assumed that the more of them that are present, the higher the likelihood of the patient having IBS. However, there have been few studies that have examined the diagnostic utility of individual symptoms in predicting a diagnosis of IBS.

A recent systematic review and meta-analysis examined the accuracy of these individual symptoms in discriminating IBS from organic lower gastro-intestinal diseases [60]. Four studies reported on the presence of passage of mucus per rectum, tenesmus, looser stools at onset of abdominal pain, more frequent stools at onset of abdominal pain and abdominal pain relieved by defaecation [61–64], and three collected data on patient-reported visible abdominal distension [62–64]. Pooled sensitivity of these individual symptom items ranged from 39 to 74%, and pooled specificity from 45 to 77%.

This suggests that individual symptoms are only modestly accurate, at best, in terms of reaching a diagnosis of IBS. This may be due to differences in the perceived connotation of individual symptom items between patients, such that standardizing the meanings of these from one patient to another is difficult. In addition, it is rare that a physician uses only one item from the clinical history in reaching a diagnosis; more often, individual items are combined with other symptoms, as well as patient characteristics, such as age and gender. It is therefore not surprising that diagnostic criteria, consisting of a combination of symptoms, were developed; these are discussed in the following sections.

### The Manning criteria

In a now seminal paper published in the *British Medical Journal* in 1978 [63], Adrian Manning and colleagues collected symptom data from 65 unselected outpatients presenting to a gastroenterology clinic with gastrointestinal symptoms and followed these individuals up in order to record the ultimate diagnosis. They reported that four symptoms: distension, relief of abdominal pain with a bowel movement, looser bowel movements with the onset of abdominal pain and more frequent bowel movements with the onset of abdominal pain were all significantly more common in patients with an ultimate diagnosis of IBS. Another two symptoms: tenesmus and passage of mucus per rectum, were also more common in those with IBS, but the difference in frequency in individuals with and without IBS for these was not statistically significant.

These symptoms became known as the Manning criteria; they are detailed in Table 1.1. As a result of their findings, the authors speculated that the use of these symptoms to positively diagnose IBS may reduce the need for investigations to reach a diagnosis. As the total number of individual symptom items reported by the patient increased, the probability of the patient being diagnosed with IBS also increased. Despite this finding, the authors did not recommend, or validate, what specific number of these criteria should be used as a cut off to diagnose IBS, although three or more are most often used in clinical practice.

The utility of the Manning criteria in diagnosing IBS has been assessed in a recent systematic review and meta-analysis [60]. This identified three

**Table 1.1** The Manning Criteria.

| Year described | Symptom items included | Minimum symptom duration required |
| --- | --- | --- |
| 1978 | Abdominal pain relieved by defaecation<br>More frequent stools with onset of pain<br>Looser stools with onset of pain<br>Mucus per rectum<br>Feeling of incomplete emptying<br>Patient-reported visible abdominal distension | No |

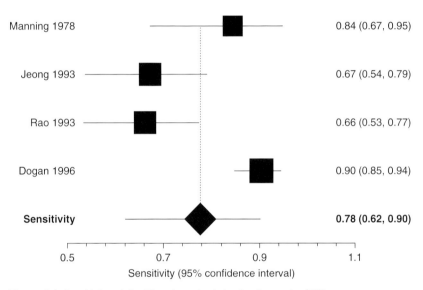

| | |
| --- | --- |
| Manning 1978 | 0.84 (0.67, 0.95) |
| Jeong 1993 | 0.67 (0.54, 0.79) |
| Rao 1993 | 0.66 (0.53, 0.77) |
| Dogan 1996 | 0.90 (0.85, 0.94) |
| **Sensitivity** | **0.78 (0.62, 0.90)** |

Sensitivity (95% confidence interval)

**Figure 1.1** Sensitivity of the Manning criteria in the diagnosis of IBS.

studies published subsequent to the original validation study [62, 64, 65]. In total, therefore, four studies containing over 500 patients have assessed the accuracy of these criteria in reaching a diagnosis of IBS. When three or more of the Manning criteria were used they performed modestly, with a pooled sensitivity for the diagnosis of IBS of 78% (Figure 1.1) and a pooled specificity of 72% (Figure 1.2). In terms of the individual studies identified, they performed best in the original report by Manning and colleagues [63], with a sensitivity of 84% and a specificity of 76%, and in a subsequent validation study conducted among 347 Turkish outpatients consulting with gastrointestinal symptoms [65], with a sensitivity of 90% and a specificity of 87%. Despite the continuing evolution of symptom-based diagnostic criteria for IBS, the Manning criteria are still in frequent use, both in clinical practice and research, more than 30 years after their original description.

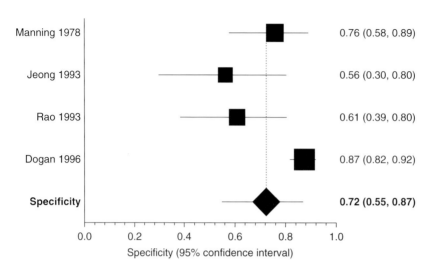

Figure 1.2 Specificity of the Manning criteria in the diagnosis of IBS.

**Table 1.2** The Kruis statistical model.

| Year described | Symptom items, signs, and laboratory investigations included | Minimum symptom duration required |
| --- | --- | --- |
| 1984 | **Symptom items (reported by the patient using a form)**<br>Abdominal pain, flatulence, or bowel irregularity<br>Description of abdominal pain as "burning, cutting, very strong, terrible, feeling of pressure, dull, boring, or 'not so bad'"<br>Alternating constipation and diarrhoea | > 2 years |
| | **Signs (each determined by the physician)**<br>Abnormal physical findings and / or history pathognomonic for any diagnosis other than IBS<br>Impression by the physician that the patient's history suggests blood in the stools | |
| | **Laboratory investigations**<br>Erythrocyte sedimentation rate > 20 mm/2 hours<br>Leucocytosis >10, 000/μL<br>Anaemia (Haemoglobin < 12 g/dL for females or < 14 g/dL for males) | |

## The Kruis statistical model

In 1984, Kruis and colleagues validated a statistical model to predict the likelihood of a patient having IBS [66]. The model used a combination of symptoms reported by the patient, signs recorded by the physician and laboratory tests (full blood count and erythrocyte sedimentation rate), with a score of 44 or more used as the cut off to define the presence of IBS. The individual items that are included in the model are detailed in Table 1.2. This model was applied to 317 consecutive outpatients seen in

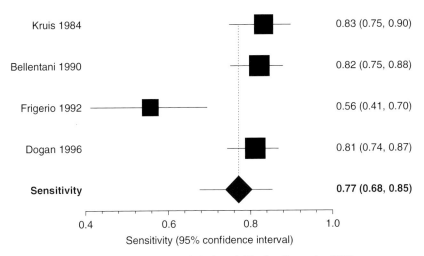

Figure 1.3 Sensitivity of the Kruis statistical model in the diagnosis of IBS.

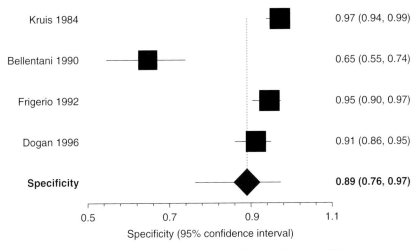

Figure 1.4 Specificity of the Kruis statistical model in the diagnosis of IBS.

a gastroenterology clinic. The authors reported that the sensitivity of their model was as high as 83% and that specificity was between 97 and 99%. Organic diseases were well-discriminated by the application of the score.

The aforementioned systematic review and meta-analysis of symptom-based definitions of IBS [60] identified a further three subsequent studies that had applied the model described by Kruis *et al.* to patients consulting with gastrointestinal symptoms [65, 67, 68]. This means that the accuracy of the Kruis model has been studied in a total of 1171 patients. The pooled sensitivity of the model in diagnosing IBS was 77% (Figure 1.3), with a pooled specificity of 89% (Figure 1.4). As with the Manning criteria, the Kruis model performed best in the original validation study [66]. The variables collected by the physician were more important than those reported by the patient, strengthening the argument for obtaining blood tests in patients consulting with suspected IBS. Combining four items self-reported by the patient with a basic history, physical examination and simple laboratory tests may hold significant appeal, as this mirrors routine clinical practice to some extent.

This greater accuracy compared with the Manning criteria may be because statistical models, such as that developed by Kruis and colleagues, reflect usual clinical practice more accurately, by combining several features from the clinical history. However, this finding could also be the result of the fact that the items in the model were validated as an integral part of the study process, with the final model being chosen on the basis that it best fit the study data. Such models require validation in populations other than the one used to generate the model – hence the need for prospective validation studies of symptom-based diagnostic criteria. Certainly in two of the three subsequent studies conducted, the Kruis model performed with similar accuracy to that reported in the original study.

One of the variables in the Kruis statistical model, symptom duration of more than two years, probably explains some of its accuracy, as this is likely to be a highly efficient way of ruling out serious underlying pathology. It would be self-evident to most physicians that any process that has been of this duration, with no organic cause detected previously, is likely to be functional in origin. Other limitations of the model include the fact that several of the symptom items were not clearly defined, such as 'irregularities of bowel habit' and 'alternating constipation and diarrhoea', whilst others are open to numerous interpretations, including the descriptions of abdominal pain and stool properties provided. In addition, despite its improved accuracy, the Kruis model seems rather unwieldy for routine clinical use.

### The Rome criteria
The groups of symptoms that, together, are thought to make up IBS tend to cluster together and have demonstrated statistically significant associations with each other in community-based factor analysis studies [69–71], lending weight to the biological plausibility of IBS as a distinct clinical entity. It was these observations that first led to a group of multinational experts convening to produce a consensus document on all of the functional gastrointestinal disorders [72]. This led to the development of the Rome process, and the first iteration of a set of new diagnostic criteria for IBS, dubbed the Rome I criteria (Table 1.3), were born. These criteria have been revised on two subsequent occasions, to produce the Rome II and Rome III criteria (Table 1.3) [73, 74].

The Rome I criteria have some similarities to those described by Manning *et al.*, although it was acknowledged that the change in stool frequency or

**Table 1.3** The Rome criteria.

| Iteration and year described | Symptom items included | Minimum symptom duration required |
|---|---|---|
| Rome I, 1990 | Abdominal pain or discomfort relieved with defaecation, or associated with a change in stool frequency or consistency, PLUS two or more of the following on at least 25% of occasions or days: Altered stool frequency Altered stool form Altered stool passage Passage of mucus Bloating or distension | ≥ 3 months |
| Rome II, 1999 | Abdominal discomfort or pain that has 2 of 3 features: Relieved with defaecation Onset associated with a change in frequency of stool Onset associated with a change in form of stool | ≥ 12 weeks (need not be consecutive) in last 1 year |
| Rome III (2006) | Recurrent abdominal pain or discomfort ≥ 3 days per month in the last 3 months associated with 2 or more of: Improvement with defaecation Onset associated with a change in frequency of stool Onset associated with a change in form of stool | Symptom onset ≥ 6 months prior to diagnosis |

form could be in either direction, rather than just more frequent and/or looser. Subsequent refinements to the Rome criteria have retained the three pain-related features originally described by Manning, but the presence of bloating or visible abdominal distension, tenesmus and passage of mucus per rectum are now no longer considered to be essential to, but may be supportive of, the diagnosis of IBS. Despite this modification, bloating is reported by up to 80% of IBS sufferers in cross-sectional surveys [75, 76]. Another difference between the various iterations of the Rome criteria and those of Manning is the requirement for a minimum duration and frequency of symptoms. This has become increasingly complex, with the Rome I criteria requiring a minimum symptom duration of at least three months, but the Rome III criteria requiring symptoms to have been present for at least six months and for the individual to have experienced symptoms on three or more days per month during the previous three months.

A recent systematic review and meta-analysis searched for studies that had attempted to validate the Rome criteria [60]. The authors identified only one study, published almost 10 years ago [77], which studied the Rome I criteria in 602 consecutive new referrals to a gastroenterology outpatient department in the United Kingdom. There were no studies identified that assessed the accuracy of either the Rome II or Rome III criteria for the diagnosis of IBS prospectively, despite the fact that the former had been published for eight years at the time this systematic review was conducted. In the study conducted by Tibble *et al.* [77], the Rome I criteria also performed only modestly, with a sensitivity of 71% and a specificity of 85% for the diagnosis of IBS.

The Rome Foundation has made great advances in our understanding of the functional gastrointestinal disorders. From a research perspective, the Rome criteria have become increasingly important over the last 20 years and have become the accepted gold-standard for diagnosing IBS. They have also been used to standardize the type of patients recruited into treatment trials for the disorder, and thereby reduce heterogeneity between study participants. This has led to an expectation that investigators conducting research in to any other aspect of IBS will use these criteria, or risk criticism of their study methodology. However, with only one published study validating any of the available iterations, this reflects poorly on the gastroenterology research community as a whole. Further validation studies assessing the accuracy of the more recent Rome III criteria are, therefore, urgently required.

A further issue that limits the usefulness of the Rome process is its rigidity. Its symptom-based classification of functional gastrointestinal disorders has become increasingly complex and the majority of these conditions are now mutually exclusive. This ignores evidence that there is considerable overlap among these various disorders. A meta-analysis demonstrated that the prevalence of IBS in individuals with functional dyspepsia was eightfold that in those without [19], and there was considerable overlap between the two conditions, no matter which of the various available symptom-based diagnostic criteria for each were used to define their presence. Another recent study examined the issue of overlap between IBS and chronic idiopathic constipation, evaluating the ability of the Rome II criteria to distinguish between the two disorders [78]. The authors suspended the mutual exclusivity of the two sets of diagnostic criteria and reported that this led to significant overlap between them, implying that IBS and chronic idiopathic constipation may be different subgroups within the same disorder. This calls into question potentially artificial divisions between the functional gastrointestinal disorders based on symptom reporting.

## A physician's opinion

It is argued that the Manning and Rome criteria are less relevant to physicians in primary care, as they have been developed primarily by gastroenterologists in secondary or tertiary care. One Scandinavian study that compared the degree of agreement between a general practitioner's diagnosis of IBS and that using the Rome II criteria reported only 58% concordance between the two [79]. A consensus panel suggested that existing diagnostic criteria were not sufficiently broad for use in primary care [80], and surveys demonstrate that few primary care physicians are aware of, or use, any of the existing diagnostic criteria to diagnose IBS, yet can still diagnose the condition with confidence using a pragmatic approach [81]. In a study conducted among Dutch general practitioners more than half thought that the cardinal feature of the condition was recurrent attacks of abdominal pain [82]. As primary care is the setting where the majority of IBS patients will present initially with symptoms, and be diagnosed and treated, this calls into question the ethos behind the use of such criteria to make the diagnosis of IBS. Unfortunately, there were no published studies reporting on the utility of a physician's opinion in making a diagnosis of IBS identified in a recent systematic review and meta-analysis [60], and guidelines for the management of IBS in primary care still advocate the use of available symptom-based diagnostic criteria [45, 83].

## Agreement between various definitions of IBS

Even though the Rome I and II criteria were derived from the Manning criteria, there are some differences between them that have already been discussed. In addition, the Rome I criteria only require the presence of one of the pain-related symptoms that make up the Manning criteria, whereas the Rome II criteria require at least two. Given the continuing evolution of definitions of IBS, it is important to assess the reproducibility of a diagnosis of IBS with one set of symptom-based diagnostic criteria compared with another. There have been several published studies that have examined this issue, with conflicting results. Overall, the prevalence of IBS appears generally higher when the Manning criteria are used to define its presence, perhaps because there is no minimum symptom duration required in order to meet diagnostic criteria [84–86]. There was generally good agreement between the Manning and Rome I criteria in two studies [85, 86], which is perhaps not surprising given the similarity of the definitions used in each. However, a third study that examined this issue reported a lower degree of concordance [84].

Agreement between Rome II criteria and those of Manning was less impressive [84, 85], and that for Rome I and Rome II criteria was of a similar magnitude [84, 85, 87]. These studies highlight that the continued refinement of the definitions of IBS reduces the overall prevalence of the disorder. This may lead to a proportion of individuals, who undoubtedly have gastrointestinal symptoms, no longer meeting diagnostic criteria for IBS when the more recent iterations of the Rome criteria are used. Instead these individuals have symptoms that are not able to be classified. This is probably not an ideal situation for either the physician or the sufferer and has led to some researchers to hypothesize that the later revisions of the

Rome criteria are too restrictive for clinical practice, and that perhaps those of Manning *et al.* should be preferred in this setting [84].

## Classification of irritable bowel syndrome

As has been discussed, when the Rome criteria were first proposed the pain-related symptoms required to fulfil a diagnosis of IBS were modified slightly from those of Manning *et al.*, to allow the change in stool form or frequency to include harder or less frequent stools, rather than only looser or more frequent stools as had originally been proposed. This adjustment has allowed the classification of IBS into subgroups based on the predominant stool pattern experienced by the patient. As a result, in the latest Rome III definition it is possible to classify IBS into diarrhoea-predominant (IBS-D), constipation-predominant (IBS-C), or those who fluctuate between the two, so-called mixed IBS (IBS-M). This is a useful approach for several reasons. Firstly, it allows the targeting of therapies by the physician towards the most troublesome symptom reported by the patient. Secondly, it aids the development of new pharmaceutical agents to treat these symptom subgroups discretely. Thirdly, it allows the investigation of patients according to these subcategories in order to explore possible underlying pathophysiological mechanisms, towards which future therapies may be directed.

From the year 2000 onwards there were a succession of randomized controlled trials of therapies for IBS that recruited patients according to the predominant stool pattern experienced [88–93]. These trials used agents acting on the 5-hydroxytryptamine receptor, which is thought to play an important role in gastrointestinal motility and sensation. Unfortunately, the drugs that were used in these trials, alosetron in IBS-D and tegaserod in IBS-C, have been withdrawn due to serious concerns about their safety. However, the principle of testing drugs in patients according to their predominant symptom has continued ever since, with drugs such as lubiprostone and linaclotide being tested in IBS-C [94, 95], the glucagon-like peptide analogue ROSE-010 being used in IBS patients with recurrent attacks of abdominal pain [96] and the efficacy of rifaximin, a non-absorbable antibiotic, being studied in patients with non-constipated IBS, but who reported troublesome bloating [97].

Whilst the classification of IBS according to stool pattern or the predominant symptom reported by the patient would seem a sensible approach, there are several potential limitations. Firstly, it has been shown that there may be a poor correlation between the stool frequency classification of the Rome criteria and diarrhoea or constipation as reported by the patient with IBS [98], leading to particular problems with the mixed stool pattern subgroup. Secondly, community-based cross-sectional surveys and case series of gastroenterology clinic patients with IBS consistently demonstrate that a significant minority of subjects with IBS, between 20 and 35%, will change their predominant stool pattern during extended follow-up [99–101]. Thirdly, in some sufferers gastrointestinal symptoms may either disappear altogether, or the symptoms alter to such an extent that the individual no longer meets diagnostic criteria for IBS, but does meet criteria for one of the other functional gastrointestinal disorders, such as dyspepsia, gastro-oesophageal reflux disease or chronic idiopathic constipation [2, 4, 101, 102]. Finally, terms such as constipation or diarrhoea are highly subjective. More objective measures such as stool weight have rarely been studied in IBS, and whether this is altered in patients with IBS-D or IBS-C is unclear [103, 104].

As a result of all this, it is therefore important that the patient with IBS is reassessed at regular intervals to ensure that they still meet criteria for IBS. If IBS criteria are still met, the physician should check whether the predominant symptom or stool pattern has changed. The inherent instability of bowel habit and of the most troublesome symptom reported that is part of the relapsing and remitting natural history of the condition suggests that relatively few patients will experience sustained relief of their symptoms with a single treatment regimen in the longer term. Despite these limitations of current classification systems for IBS, this approach remains a useful strategy for directing therapy, as well as for the testing of novel treatment agents in order to identify subgroups of patients which are likely to derive the most benefit.

## Conclusions

Irritable bowel syndrome is a highly prevalent condition in the community. Defining the condition using symptom-based criteria, in order to encourage physicians to make a positive diagnosis of IBS, thereby reducing inappropriate invasive investigation in patients who clearly meet these criteria, remains an important part of the management process. However, available symptom-based criteria perform only modestly in most cases. In addition, the current gold-standard for defining IBS, the Rome criteria, has not been extensively validated in prospective studies. This is concerning and needs to be addressed. In the absence of an accurate biomarker for the condition, we require either more studies recruiting groups of patients with gastrointestinal symptoms undergoing lower gastrointestinal investigation that apply the current diagnostic criteria to assess their accuracy in making a diagnosis of IBS, or studies that assess newer and potentially more accurate ways of detecting the condition. Ideally, any novel definitions that are developed should be equally applicable to physicians in primary and secondary care settings.

In terms of the classification of IBS, establishing the patient's predominant or most troublesome symptom is an important part of the effective management of the condition, and therapy should be tailored accordingly. However, the fluctuating nature of IBS should be borne in mind. Patients should be reassessed at regular intervals to ensure that they have not become asymptomatic, changed their predominant symptom or developed an alternative functional gastrointestinal disorder, and hence that the treatment that is being delivered is still appropriate. Further research based on these subgroups of IBS patients may allow us to discover new pathophysiological mechanisms that underlie this heterogeneous disorder, as well as develop new and more effective therapies against it.

## References

1 Agreus L, Svardsudd K, Nyren O et al. Irritable bowel syndrome and dyspepsia in the general population: Overlap and lack of stability over time. Gastroenterology 1995; 109:671–680.

2 Agreus L, Svardsudd K, Talley NJ et al. Natural history of gastroesophageal reflux disease and functional abdominal disorders. Am J Gastroenterol 2001;96:2905–2914.

3 Ford AC, Forman D, Bailey AG et al. Irritable bowel syndrome: A 10-year natural history of symptoms, and factors that influence consultation behavior. Am J Gastroenterol 2008;103:1229–1239.

4 Halder SLS, Locke III GR, Schleck CD et al. Natural history of functional gastrointestinal disorders: A 12-year longitudinal population-based study. Gastroenterology 2007;133:799–807.

5 Agreus L, Talley NJ, Svardsudd K et al. Identifying dyspepsia and irritable bowel syndrome: The value of pain or discomfort, and bowel habit descriptors. Scand J Gastroenterol 2000;35:142–151.

6 Hillila MT and Farkkila MA. Prevalence of irritable bowel syndrome according to different diagnostic criteria in a non-selected adult population. Aliment Pharmacol Ther 2004;20:339–345.

7 Hungin APS, Whorwell PJ, Tack J et al. The prevalence, patterns and impact of irritable bowel syndrome: An international survey of 40 000 subjects. Aliment Pharmacol Ther 2003;17:643–650.

8 Sperber AD, Shvartzman P, Friger M et al. Unexpectedly low prevalence rates of IBS among adult Israeli Jews. Neurogastroenterol Motil 2005;17:207–211.

9 Thompson WG, Irvine EJ, Pare P et al. Functional gastrointestinal disorders in Canada: First population-based survey using Rome II criteria with suggestions for improving the questionnaire. Dig Dis Sci 2002;47:225–235.

10 Lau EM, Chan FK, Ziea ET et al. Epidemiology of irritable bowel syndrome in Chinese. Dig Dis Sci 2002;47:2621–2624.

11 Hungin AP, Chang L, Locke GR et al. Irritable bowel syndrome in the United States: Prevalence, symptom patterns and impact. Aliment Pharmacol Ther 2005;21:1365–13675.

12 Howell S, Talley NJ, Quine S et al. The Irritable Bowel Syndrome has Origins in the Childhood Socioeconomic Environment. Am J Gastroenterol 2004;99:1572–1578.

13 Wilson S, Roberts L, Roalfe A et al. Prevalence of irritable bowel syndrome: A community survey. Br J Gen Pract 2004;54:495–502.

14 Minocha A, Chad W, Do W *et al*. Racial differences in epidemiology of irritable bowel syndrome alone, un-investigated dyspepsia alone, and 'overlap syndrome' among African Americans compared to Caucasians: A population-based study. *Dig Dis Sci* 2006;51:218–226.

15 Gwee KA, Wee S, Wong ML *et al*. The prevalence, symptom characteristics, and impact of irritable bowel syndrome in an Asian urban community. *Am J Gastroenterol* 2004;99:924–931.

16 Lule GN and Amayo EO. Irritable bowel syndrome in Kenyans. *East Afr Med J* 2002;79:360–363.

17 Drossman DA, Li Z, Andruzzi E *et al*. U.S. householder survey of functional gastrointestinal disorders. Prevalence, sociodemography, and health impact. *Dig Dis Sci* 1993;38:1569–1580.

18 Jung HK, Halder SL, McNally M *et al*. Overlap of gastro-oesophageal reflux disease and irritable bowel syndrome: Prevalence and risk factors in the general population. *Aliment Pharmacol Ther* 2007;26:453–461.

19 Ford AC, Marwaha A, Lim A *et al*. Systematic review and meta-analysis of the prevalence of irritable bowel syndrome in individuals with dyspepsia. *Clin Gastroenterol Hepatol* 2010;8:401–409.

20 Riedl A, Schmidtmann M, Stengel A *et al*. Somatic comorbidities of irritable bowel syndrome: A systematic analysis. *J Psychosom Res* 2008;64:573–582.

21 Cann PA, Read NW, Brown C *et al*. Irritable bowel syndrome: Relationship of disorders in the transit of a single solid meal to symptom patterns. *Gut* 1983;24:405–411.

22 McKee DP and Quigley EM. Intestinal motility in irritable bowel syndrome: Is IBS a motility disorder? Part 1. Definition of IBS and colonic motility. *Dig Dis Sci* 1993;38:1761–1762.

23 Moriarty KJ and Dawson AM. Functional abdominal pain: Further evidence that whole gut is affected. *BMJ* 1982;284:1670–1672.

24 Trimble KC, Farouk R, Pryde A *et al*. Heightened visceral sensation in functional gastrointestinal disease is not site-specific. Evidence for a generalized disorder of gut sensitivity. *Dig Dis Sci* 1995;40:1607–1613.

25 Bonaz B, Baciu M, Papillon E *et al*. Central processing of rectal pain in patients with irritable bowel syndrome: An fMRI study. *Am J Gastroenterol* 2002;97:654–661.

26 Mertz H, Morgan V, Tanner G *et al*. Regional cerebral activation in irritable bowel syndrome and control subjects with painful and nonpainful rectal distention. *Gastroenterology* 2000;118:842–848.

27 Chadwick V, Chen W, Shu D *et al*. Activation of the mucosal immune system in irritable bowel syndrome. *Gastroenterology* 2002;122:1778–1783.

28 Wang LH, Fang XC and Pan GZ. Bacillary dysentery as a causative factor of irritable bowle syndrome and its pathogenesis. *Gut* 2004;53:1096–1101.

29 Marshall JK, Thabane M, Garg AX *et al*. Intestinal permeability in patients with irritable bowel syndrome after a waterborne outbreak of acute gastroenteritis in Walkerton, Ontario. *Aliment Pharmacol Ther* 2004;20:1317–1322.

30 Kassinen A, Krogius-Kurikka L, Makivuokko H *et al*. The fecal microbiota of irritable bowel syndrome patients differs significantly from that of healthy subjects. *Gastroenterology* 2007;133:24–33.

31 Henningsen P, Zimmermann T and Sattel H. Medically unexplained physical symptoms, anxiety and depression: A meta-analytic review. *Psychosom Med* 2003;65:528–533.

32 Kalantar JS, Locke GR, Zinsmeister AR *et al*. Familial aggregation of irritable bowel syndrome: A prospective study. *Gut* 2003;52:1703–1707.

33 Talley NJ, Gabriel SE, Harmsen WS *et al*. Medical costs in community subjects with irritable bowel syndrome. *Gastroenterology* 1995;109:1736–1741.

34 Koloski NA, Talley NJ and Boyce PM. Epidemiology and health care seeking in the functional GI disorders: A population-based study. *Am J Gastroenterol* 2002;97:2290–2299.

35 Koloski NA, Talley NJ, Huskic SS *et al.* Predictors of conventional and alternative health care seeking for irritable bowel syndrome and functional dyspepsia. *Aliment Pharmacol Ther* 2003;17:841–851.

36 Harvey RF, Salih SY and Read AE. Organic and functional disorders in 2000 gastro-enterology outpatients. *Lancet* 1983;321:632–634.

37 Chey WD, Nojkov B, Rubenstein JH *et al.* The yield of colonoscopy in patients with non-constipated irritable bowel syndrome: Results from a prospective, controlled US trial. *Am J Gastroenterol* 2010;105:859–865.

38 Ford AC, Spiegel BMR, Talley NJ *et al.* Small intestinal bacterial overgrowth in irritable bowel syndrome: Systematic review and meta-analysis. *Clin Gastroenterol Hepatol* 2009;7:1279–1286.

39 Ford AC, Chey WD, Talley NJ *et al.* Yield of diagnostic tests for coeliaccoeliac disease in subjects with symptoms suggestive of irritable bowel syndrome: Systematic review and meta-analysis. *Arch Intern Med* 2009;169:651–658.

40 Leeds JS, Hopper AD, Sidhu R *et al.* Some patients with irritable bowel syndrome may have exocrine pancreatic insufficiency. *Clin Gastroenterol Hepatol* 2010;8:433–438.

41 Wedlake L, A'Hern R, Russell D *et al.* Systematic review: The prevalence of idiopathic bile acid malabsorption as diagnosed by SeHCAT scanning in patients with diarrhoea-predominant irritable bowel syndrome. *Aliment Pharmacol Ther* 2009;30:707–717.

42 Lembo AJ, Neri B, Tolley J *et al.* Use of serum biomarkers in a diagnostic test for irritable bowel syndrome. *Aliment Pharmacol Ther* 2009;29:834–842.

43 American College of Gastroenterology IBS Task Force. An evidence-based position statement on the management of irritable bowel syndrome. *Am J Gastroenterol* 2009;104 (suppl I):S1–S7.

44 Drossman DA, Camilleri M, Mayer EA *et al.* AGA technical review on irritable bowel syndrome. *Gastroenterology* 2002;123:2108–2131.

45 National Institute for Health and Clinical Excellence. Irritable bowel syndrome in adults: Diagnosis and management of irritable bowel syndrome in primary care. http://www.nice.org.uk/nicemedia/live/11927/39622/39622.pdf (accessed 6 October 2012).

46 Spiller R, Aziz Q, Creed FEA *et al.* Guidelines on the irritable bowel syndrome: Mechanisms and practical management. *Gut* 2007;56:1770–1798.

47 May C, Allison G, Chapple A *et al.* Framing the doctor-patient relationship in chronic illness: A comparative study of general practitioners' accounts. *Sociol Health Illn* 2004;26:135–158.

48 Adeniji OA, Barnett CB and Di Palma JA. Durability of the diagnosis of irritable bowel syndrome based on clinical criteria. *Dig Dis Sci* 2004;49:572–574.

49 Owens DM, Nelson DK and Talley NJ. The irritable bowel syndrome: Long-term prognosis and the physician-patient interaction. *Ann Intern Med* 1995;122:107–112.

50 Sandler RS, Everhart JE, Donowitz M *et al.* The burden of selected digestive diseases in the United States. *Gastroenterology* 2002;122:1500–1511.

51 Ford AC and Moayyedi P. Meta-analysis: Factors affecting placebo response rate in irritable bowel syndrome. *Aliment Pharmacol Ther* 2010;32:144–158.

52 Ford AC, Talley NJ, Spiegel BMR *et al.* Effect of fibre, antispasmodics, and peppermint oil in irritable bowel syndrome: Systematic review and meta-analysis. *BMJ* 2008;337:1388–1392.

53 Ford AC, Talley NJ, Schoenfeld PS *et al.* Efficacy of antidepressants and psychological therapies in irritable bowel syndrome: Systematic review and meta-analysis. *Gut* 2009;58:367–378.

54 Moayyedi P, Ford AC, Brandt LJ *et al.* The efficacy of probiotics in the treatment of irritable bowel syndrome: A systematic review. *Gut* 2010;59:325–332.

55 Martin R, Barron JJ and Zacker C. Irritable bowel syndrome: toward a cost-effective management approach. *Am J Manag Care* 2001;7:S268–S275.

56 Longstreth GF and Yao JF. Irritable bowel syndrome and surgery: A multivariate analysis. *Gastroenterology* 2004;126:1665–1673.

57 Brown PW. The irritable bowel syndrome. *Rocky Mt Med J* 1950;47:343–346.

58 Chaudhary NA and Truelove SC. The irritable colon syndrome. A study of the clinical features, predisposing causes, and prognosis in 130 cases. *Q J Med* 1962;31:307–322.

59 Waller SL and Misiewicz JJ. Prognosis in the irritable-bowel syndrome. A prospective study. *Lancet* 1969;2:754–756.

60 Ford AC, Talley NJ, Veldhuyzen Van Zanten SJ *et al.* Will the history and physical examination help establish that irritable bowel syndrome is causing this patient's lower gastrointestinal tract symptoms? *JAMA* 2008;300:1793–1805.

61 Hammer J, Eslick GD, Howell SC *et al.* Diagnostic yield of alarm features in irritable bowel syndrome and functional dyspepsia. *Gut* 2004;53:666–672.

62 Jeong H, Lee HR, Yoo BC *et al.* Manning criteria in irritable bowel syndrome: Its diagnostic significance. *Korean J Intern Med* 1993;8:34–39.

63 Manning AP, Thompson WG, Heaton KW *et al.* Towards positive diagnosis of the irritable bowel. *BMJ* 1978;277:653–654.

64 Rao KP, Gupta S, Jain AK *et al.* Evaluation of Manning's criteria in the diagnosis of irritable bowel syndrome. *J Assoc Physicians India* 1993;41:357–363.

65 Dogan UB and Unal S. Kruis scoring system and Manning's criteria in diagnosis of irritable bowel syndrome: Is it better to use combined? *Acta Gastroenterol Belg* 1996;59:225–228.

66 Kruis W, Thieme CH, Weinzierl M et al. A diagnostic score for the irritable bowel syndrome. Its value in the exclusion of organic disease. *Gastroenterology* 1984;87:1–7.

67 Bellentani S, Baldoni P, Petrella S *et al.* A simple score for the identification of patients at high risk of organic diseases of the colon in the family doctor consulting room. *Fam Pract* 1990;7:307–312.

68 Frigerio G, Beretta A, Orsenigo G *et al.* Irritable bowel syndrome. Still far from a positive diagnosis. *Dig Dis Sci* 1992;37:164–167.

69 Talley NJ, Boyce P and Jones M. Identification of distinct upper and lower gastrointestinal symptom groupings in an urban population. *Gut* 1998;42:690–695.

70 Taub E, Cuevas JL, Cook EW *et al.* Irritable bowel syndrome defined by factor analysis. Gender and race comparisons. *Dig Dis Sci* 1995;40:2647–2655.

71 Whitehead WE, Crowell MD, Bosmajian L *et al.* Existence of irritable bowel syndrome supported by factor analysis of symptoms in two community samples. *Gastroenterology* 1990;98:336–340.

72 Drossman DA, Thompson WG and Talley NJ. Identification of sub-groups of functional gastrointestinal disorders. *Gastroenterology Intl* 1990;3:159–172.

73 Longstreth GF, Thompson WG, Chey WD *et al.* Functional bowel disorders. *Gastroenterology* 2006;130:1480–1491.

74 Thompson WG, Longstreth GF, Drossman DA *et al.* Functional bowel disorders and functional abdominal pain. *Gut* 1999;45(suppl II):II43–II47.

75 Chang L, Lee OY, Naliboff B *et al.* Sensation of bloating and visible abdominal distension in patients with irritable bowel syndrome. *Am J Gastroenterol* 2001;96:3341–3347.

76 Ringel Y, Williams RE, Kalilani L *et al.* Prevalence, characteristics, and impact of bloating symptoms in patients with irritable bowel syndrome. *Clin Gastroenterol Hepatol* 2009;7:68–72.

77  Tibble JA, Sigthorsson G, Foster R *et al*. Use of surrogate markers of inflammation and Rome criteria to distinguish organic from nonorganic intestinal disease. *Gastroenterology* 2002;123:450–460.

78  Wong RK, Palsson O, Turner MJ *et al*. Inability of the Rome III criteria to distinguish functional constipation from constipation-subtype irritable bowel syndrome. *Am J Gastroenterol* 2010;105:2228–2234.

79  Vandvik PO, Aabakken L and Farup PG. Diagnosing irritable bowel syndrome: Poor agreement between general practitioners and the Rome II criteria. *Scand J Gastroenterol* 2004;39:448–453.

80  Rubin G, de Wit N, Meineche-Schmidt V *et al*. The diagnosis of IBS in primary care: Consensus development using nominal group technique. *Fam Pract* 2006;23:687–692.

81  Thompson WG, Heaton KW, Smyth GT *et al*. Irritable bowel syndrome: The view from general practice. *Eur J Gastroenterol Hepatol* 1997;9:689–692.

82  Bijkerk CJ, de Wit NJ, Stalman WA *et al*. Irritable bowel syndrome in primary care: The patients' and doctors' views on symptoms, etiology and management. *Can J Gastroenterol* 2003;17:363–368.

83  Paterson WG, Thompson WG, Vanner SJ *et al*. Recommendations for the management of irritable bowel syndrome in family practice. *IBS Consensus Conference Participants. CMAJ* 1999;161:154–160.

84  Boyce PM, Koloski NA and Talley NJ. Irritable bowel syndrome according to varying diagnostic criteria: Are the new Rome II criteria unnecessarily restrictive for research and practice? *Am J Gastroenterol* 2000;95:3176–3183.

85  Mearin F, Badia X, Balboa A *et al*. Irritable bowel syndrome prevalence varies enormously depending on the employed diagnostic criteria: Comparison of Rome II versus previous criteria in a general population. *Scand J Gastroenterol* 2001;36:1155–1161.

86  Saito YA, Locke GR, Talley NJ *et al*. A comparison of the Rome and Manning criteria for case identification in epidemiological investigations of irritable bowel syndrome. *Am J Gastroenterol* 2000;95:2816–2824.

87  Mearin F, Roset M, Badia X *et al*. Splitting irritable bowel syndrome: From original Rome to Rome II criteria. *Am J Gastroenterol* 2004;99:122–130.

88  Muller-Lissner SA, Fumagalli I, Bardhan KD *et al*. Tegaserod, a 5-HT$_4$ receptor partial agonist, relieves symptoms in irritable bowel syndrome patients with abdominal pain, bloating and constipation. *Aliment Pharmacol Ther* 2001;15:1655–1666.

89  Novick J, Miner P, Krause R *et al*. A randomized, double-blind, placebo-controlled trial of tegaserod in female patients suffering from irritable bowel syndrome with constipation. *Aliment Pharmacol Ther* 2002;16:1877–1888.

90  Kellow J, Lee OY, Chang FY *et al*. An Asia-Pacific, double-blind, placebo-controlled, randomised study to evaluate the efficacy, safety, and tolerability of tegaserod in patients with irritable bowel syndrome. *Gut* 2003;52:671–676.

91  Camilleri M, Northcutt AR, Kong S *et al*. Efficacy and safety of alosetron in women with irritable bowel syndrome: A randomised, placebo-controlled trial. *Lancet* 2000;355:1035–1040.

92  Bardhan KD, Bodemar G, Geldof H *et al*. A double-blind, randomized, placebo-controlled dose-ranging study to evaluate the efficacy of alosetron in the treatment of irritable bowel syndrome. *Aliment Pharmacol Ther* 2000;14:23–34.

93  Camilleri M, Chey WY, Mayer EA *et al*. A randomized controlled clinical trial of the serotonin type 3 receptor antagonist alosetron in women with diarrhea-predominant irritable bowel syndrome. *Arch Intern Med* 2001;161:1733–1740.

94  Drossman DA, Chey WD, Johanson JF *et al*. Clinical trial: lubiprostone in patients with constipation-associated irritable bowel syndrome - results of two randomized, placebo-controlled studies. *Aliment Pharmacol Ther* 2009;29:329–341.

95 Johnston JM, Kurtz CB, MacDougall JE *et al.* Linaclotide improves abdominal pain and bowel habits in a phase IIb study of patients with irritable bowel syndrome and constipation. *Gastroenterology* 2010;139:1877–1886.

96 Hellstrom PM, Hein J, Bytzer P *et al.* Clinical trial: The glucagon-like peptide-1 analogue ROSE-010 for management of acute pain in patients with irritable bowel syndrome: A randomized, placebo-controlled, double-blind study. *Aliment Pharmacol Ther* 2009;29:198–206.

97 Pimentel M, Lembo A, Chey WD *et al.* Rifaximin therapy for patients with irritable bowel syndrome without constipation. *N Engl J Med* 2011;364:22–32.

98 Mearin F, Balboa A, Badia X *et al.* Irritable bowel syndrome subtypes according to bowel habit: Revisiting the alternating subtype. *Eur J Gastroenterol Hepatol* 2003; 15:165–172.

99 Drossman DA, Morris CB, Hu Y *et al.* A prospective assessment of bowel habit in irritable bowel syndrome in women: Defining an alternator. *Gastroenterology* 2005;128:580–589.

100 Mearin F, Baro E, Roset M *et al.* Clinical patterns over time in irritable bowel syndrome: Symptom instability and severity variability. *Am J Gastroenterol* 2004;99:113–121.

101 Williams RE, Black CL, Kim HY *et al.* Stability of irritable bowel syndrome using a Rome II-based classification. *Aliment Pharmacol Ther* 2006;23:197–205.

102 Ford AC, Forman D, Bailey AG *et al.* Fluctuation of gastrointestinal symptoms in the community: A 10-year longitudinal follow-up study. *Aliment Pharmacol Ther* 2008;28: 1013–1020.

103 Oettle GJ and Heaton KW. Is there a relationship between symptoms of the irritable bowel syndrome and objective measurements of large bowel function? A longitudinal study. *Gut* 1987;28:146–149.

104 Eastwood MA, Walton BA, Brydon WG *et al.* Faecal weight, constituents, colonic motility, and lactose intolerance in the irritable bowel syndrome. *Digestion* 1984;30:7–12.

## CHAPTER 2

# Epidemiology of Irritable Bowel Syndrome

*Stefan Müller-Lissner*

Park-Klinik Weissensee, Berlin, Germany

---

**Key points**

- Prevalence of IBS lies mostly between 5 and 15 % of the population.
- No apparent differences between the various regions of the world from which data are available.
- Slightly more women afflicted.
- In most patients, IBS remains stable over time.
- Infectious diarrhoea is the best defined risk factor.

---

## Introduction

The study of the epidemiology of irritable bowel syndrome (IBS) is hampered by several factors: for example (i) IBS is defined by symptoms and not by objective findings; (ii) these symptoms may vary over time and there may be a shift of symptomatology from IBS to other functional disorders [1]; and (iii) only a proportion of patients seeks medical help.

## Methodology

In this study, relevant publications were identified by repeated PubMed searches, the last performed in early 2011, and by hand search of the reference list of the respective publications.

## Prevalence in various populations

Nearly 50 papers with extractable data on the prevalence of IBS could be identified. These papers addressed different populations from all over the

---

*Irritable Bowel Syndrome: Diagnosis and Clinical Management*, First Edition.
Edited by Anton Emmanuel and Eamonn M.M. Quigley.
© 2013 John Wiley & Sons, Ltd. Published 2013 by John Wiley & Sons, Ltd.

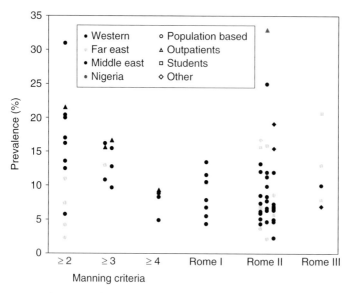

**Figure 2.1** Prevalence rates from the original studies on IBS epidemiology [1–47]. [Data are grouped according to the criteria applied to define IBS. Older studies used the Manning criteria, and IBS was diagnosed when at least two, three or four criteria were fulfilled, respectively. The data are grouped according to geographic region; forms of symbols are used to differentiate between different modes of data gathering. 'Western' denotes studies from North America and Europe, 'Far East' from Singapore, Malaysia, Korea, and China, 'Middle East' from Turley, Iran, Pakistan, and Bangladesh, respectively. 'Outpatients' denotes prevalence of IBS in samples from GP lists [19, 22] or among patients presenting for other reasons than IBS [25]. 'Other' denotes sampling by advertising or alike [21, 33]. All four samples consisting of students originate from the Far East [7, 23, 39, 47].]

world, used different diagnostic criteria, and the samples were of varying size. These data are summarized in Figure 2.1. The older studies applied the Manning criteria. As expected, the prevalence of IBS decreased the more Manning criteria that were required to be fulfilled to establish the diagnosis. Most of the older studies were done in the Western world. As can be seen from Figure 2.1, papers from Asia became more frequent in recent years following the publication of the second and third versions of the Rome criteria. The estimated prevalence of IBS covers a wide range, from less than 3% to more than 30% of the population investigated. One wonders, therefore, how this enormous spread of results can be explained.

## Type of diagnostic criteria

Some of the studies analysed the same patient sample with different diagnostic criteria (Figure 2.2). While it is obvious that more patients are classified as suffering from IBS when only two of the Manning criteria [48] have to

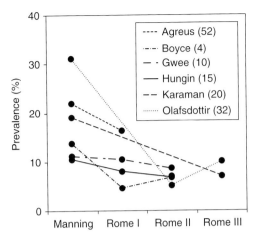

**Figure 2.2** Prevalence estimates of IBS in those studies analysing the same patient sample with more than one diagnostic tool [4, 10, 15, 20, 32, 52].

be fulfilled, there does not seem to be a systematic increase or decrease, respectively, in the number of IBS diagnoses whether Rome I, Rome II, or Rome III criteria are applied [49–51]. The type of diagnostic criteria used does therefore not explain the large spread of data from Figure 2.1.

## Recruitment of patients

Most of the studies used some kind of population based recruitment of participants, be it on the basis of resident lists, randomly selected telephone numbers or alike. Two studies used patient lists of General Practitioners [19, 22], a third study a sample of patients presenting for a problem other than IBS [25]. The latter originating from Nigeria exhibited the highest percentage of IBS patients (33%) and should be regarded with particular caution. Four studies from the Far East looked at students [7, 23, 39, 47]. Other studies made a 'systematic sampling of people in a city center' [20] or recruited by advertisements [21]. Both methods are in danger of a selection bias. However, when looking at Figure 1 it does not become apparent that the sampling technique had a systematic influence on the estimated IBS prevalence. Likewise the origin of the studies from the Western world, Middle East including Turkey, and Far East is without obvious effect on IBS prevalence.

## Age

The prevalence of IBS seems to slightly decline from the third decade to the higher age groups [16]. However, this has not been confirmed in all studies, at least not in females [31].

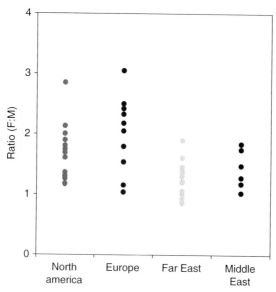

**Figure 2.3** Gender (F:M) ratio from the different studies. [When more than one diagnostic criterion was applied within the same study, the Rome II results were used. Data are grouped according to the geographic region. Numerically higher ratios are reported from the Western world [2–8, 10–15, 17–24, 26–28, 31–37, 39–43, 45–47, 53].]

## Sex differences

It seems to be common knowledge that IBS is more prevalent in females than in males. When looking at Figure 2.3 it seems apparent that this is particularly true for populations in the Western hemisphere. While the female to male ratio in North America and Europe is spread around two, it is about 1.2 in the Far East, about 1.5 in the Middle East, and close to one in Nigeria [25]. It seems conceivable that cultural differences between different regions of the world may play a role for this phenomenon. However, a meta-analysis was unable to establish a statistically significant difference between the figures of the regions.

## Reporters and non-reporters

It has also been known for quite a long time that many people in the community fulfil the criteria for IBS – whichever these are – but do not consult a health professional for these symptoms. Such people are called non-reporters, non-consulters or non-patients. The proportion of reporters also differs considerably between studies (Figure 2.4). There are no obvious differences between the respective rates from different regions of the world.

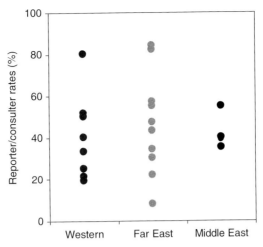

**Figure 2.4** Reporter/Consulter rates from the different studies. [Data are grouped according to the geographic region. There are no obvious differences; rates cluster around 40% [2–8, 10–14, 17–28, 31, 33–37, 39–42, 45, 46, 54–56].]

The mean proportion of reporters is around 40%, that is only two out of five people with IBS symptoms seek medical advice for this problem.

## Subtypes of IBS

The Rome III criteria incorporate an assessment of stool consistency as part of the subclassification of IBS [49–51]. On the basis of the form or appearance of the stools subtypes of IBS have been defined, namely constipation-predominant IBS, diarrhoea-predominant IBS and mixed IBS [51]. Quantification of consistency is usually done by the Bristol Stool Form Scale developed by Ken Heaton, the father of the Manning criteria [57]. Figure 2.5 visualizes the proportion of IBS subtypes in the studies where this distinction had been made. Again it does not seem possible to ascribe different patterns to geographic or cultural regions of the world.

## Fluctuation in severity

It is a common phenomenon in chronic diseases that the severity and/or frequency of a particular symptom or group of symptoms vary over time. Since patients usually do not present themselves to a doctor at a random time point but at the summit of symptom severity, a subsequent improvement is to be expected independent of any therapeutic measures which may be instituted [59]. This phenomenon is called 'regression towards the

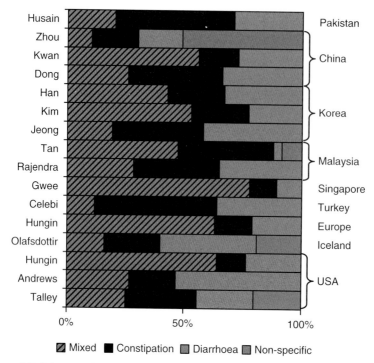

**Figure 2.5** Subtypes of IBS according to stool form. [The name of the first author and the country of origin are denoted at the left and right borders of the figure, respectively. No consistent pattern is apparent [2, 5, 7, 10, 11, 15–18, 23, 24, 32, 35, 42, 47, 58].]

mean' and has to be taken into account in therapeutic trials when trying to quantify the placebo effect. Waxing and waning of symptoms is a common feature also in IBS and is taken into account in the Rome criteria [51].

## Follow up

Only a few studies have followed a cohort of IBS patients longer than the duration of a therapeutic drug trial. A study of 400 IBS patients from Spain found only a minor improvement after a one year follow up [29]. This seems still compatible with a regression towards the mean. In a Swedish study in IBS patients the assessment was repeated after seven years [1]. From the original 1290 patients 1065 responded. In slightly more than half of these patients the symptoms had remained similar over the observation period, a quarter experienced only minor symptoms, 20% had become asymptomatic and a further 20% had switched to reflux disease or functional dyspepsia. Similar results were obtained in a study from Olmsted County with a follow up of 12 years [60]. In a study from Iceland the prevalence of IBS was 10% according to the Rome III criteria. After a ten year observation period, more than half of these patients no longer fulfilled the definition of IBS, while 8.7% of the total sample developed symptoms fulfilling the definition (incidence) [32].

## Post-infectious IBS

An interesting subgroup of the total IBS population is comprised of post-infectious IBS [61]. It develops in about 10% of people afflicted by an acute gastrointestinal infection [62] and is more likely than sporadic IBS to feature diarrhoea predominance [63]. Psychological traits such as anxiety, depression, somatisation and neuroticism were identified as risk factors for the development of post-infectious IBS symptoms [64]. These traits remained similar when re-evaluated three months after the acute illness and, hence, were probably not the consequence of the bowel infection.

Epidemic infectious diarrhoea after the contamination of a municipal water supply by *Escherichia coli* 0157:H7 and *Campylobacter jejuni* gastro-enteritis provided an excellent opportunity to study the development of post-infectious IBS [63]. Rome I criteria were met by 27.5% of subjects with self-reported gastroenteritis and 10.1% of controls. Independent risk factors for the development of post-infectious IBS included younger age, female sex, bloody stools, abdominal cramps, weight loss and prolonged diarrhoea. The likelihood of having IBS symptoms declined from a pooled odds ratio of 7.58 at three months after the index infection to 3.85 after 24–36 months [62].

## Other risk factors

Apart from gastrointestinal infections other risk factors for IBS have been identified, in particular, psychological traits. Somatisation, or health care seeking, may be learned in childhood if parents reinforce somatic complaints in their child, complain themselves of somatic symptoms, often seek health care, use sickness to avoid work or use sickness in conflict situations. This is called 'learned illness behaviour' and is a risk factor for IBS complaints in later life [65, 66]. Likewise, perceived stress and reported life events have been reported to be risk factors for IBS [6–70] but this has not been confirmed in all studies [71, 72].

Though there is a higher concordance for IBS in monozygotic than in dizygotic twins, the proportion of dizygotic twins with IBS who have mothers with IBS is greater than the proportion of dizygotic twins with IBS who have cotwins with IBS. Hence, while heredity appears to contribute to IBS, social learning may exert an equal or even greater influence [73].

An urban population seems to be at higher risk for IBS than a rural population, the prevalence being about twice as high [45].

## Summary

In summary, reported prevalence rates cover a wide range and the reason for this is not obvious. There is a trend towards a female predominance, at least in the Western world. Otherwise, neither geographical nor cultural factors seem to play a major role. IBS is stable over time for the majority of afflicted people. The most potent risk factor for the development of IBS symptoms is a gastrointestinal infection, such as traveller's diarrhoea, but psychological traits also play a role.

## Acknowledgement

I am grateful to Peter Schlattmann, PhD, Institut für Medizinische Statistik, Informatik und Dokumentation, University of Jena, for the statistical analysis of potential sex differences.

## References

1  Agreus L, Svardsudd K, Nyren O and Tibblin G. Irritable bowel syndrome and dyspepsia in the general population: overlap and lack of stability over time. *Gastroenterology* 1995;109:671–680.
2  Andrews EB, Eaton SC, Hollis KA *et al.* Prevalence and demographics of irritable bowel syndrome: results from a large web-based survey. *Aliment Pharmacol Ther.* 2005 15;22:935–942.
3  Boekema PJ, van Dam van Isselt EF, Bots ML and Smout AJ. Functional bowel symptoms in a general Dutch population and associations with common stimulants. *Neth J Med* 2001;59:23–30.
4  Boyce PM, Koloski NA and Talley NJ. Irritable bowel syndrome according to varying diagnostic criteria: are the new Rome II criteria unnecessarily restrictive for research and practice? *Am J Gastroenterol* 2000;95:3176–3183.
5  Celebi S, Acik Y, Deveci SE *et al.* Epidemiological features of irritable bowel syndrome in a Turkish urban society. *J Gastroenterol Hepatol* 2004;19:738–743.
6  Dapoigny M, Bellanger J, Bonaz B *et al.* Irritable bowel syndrome in France: a common, debilitating and costly disorder. *Eur J Gastroenterol Hepatol* 2004;16:995–1001.
7  Dong YY, Zuo XL, Li CQ *et al.* Prevalence of irritable bowel syndrome in Chinese college and university students assessed using Rome III criteria. *World J Gastroenterol* 2010;16:4221–4226.
8  Drossman DA, Li Z, Andruzzi E *et al.* US householder survey of functional gastrointestinal disorders. Prevalence, sociodemography, and health impact. *Dig Dis Sci* 1993; 38:1569–1580.

9 Ghoshal UC, Abraham P, Bhatt C *et al*. Epidemiological and clinical profile of irritable bowel syndrome in India; Report of the Indian Society of Gastroenterology Task Force. *Indian J. Gastroenterol* 2008;27:22–28.

10 Gwee KA, Wee S, Wong ML and Png DJ. The prevalence, symptom characteristics, and impact of irritable bowel syndrome in an Asian urban community. *Am J Gastroenterol* 2004;99:924–931.

11 Han SH, Lee OY, Bae SC *et al*. Prevalence of irritable bowel syndrome in Korea: population-based survey using the Rome II criteria. *J Gastroenterol Hepatol* 2006; 21:1687–1692.

12 Hillila MT and Farkkila MA. Prevalence of irritable bowel syndrome according to different diagnostic criteria in a nonselected adult population. *Aliment Pharmacol Ther* 2004;20:339–345.

13 Ho KY, Kang JY and Seow A. Prevalence of gastrointestinal symptoms in a multiracial Asian population, with particular reference to reflux-type symptoms. *Am J Gastroenterol* 1998;93:1816–1822.

14 Hoseini-Asl MK and Amra B. Prevalence of irritable bowel syndrome in Shahrekord, Iran. *Indian J Gastroenterol* 2003;22:215–216.

15 Hungin AP, Chang L, Locke GR, Dennis EH and Barghout V. Irritable bowel syndrome in the United States: prevalence, symptom patterns and impact. *Aliment Pharmacol Ther* 2005 1;21:1365–1375.

16 Hungin AP, Whorwell PJ, Tack J and Mearin F. The prevalence, patterns and impact of irritable bowel syndrome: an international survey of 40 000 subjects. *Aliment Pharmacol Ther* 2003;17:643–650.

17 Husain N, Chaudhry IB, Jafri F *et al*. A population-based study of irritable bowel syndrome in a non-Western population. *Neurogastroenterol Motil* 2008;20:1022–1029.

18 Jeong JJ, Choi MG, Cho YS *et al*. Chronic gastrointestinal symptoms and quality of life in the Korean population. *World J Gastroenterol* 2008 7;14:6388–6394.

19 Jones R and Lydeard S. Irritable bowel syndrome in the general population. *BMJ* 1992;304:87–90.

20 Karaman N, Turkay C and Yonem O. Irritable bowel syndrome prevalence in city center of Sivas. *Turk J Gastroenterol* 2003; 14: 128–131.

21 Katsinelos P, Lazaraki G, Kountouras J *et al*. Prevalence, bowel habit subtypes and medical care-seeking behaviour of patients with irritable bowel syndrome in Northern Greece. *Eur J Gastroenterol Hepatol* 2009;21:183–189.

22 Kennedy TM, Jones RH, Hungin APS, O'Flanagan H and Kelly P. Irritable bowel syndrome, gastro-oesophageal reflux, and bronchial hyper-responsiveness in the general population. *Gut* 1998;43:770–774.

23 Kim YJ and Ban DJ. Prevalence of irritable bowel syndrome, influence of lifestyle factors and bowel habits in Korean college students. *Int J Nurs Stud* 2005;42: 247–254.

24 Kwan AC, Hu WH, Chan YK *et al*. Prevalence of irritable bowel syndrome in Hong Kong. *J Gastroenterol Hepatol* 2002;17:1180–1186.

25 Ladep NG, Okeke EN, Samaila AA *et al*. Irritable bowel syndrome among patients attending General Outpatients' clinics in Jos, Nigeria. *Eur J Gastroenterol Hepatol* 2007;19:795–799.

26 Lau EM, Chan FK, Ziea ET *et al*. Epidemiology of irritable bowel syndrome in Chinese. *Dig Dis Sci* 2002;47:2621–2624.

27 Li FX, Patten SB, Hilsden RJ and Sutherland LR. Irritable bowel syndrome and health-related quality of life: a population-based study in Calgary, Alberta. *Can J Gastroenterol* 2003;17:259–263.

28  Masud MA, Hasan M and Khan AK. Irritable bowel syndrome in a rural community in Bangladesh: prevalence, symptoms pattern, and health care seeking behavior. *Am J Gastroenterol* 2001;96:1547–1552.

29  Mearin F, Badia X and Balboa A. Irritable bowel syndrome prevalence varies enormously depending on the employed diagnostic criteria: comparison of Rome 2 versus previous criteria in a general population. *Scand J Gastroenterol* 2001;36:1155–1161.

30  Miwa H. Prevalence of irritable bowel syndrome in Japan: internet survey using Rome III criteria. *Patient Preference Adherence* 2008;2:143–147.

31  Oesterberg E, Blomquist L, Krakau I *et al*. A population based study of irritable bowel syndrome and mental health. *Scand J Gastroenterol* 2000;35:264–268.

32  Olafsdottir LB, Gudjonsson H, Jonsdottir H and Thjodleifsson B. Stability of the irritable bowel syndrome and subgroups as measured by three diagnostic criteria – a 10-year follow-up study. *Aliment Pharmacol Ther* 2010;32:670–680.

33  Park KS, Ahn SH, Hwang JS *et al*. A survey about irritable bowel syndrome in South Korea: prevalence and observable organic abnormalities in IBS patients. *Dig Dis Sci* 2008;53:704–711.

34  Perveen I, Hasan M, Masud MA *et al*. Irritable bowel syndrome in a Bangladeshi urban community: prevalence and health care seeking pattern. *Saudi J Gastroenterol* 2009;15:239–243.

35  Rajendra S and Alahuddin S. Prevalence of irritable bowel syndrome in a multiethnic Asian population. *Aliment Pharmacol Ther* 2004;19:704–706.

36  Saito YA, Locke GR, Talley NJ *et al*. A comparison of the Rome and Manning criteria for case identification in epidemiological investigations of irritable bowel syndrome. *Am J Gastroenterol* 2000;95:2816–2824.

37  Saito YA, Talley NJ, Melton J *et al*. The effect of new diagnostic criteria for irritable bowel syndrome on community prevalence estimates. *Neurogastroenterol Motil* 2003;15:687–694.

38  Shah SS, Bhatia SJ and Mistry FP. Epidemiology of dyspepsia in Mumbai. *Indian J. Gastroenterol* 2001;20:103–106.

39  Shen L, Kong H and Hou X. Prevalence of irritable bowel syndrome and its relationship with psychological stress status in Chinese university students. *J Gastroenterol Hepatol* 2009;24:1885–1890.

40  Talley NJ, Zinsmeister AR, Van Dyke C and Melton LJ III. Epidemiology of colonic symptoms and the irritable bowel syndrome. *Gastroenterology* 1991;101:927–934.

41  Talley NJ, O'Keefe EA, Zinsmeister AR and Melton LJ III. Prevalence of gastrointestinal symptoms in the elderly: a population-based study. *Gastroenterology* 1992;102:895–901.

42  Talley NJ, Zinsmeister AR and Melton LJ III. Irritable bowel syndrome in a community: symptom subgroups, risk factors, and health care utilization. *Am J Epidemiol* 1995; 142:76–83.

43  Thompson WG and Heaton KW. Functional bowel disorders in apparently healthy people. *Gastroenterology* 1980;79:283–288.

44  Thompson WG, Irvine EJ, Pare P, Ferrazzi S and Rance L. Functional gastrointestinal disorders in Canada: first population-based survey using Rome II criteria with suggestions for improving the questionnaire. *Dig Dis Sci* 2002;47:225–235.

45  Usai P, Manca R, Lai MA et al. Prevalence of irritable bowel syndrome in Italian rural and urban areas. *Eur J Intern Med* 2010;21:324–326.

46  Xiong LS, Chen MH, Chen HX et al. A population-based epidemiologic study of irritable bowel syndrome in South China: stratified randomized study by cluster sampling. *Aliment Pharmacol Ther* 2004;19:1217–11224.

47  Zhou H, Li D, Cheng G *et al*. An epidemiologic study of irritable bowel syndrome in adolescents and children in South China: a school-based study. *Child: care, health and development* 2010;36:781–786.

48  Manning AP, Thompson WG, Heaton KW and Morris AF: Towards positive diagnosis of the irritable bowel. *BMJ* 1978,2:653–654.

49  Thompson WG, Creed F, Drossman DA et al. Functional bowel disorders and chronic functional abdominal pain. *Gastroenterology International* 1992;5:75–91.

50  Thompson WG, Longstreth GF, Drossman DA *et al*. Functional bowel disorders and functional abdominal pain. *Gut* 1999;45(Suppl. 2):II43–II47.

51  Longstreth GF, Thompson WG, Chey WD *et al*. Functional Bowel Disorders. *Gastroenterology* 2006 130:1480–1491.

52  Agreus L, Talley NJ, Svardsudd K *et al*. Identifying dyspepsia and irritable bowel syndrome: The value of pain or discomfort, and bowel habit descriptors. *Scand J Gastroenterol* 2000; 35:142–151.

53  Ruigomez A, Wallander MA, Johansson S and Garcia Rodriguez LA. One-year follow-up of newly diagnosed irritable bowel syndrome patients. *Aliment Pharmacol Ther* 1999;13:1097–1102.

54  Frexinos J, Denis P, Allemand H *et al*. Etude descriptive des symptomes fonctionelles digestives dans la population generale francaise. *Gastroenterol Clin Biol* 1998;22:85–791.

55  Hu WHC, Wong WM, Lam CLK *et al*. Anxiety but not depression determines health care-seeking behaviour in Chinese patients with dyspepsia and irritable bowel syndrome: a population-based study. *Aliment Pharmacol Therap* 2002;16:2081–2088.

56  Lu CL, Chen CY, Lang HC *et al*. Current patterns of irritable bowel syndrome in Taiwan: the Rome II questionnaire on a Chinese population. *Aliment Pharmacol Ther* 2003;18:1159–1169.

57  Lewis SJ and Heaton KW. Stool form scale as a useful guide to intestinal transit time. *Scand J Gastroenterol* 1997; 32:920–924.

58  Tan YM, Goh KL, Muhidayah R *et al*. Prevalence of irritable bowel syndrome in young adult Malaysians: a survey among medical students. *J Gastroenterol Hepatol* 2003;18:1412–1416.

59  Ragnarsson G and Bodemar G. Pain is temporally related to eating but not to defecation in the irritable bowel syndrome (IBS). Patients' description of diarrhoea, constipation and symptom variation during a prospective 6-week study. *Eur J Gastroenterol Hepatol* 1998;10:415–421.

60  Halder SL, Locke GR, Schleck CD *et al*. Natural history of functional gastrointestinal disorders: a 12-year longitudinal population-based study. *Gastroenterology* 2007;133: 799–807.

61  Halvorson HA, Schlett CD and Riddle MS. Postinfectious irritable bowel syndrome – a meta-analysis. *Am J Gastroenterol* 2006;101:1894–1899.

62  Thabane M, Simunovic M, Akhtar-Danesh N *et al*. An outbreak of acute bacterial gastroenteritis is associated with an increased incidence of irritable bowel syndrome in children. *Am J Gastroenterol* 2010;105:933–939.

63  Marshall JK, Thabane M, Garg AX *et al*. Incidence and Epidemiology of Irritable Bowel Syndrome After a Large Waterborne Outbreak of Bacterial Dysentery. *Gastroenterology* 2006;131:445–450.

64  Gwee KA, Graham JC, McKendrick MW *et al*. Psychometric scores and persistence of irritable bowel after infectious diarrhoea. *Lancet* 1996(Jan 20);347(8995):150v3.

65  Sandler RS, Drossman DA, Nathan HP and McKee DC. Symptom complaints and health care seeking behavior in subjects with bowel dysfunction. *Gastroenterology* 1984;87:314–318.

66  Whitehead WE, Winget C, Fedoravicius AS *et al*. Learned illness behaviour in patients with irritable bowel syndrome and peptic ulcer. *Dig Dis Sci* 1982;27:202–208.

67  Dancey CP, Taghavi M and Fox RJ. The relationship between daily stress and symptoms of irritable bowel: a time-series approach. *J Psychosom Res* 1998;44:537–545.

68 Drossman DA, Sandler RS, McKee DC and Lovitz AJ. Bowel patterns among subjects not seeking health care. Use of a questionnaire to identify a population with bowel dysfunction. *Gastroenterology* 1982;83:529–534.

69 Levy RL, Cain KC, Jarrett M and Heitkemper MM. The relationship between daily life stress and gastrointestinal symptoms in women with irritable bowel syndrome. *J Behav Med* 1997;20:177–193.

70 Whitehead WE, Crowell MD, Robinson JC *et al.* Effects of stressful life events on bowel symptoms: subjects with irritable bowel syndrome compared with subjects without bowel dysfunction. *Gut* 1992;33:825–830.

71 Drossman DA, McKee DC, Sandler RS *et al.* Psychosocial factors in the irritable bowel syndrome. A multivariate study of patients and nonpatients with irritable bowel syndrome. *Gastroenterology* 1988;95:701–708.

72 Suls J, Wan CK and Blanchard EB. A multilevel data-analytic approach for evaluation of relationships between daily life stressors and symptomatology: patients with irritable bowel syndrome. *Health Psychol* 1994;13:103–113.

73 Levy RL, Jones KR, Whitehead WE *et al.* Irritable bowel syndrome in twins: heredity and social learning both contribute to etiology. *Gastroenterology* 2001;121:799–804.

# Multiple Choice Questions

1  IBS may be subclassified into
   **A**  C-IBS, D-IBS, M-IBS.
   **B**  inflammatory IBS and non-inflammatory IBS.
   **C**  IBS with and without abdominal discomfort.
   **D**  acute IBS and chronic IBS.

Answer: A

2  The prevalence of IBS
   **A**  is remarkably similar in all studies irrespective of location of study
        or the nature of the study population.
   **B**  decreases when the Rome II instead of the Rome I criteria are applied.
   **C**  covers a wide range around an average of approximately 10%.
   **D**  increases in older age groups.

Answer: C

3  A risk factor to develop IBS is
   **A**  male sex.
   **B**  overprotective parents.
   **C**  a history of frequent urinary tract infections.
   **D**  being of East Asian origin.

Answer: B

4  The symptoms of IBS
   **A**  predictably deteriorate over time.
   **B**  predictably improve or even disappear over time.
   **C**  are sufficiently severe to lead nearly all afflicted patients to seek
        medical help.
   **D**  are common in the community among individual who do not seek
        medical help for their complaints.

Answer: D

**5** Post-infectious IBS
   **A** develops in more than half of patients with bacterial diarrhoea.
   **B** is not influenced by the presence or absence of psychological traits.
   **C** persists for the life of the individual.
   **D** its occurrence becomes more likely the more severe the initial diar-
   rhoeal illness is.

Answer: D

# CHAPTER 3

# Global Impact of Irritable Bowel Syndrome

*Eamonn M.M. Quigley*
Alimentary Pharmabiotic Centre, University College Cork and Cork University Hospital,
Cork, Ireland

---

**Key points**

- IBS is a global issue, although its true prevalence in many regions remains to be defined.
- IBS can exert a substantial impact on the individual and impair quality of life.
- The socio-economic impact of IBS is likely to be considerable, not only in terms of work and education but also on healthcare expenditure.
- Healthcare costs related to IBS are driven by a failure to recognize it as a distinct clinical entity, overzealous performance of unnecessary tests and poor therapeutic results.
- Healthcare costs may be subject to considerable local and regional influences which remain, in large part, unexplored.
- Future research in IBS should be more aware of the global dimensions of IBS and its impact.

---

## Global prevalence of IBS

Chapter 2 has dealt in detail with the epidemiology of IBS and has illustrated how global IBS truly is [1]. The global map of IBS is far from complete and, even where incidence and/or prevalence data are available, major challenges confront those who attempt to perform comparative studies. Among the factors that complicate such international or inter-regional studies are variations in the diagnostic criteria employed, the physical location of the study (i.e. whether performed in a hospital or clinic, in a primary care setting, in a health screening population or, truly, in the community), geographic location (i.e. urban vs rural), ethnicity, gender and age distribution, as well as social stratification of the population sample studied, personal, social and cultural influences, access to health care and local healthcare resources and, finally, the actual time of the study.

In the context of describing IBS global prevalence and impact, the impact of the definition(s) used to define this common syndrome deserves re-emphasis.

---

*Irritable Bowel Syndrome: Diagnosis and Clinical Management*, First Edition.
Edited by Anton Emmanuel and Eamonn M.M. Quigley.
© 2013 John Wiley & Sons, Ltd. Published 2013 by John Wiley & Sons, Ltd.

Although the Rome criteria have come to be regarded as the standard for defining IBS for clinical trials [2], they have not been as widely used in clinical practice, although strategies to promote their use are being developed [3]. Meanwhile, clinicians across the world employ clinical approaches more reminiscent of the Manning criteria [4] and the approach of Kruis and colleagues [5]. The latter is especially relevant to clinical practice by combining symptoms with some 'simple' laboratory tests. The issue of IBS definition is emphasized by the observation that epidemiological studies that used broader diagnostic criteria (e.g. 'diagnosed by physician' or Manning criteria) generally have produced higher prevalence figures compared with more restrictive criteria (e.g. Rome II) [6–18]. Furthermore, there is evidence that the criterion used may influence the demographics of a given IBS population; in Asia, for example, Rome III selects more females than Rome II [19]. Many other factors contribute to variations in IBS prevalence, demographics, presentation and impact both between and within populations such as study location [20, 21] and consultation and referral rates. The latter vary tremendously throughout the world [9, 22–31], with anywhere from 18 to 50% of sufferers seeking some form of medical attention and an even smaller percentage reaching a gastroenterologist, but the predictors for health-care seeking may vary on a global basis. Thus, while female gender is associated with seeking medical attention for IBS in the West [22], males may dominate among health-care seekers in the Indian subcontinent, as indicated in a community survey in Pakistan [30] and as can be inferred by striking differences in gender ratios for IBS between community and clinic-based surveys in India [32–34]. Furthermore, there is considerable evidence to indicate that 'consulters' differ in many ways from their 'nonconsulting' brethren in the community [35–43].

## Global impact of IBS

Studies from Europe and North America have extensively documented the impact of IBS on a variety of measures of quality of life [44–46] and have delineated, in some detail, the factors that contribute, in a given patient, to a greater or lesser impact of IBS symptoms on that individual's daily life [46–50]. It is clear that IBS has a similar impact on quality of life in the rest of the world although details on the factors that influence such impairment are less well defined [42, 51–56].

The socio-economic impact of IBS has also been examined, documenting both direct healthcare costs attributable to the assessment and management of IBS symptoms and indirect costs related to work absenteeism and presenteeism (reduced productivity among those at work) [46]. Relatively little is known of these important consequences of IBS in the rest of the world.

The spectre of missing a 'significant' lesion, such as cancer, and incurring the medico-legal consequences is an important driver of often unnecessary investigations and, thereby, medical costs in IBS. In Mexico, patients with IBS consume considerable amounts of such medical resources as laboratory tests and imaging studies, especially in the private sector, and it has been estimated that considerable savings (in the region of 90–94%) could be generated by limiting, in the appropriate clinical setting, investigations to such 'simple' tests as full blood count, erythrocyte sedimentation rate, blood chemistry, thyroid function and stool examination for ova and parasites and occult blood in the younger IBS patient. Similarly, limiting colonoscopy to those older than 50 years of age. Such a strategy would result in savings of between 56 and 63% [57].

While there is a reasonable amount of data on the natural history of IBS in the West, few such studies have examined the evolution of symptoms over time, the integrity of the diagnosis (and thus the likelihood of other diagnoses being made), mortality or morbidity in long-term follow up studies in other communities.

A serious (and not very well described) impact of IBS relates to its potential to impair the patient–doctor relationship. This is especially the case in primary care, where if symptom control is not effectively managed, the patient may doubt the clinician's credibility or diagnostic ability and, consequently, seek further opinions [58].

## Impact of comorbidity

A variety of gastrointestinal (functional dyspepsia, GERD [gastro-oesophageal reflux disease], noncardiac chest pain) and nongastrointestinal disorders (anxiety, depression, fibromyalgia, chronic pelvic pain, chronic fatigue etc.) have been linked with IBS in the Western literature and have been well documented in the rest of the world [59–67]. What is striking is the relative consistency of these associations wherever they have been examined throughout the world.

These associations are dealt with in detail elsewhere in this book; what is important to emphasize here is the impact that these comorbidities have on quality of life (QOL), consultation rates and use of medical resources. Thus Spiegel and colleagues, in the United States, found that extra-intestinal rather than intestinal symptoms were the main drivers of impaired QOL [68] and Rey and colleagues, in Spain, noted that hypochondriasis and anxiety were the patient factors most closely associated with impaired quality of life [69]. Furthermore, in Sweden, Ringstrom and colleagues noted that, whereas symptom severity alone was not predictive of consulting behaviour, consulters to primary, secondary and tertiary care had poorer

HRQOL (health-related quality of life), more severe psychological symptoms, higher levels of GI-specific anxiety and less adequate coping resources [43].

## Economic consequences of patient assessment

It stands to reason that any factor that promotes consulting behaviour will, in turn, escalate healthcare costs related to IBS. Similarly, a reluctance to make a clinical diagnosis of IBS on the basis of symptoms alone, or a relative lack of awareness of the existence of IBS as a distinct clinical entity, will promote more detailed, expensive and often unnecessary testing. Unfortunately, and despite the availability of detailed algorithms for the evaluation of IBS in the West [3], the clinician confronted with the patient with IBS-type symptoms elsewhere in the world has little guidance to assist him or her. Before one considers any diagnostic or therapeutic strategy, a major barrier that must be overcome in any attempt to develop global approaches is that of fully understanding symptoms and what they mean to the individual sufferer and/or patient in a given geographic, ethnic or cultural context. Not only do the relative prevalence and impact of the various symptoms that comprise IBS differ between regions of the world [70, 71], but also commonly applied diagnostic criteria assume that the clinical presentation of IBS is relatively homogenous.

While definitive approaches to the diagnosis of IBS are widely advocated and the futility of further testing illustrated by some studies and many reviews and guidelines, it is still common practice for the physician who first encounters the patient with suspected IBS to embark on a greater or lesser degree of laboratory and other investigation. Such tests may include full blood count, serum biochemistry profiles, ESR or CRP, tests of thyroid function as well as stool testing for occult blood and pathogens, ova or parasites; yet the evidence base to support this approach is scanty [44, 45, 72–77]. Even more expense is generated by the performance of imaging and endoscopy; here again there is little or no evidence base to support the use of contrast studies, ultrasonography or computerized tomography on the one hand, or colonoscopy, on the other, in the evaluation of IBS [78]. Furthermore, the use of radiological studies may result in excessive radiation exposure [79]. Considerable costs could be saved if testing was confined to those situations where they are indicated by patient features or presenting symptoms and where tests are relevant to local disease prevalence. Here again limitations must be confronted and, specifically, those of so-called 'alarm' symptoms [80].

In attempting to understand the potential impact of IBS on healthcare systems from a global perspective, attention must be paid to local and regional conditions that can influence testing strategies. In any given context clinicians will seek to exclude that which is common and may mimic IBS symptomatology and those conditions that they most fear 'missing'. With regard to the former concern, coeliac disease will be an important consideration in some areas whereas enteric infections and infestations will loom large in the differential diagnosis in others. In Uruguay and Argentina, where the background prevalence of coeliac disease is approximately 1%, serological screening for gluten-sensitive enteropathy is regarded as cost effective (Olano C, personal communication). This is an evolving issue, as rates of coeliac disease are now recognized as being much higher than previously thought in many parts of the world [9, 10]. Although some recent studies have questioned the assumption that coeliac disease is more common among those with nonconstipated IBS [81], such is the prevalence of coeliac disease in Europe and North America, and so non-specific are its presenting features nowadays, that this author contends that routine serological testing is justified among all with known or suspected IBS. Routine parasitological investigation is recommended only in those regions in which the prevalence of parasitic infestation in adults is high. Even then, these results need to be interpreted with caution. For example, while Entamoeba histolytica cysts are commonly found in the Middle East in faecal samples from both healthy subjects and IBS patients, these are noninvasive, do not lead to symptoms and should not, as is, unfortunately, often the case, lead to the prescription of anti-amoebic chemotherapy, a major waste of precious healthcare monies.

With regard to the second anxiety, that of 'missing something serious', background age-related rates for inflammatory bowel disease, colon cancer and other 'organic' conditions, coupled with the demographics of an individual patient, appear to heavily influence the approach to testing, as will access to care and availability of diagnostic modalities. In more affluent societies, elevated levels of physician anxiety (exacerbated, perhaps, by a litigious environment) coupled with the availability of sophisticated but expensive diagnostic hardware, result in excessive expenditures. There are several other examples of wasted effort in the assessment of IBS. For example, although rates of lactose intolerance (which may produce symptoms that may mimic those of IBS) vary considerably between different ethnic groups, the yield from lactose tolerance testing and the institution of lactose-free diets among those that truly have IBS, is minimal. The status of other approaches, such as defining the presence of small intestinal bacterial overgrowth [82] or bile acid malabsorption [83], is also unclear; here again, the indiscriminate use of such tests could add even further to the costs associated with IBS.

Cultural factors and patient expectations undoubtedly influence physician decision making in the assessment of the patient with IBS: a reluctance to accept that an illness which has such a detrimental impact on their daily life merits little or no investigation and the degree of reassurance gained by some through direct visualization of their gastrointestinal tract (by endoscopy), abdominal organs (by ultrasound) or overall well-being (by blood tests) may vary between cultures. Although negative test results seem to have little or no positive impact on patient well-being in the West, this may not apply elsewhere.

Depression and anxiety are common among IBS subjects and psychological factors may be associated with, amplify the symptom experience of, and, as already mentioned, contribute to impairment in quality of life and excessive use of healthcare resources in IBS [61–64]. However, there continues to be a considerable reluctance among gastroenterologists, in particular, to explore the potential contribution of these common co-morbidities. Clinicians must recognize the role of psychological factors and improve the assessment of psychological comorbidities; otherwise considerable time, effort and expense will be wasted on fruitless testing and inappropriate therapies. However, the approach to the detection, assessment and management of psychiatric comorbidity varies tremendously; from a virtually standard recourse to psychiatric consultation in Russia to a more common reluctance to engage with psychiatric colleagues except on a very selective basis in the West. Furthermore, in some cultures, the concept that IBS might have a psychological component and that formal psychological assessment and treatment approaches might be useful may be very unacceptable because of the stigma that surrounds any implication that they may be 'crazy' or 'mentally ill'. A denial by patient and clinician alike of the impact of anxiety and/or depression, if present, will undoubtedly further impact on quality of life, natural history and ultimate prognosis.

## Economic impact of management strategies

To understand the economic impact resulting from the various approaches to the management of IBS is a daunting task. It should come as no surprise that an inventory of the different approaches to the management of IBS around the world has not been compiled and, indeed, may be nigh impossible to achieve given the tremendous range of therapies, many not prescribed by medical practitioners, that are employed worldwide. Given the role of food in the precipitation of IBS symptoms (Chapter 8), the impact of variations in dietary habits and intake between different parts of the world deserves attention but has been scarcely addressed. It stands to reason that the management of IBS will be influenced by several factors including, but not restricted to, the range of therapeutic agents available (based on regulatory environment), culture (some cultures will have much more recourse to complementary therapies and alternative practitioners and other practices), access to care and other resource issues, as well as perceived or real differences in aetiology (e.g. use of antibiotics or antiparasitics).

In central Mexico, for example, over 50% of IBS subjects used some form of complementary and alternative medicine (CAM), with herbal medicine being the type most commonly used [84]. The use of complementary and alternative medicine in IBS [85] is common in many parts of the world, although little work has been done to investigate these approaches and their real impact. In Russia, spa therapy, homeopathy, herbal medicines and acupuncture are commonly employed. In Sub-Saharan Africa where a variety of dietary changes, dietary supplements and herbal medicines are commonly employed, sufferers commonly have recourse to traditional religious practices, such as making offerings to their ancestors, in an attempt to alleviate symptoms. Physician referral is, therefore, often delayed, as is the diagnosis of disorders such as cancer. In Uruguay, Yerba Mate tea, an infusion made from the leaves of the tree *ilex paraguariensis*, is commonly used as a remedy for constipation. In Western Europe and North America suffers commonly resort to a variety of 'allergy tests' of little or no validity and commence exclusion diets often featuring removal of wheat products as a consequence.

It is evident from a perusal of the literature that a given physician's approach to the use of various agents in the management of IBS owes as much to personal attitudes/beliefs as it does to clinical evidence of efficacy. For many of these compounds, the evidence base in the West, where most of these studies have been performed, is shaky; in the rest of the world, where IBS may well be quite different, evidence is either scanty or nonexistent. As a consequence, in many instances, the use of pharmacological agents in IBS is based primarily on studies performed in the West.

In some regions, there is a growing trend to use narcotics to manage pain in IBS patients and this trend is concerning. Long-term use of narcotics can cause increased sensitivity to visceral pain and disordered motility and, therefore, may worsen rather than solve the problem [86]. It is also of interest to note the high frequency with which acid-suppressive drugs, and proton pump inhibitors (PPIs), in particular [87], are prescribed for IBS.

It is evident from many surveys that many IBS sufferers self-medicate with the range of over-the-counter agents available to them varying widely from country to country. Nevertheless, probiotics, high-fibre products and 'antiflatulence' preparations, often containing activated charcoal or simethicone, seem to be commonly used. The 'real' costs of IBS, which do not usually take account of the monies spent by sufferers on these therapies are, in all likelihood, therefore, a gross underestimate.

## Conclusion

Although the available data are far from complete and fraught with issues that limit comparisons and definite conclusions, some trends seem clear: IBS is common worldwide and, with the possible exception of some Asian populations [71, 75], is most common among young adult females. One other theme is consistent: the impact of IBS on the sufferer is considerable worldwide and its comorbidities many [78]. Socio-economic costs, although poorly defined in most countries and regions, are likely to be considerable and owe much to the diagnostic uncertainty that surrounds IBS and the lack of universally effective therapeutic strategies. Yet, there is much to learn: of why IBS prevalence varies between populations and what risk factors may determine its occurrence in different regions. Above all, much effort needs to be expended on understanding the symptom complex that is called IBS in the West, how it is expressed in other parts of the world and in non-English languages and what impact it has on the individual, their family and society at large in various locations. Only then can the true global impact of IBS be defined; an outcome that must result in optimal and locally-tailored approaches to the definition, assessment and management of IBS.

# References

1 World Gastroenterology Organisation Global Guideline – Irritable Bowel Syndrome: A Global Perspective. 20 April 2009. http://www.worldgastroenterology.org/irritable-bowel-syndrome.html (accessed 8 October 2012).

2 Longstreth GF, Thompson WG, Chey WD et al. Functional bowel disorders. *Gastroenterology* 2006;130:1480–1491.

3 Spiller RC and Thompson WG. Bowel Disorders. *Am J Gastroenterol* 2010;105:775–785.

4 Manning AP, Thompson WG, Heaton KW and Morris AF. Towards positive diagnosis of the irritable bowel. BM J 1978;2:653–654.

5 Kruis W, Thieme C, Weinzierl M et al. A diagnostic score for the irritable bowel syndrome. Its value in the exclusion of organic disease. *Gastroenterology* 1984;87:1–7.

6 Boyce PM, Koloski NA and Talley NJ. Irritable bowel syndrome according to varying diagnostic criteria: are the new Rome II criteria unnecessarily restrictive for research and practice? *Am J Gastroenterol* 2000;95:3176–3183.

7 Pan GZ, Lu S, Ke M et al. Epidemiologic study of the irritable bowel syndrome in Beijing: stratified, randomized study by cluster sampling. *Chin Med J* (Engl) 2000;113:35–39.

8 Mearin F, Badia X, Balboa A et al. Irritable bowel syndrome prevalence varies enormously depending on the employed diagnostic criteria: comparison of Rome II versus previous criteria in a general population. *Scand J Gastroenterol* 2001;36:1155–1161.

9 Hungin AP, Whorwell PJ, Tack J and Mearin F. The prevalence, patterns and impact of irritable bowel syndrome: an international survey of 40 000 subjects. *Aliment Pharmacol Ther* 2003;17:643–650.

10 Xiong LS, Chen MH, Chen HX et al. A population-based epidemiologic study of irritable bowel syndrome in South China: stratified randomized study by cluster sampling. *Aliment Pharmacol Ther* 2004;19:1217–1224.

11 Gwee KA, Wee S, Wong ML and Png DJ. The prevalence, symptom characteristics, and impact of irritable bowel syndrome in an Asian urban community. *Am J Gastroenterol* 2004;99:924–931.

12 Sperber AD, Shvartzman P, Friger M and Fich A. A comparative reappraisal of the Rome II and Rome III diagnostic criteria: are we getting closer to the 'true' prevalence of irritable bowel syndrome? *Eur J Gastroenterol Hepatol* 2007;19:441–447.

13 Miwa H. Prevalence of irritable bowel syndrome in Japan: internet survey using Rome III criteria. *Patient Preference Adherence* 2008;2:143–147.

14 Dorn SD, Morris CB, Hu Y *et al.* Irritable bowel syndrome subtypes defined by Rome II and Rome III criteria are similar. *J Clin Gastroenterol* 2009;43:214–220.

15 Gwee K-A and Ghoshal UC. The Rome criteria divides, distorts and dilutes the prevalence of irritable bowel syndrome. *Saudi J Gastroenterol* 2010;16:143–4.

16 Olafsdottir LB, Gudjonsson H, Jonsdottir HH and Thjodleifsson B. Stability of the irritable bowel syndrome and subgroups as measured by three diagnostic criteria – a 10-year follow-up study. *Aliment Pharmcol Ther* 2010;32:670–680.

17 Park DW, Lee OY, Shim LG *et al.* The differences in prevalence and sociodemographic characteristics of irritable bowel syndrome according to Rome II and Rome III. *J Neurogastroenterol Motil* 2010;16:186–193.

18 Devanarayana NM, Adhikari C, Pannala W and Rajindrajith S. Prevalence of functional gastrointestinal diseases in a cohort of Sri Lankan adolescents: comparison between Rome II and Rome III criteria. *J Trop Pediatr* 2011;57:34–39.

19 Lee OY. Prevalence and risk factors of irritable bowel syndrome in Asia. *J Neurogastroenterol Motil* 2010;16:47–51.

20 Lix LM, Yogendran MS, Shaw SY *et al.* Comparing administrative and survey data for ascertaining cases of irritable bowel syndrome: a population-based investigation. *BMC Health Services Res* 2010;10:31.

21 Rubin G, De Wit N, Meineche-Schmidt V *et al.* The diagnosis of IBS in primary care: consensus development using nominal group technique. *Family Practice* 2006;23: 687–692.

22 Cremonini F and Talley NJ. Irritable bowel syndrome: epidemiology, natural history, health care seeking and emerging risk factors. *Gastroenterol Clin N Am* 2005;34: 189–204.

23 Rey E and Talley NJ. Irritable bowel syndrome: novel views on the epidemiology and potential risk factors. *Dig Liver Dis* 2009;41:772–780.

24 Masud MA, Hasan M and Khan AK. Irritable bowel syndrome in a rural community in Bangladesh: prevalence, symptoms pattern, and health care seeking behavior. *Am. J. Gastroenterol* 2001;96:1547–5152.

25 Kwan AC, Hu WH, Chan YK *et al.* Prevalence of irritable bowel syndrome in Hong Kong. *J Gastroenterol Hepatol* 2002;17:1180–1186.

26 Lu CL, Chen CY, Lang HC *et al.* Current patterns of irritable bowel syndrome in Taiwan: the Rome II questionnaire on a Chinese population. *Aliment Pharmacol Ther* 2003;18:1159–1169.

27 Wilson S, Roberts L, Roalfe A *et al.* Prevalence of irritable bowel syndrome: a community survey. *Br J Gen Pract* 2004;54:495–502.

28 Andrews EB, Eaton SC, Hollis KA *et al.* Prevalence and demographics of irritable bowel syndrome: results from a large web-based survey. *Aliment Pharmacol Ther* 2005;22:935–942.

29 Zuckerman MJ, Nguyen G, Ho H *et al.* A survey of irritable bowel syndrome in Vietnam using the Rome criteria. *Dig Dis Sci* 2006;51:946–951.

30 Jafri W, Yakoob J, Jafri N *et al.* Irritable bowel syndrome and health seeking behavior in different communities in Pakistan. *J Pak Med Assoc* 2007;57:285–287.

31 Moghimi-Dehkordi B, Vahedi M, Pourhoseingholi MA *et al.* Economic burden attributable to functional bowel disorders in Iran: a cross-sectional population-based study. *J Dig Dis* 2011;12:384–392.

32 Ghoshal UC, Abraham P, Bhatt C *et al.* Epidemiological and clinical profile of irritable bowel syndrome in India: report of the Indian Society of Gastroenterology Task Force. *Indian J Gastroenterol* 2008;27:22–28.

33  Makharia GK, Verma AK, Amarchand R, Goswami A, Singh P, Agnithori A, Suhail F, Krishnan A. Prevalence of irritable bowel syndrome: a community-based study from northern India. *J Neurogastroenterol Motil* 2011;17:82–87.

34  Shah SS, Bhatia SJ and Mistry FP. Epidemiology of dyspepsia in the general population in Mumbai. *Indian J. Gastroenterol* 2001;20:103–106.

35  Agreus L Socio-economic factors, health care consumption and rating of abdominal symptom severity. A report from the abdominal symptom study. *Fam Prac* 1993;10: 152–163.

36  Simrén M, Abrahamsson H, Svedlund J, Björnsson ES. Quality of life in patients with irritable bowel syndrome seen in referral centers versus primary care: The impact of gender and predominant bowel pattern. *Scand J Gastroenterol* 2001;36:545–552.

37  Jun DW, Lee OY, Jo GL *et al.* The comparison of irritable bowel syndrome between consulters and non-consulters. *Korean J Gastrointest Motil* 2005;11:50–57.

38  Ålander T, Svärdsudd K and Agréus L. Functional gastointestinal disorder is associated with increased non-gastrointestinal healthcare consumption in the general population. *Int J Clin Prac* 2008;62:234–240.

39  Kettell J, Jones R and Lydeard S. Reasons for consultation in irritable bowel syndrome: symptoms and patient characteristics. *Br J Gen Pract* 1992;42:459–461.

40  Heaton KW, O'Donnell LJ, Braddon FE *et al.* Symptoms of irritable bowel syndrome in a British urban community: consulters and nonconsulters. *Gastroenterology* 1992;102:1962–1967.

41  Koloski NA, Talley NJ, Huskic SS and Boyce PM. Predictors of conventional and alternative health care seeking for irritable bowel syndrome and functional dyspepsia. *Aliment Pharmacol Ther* 2003;17:841–851.

42  Si JM, Wang LJ, Chen SJ *et al.* Irritable bowel syndrome consulters in Zhejiang province: the symptoms pattern, predominant bowel habit subgroups and quality of life. *World J Gastroenterol* 2004;10:1059–1064.

43  Ringström G, Abrahamsson H, Strid H and Simrén M. Why do subjects with irritable bowel syndrome seek health care for their symptoms? *Scand J Gastroenterol* 2007;42:1194–1203.

44  Brandt LJ, Bjorkman D, Fennerty MB *et al.* Systematic review on the management of irritable bowel syndrome in North America. *Am J Gastroenterol* 2002;97(Suppl II): S7–S26.

45  Valenzuela J, Alvarado J, Cohen H *et al.* Un consenso latinoamericano sobre el syndrome del intestine irritable. *Gastroenterol Hepatol* 2004;27:325–343.

46  Agarwal N and Spiegel BM. The effect of irritable bowel syndrome on health-related quality of life and health care expenditures. *Gastroenterol Clin North Am* 2011;40:11–19.

47  Simrén M, Svedlund J, Posserud I *et al.* Health-related quality of life in patients attending a gastroenterology outpatient clinic: Functional disorders versus organic disorders. *Clin Gastroenterol Hepatol* 2006;4:187–195.

48  Simren M, Svedlund J, Posserud I *et al.* Health-related quality of life in patients attending a gastroenterology outpatient clinic: functional disorders versus organic disorders. *Clin Gastroenterol Hepatol* 2006;4:187–195.

49  Spiegel B, Harris L, Lucak S *et al.* Developing valid and reliable health utilities in irritable bowel syndrome: results from the IBS PROOF Cohort. *Am J Gastroenterol* 2009;104:1984–1991.

50  Hansel SL, Umar SB, Lunsford TN *et al.* Personality Traits and Impaired Health-Related Quality of Life in Patients with Functional Gastrointestinal Disorders. *Clin Gastroenterol Hepatol* 2010;8:220–222.

51  Jeong JJ, Choi MG, Cho YS *et al.* Chronic gastrointestinal symptoms and quality of life in the Korean population. *World J Gastroenterol* 2008;14:6388–6394.

52  Quality of life at dyspepsia and irritable bowel syndrome: population-based studies. *Eksp Klin Gastroenterol* 2010;(3):27–31.

53  Hungin AP, Chang L, Locke GR *et al*. Irritable bowel syndrome in the United States: prevalence, symptom patterns and impact. *Aliment Pharmacol Ther* 2005;21:1365–1375.

54  Park JM, Choi M-G, Kim YS *et al*. Quality of life of patients with irritable bowel syndrome in Korea. *Qual Life Res* 2009;18:435–436.

55  Schmulson M, Ortiz O, Mejia-Arangure JM *et al*. Further validation of the IBS-QOL: Female Mexican IBS patients have poorer quality of life than females from North Carolina. *Dig Dis Sci* 2007;52:2950–2955.

56  Schmulson M, Robles G, Kershenobich D *et al*. Los pacientes con trastornos funcionales digestivos (TFD) tienen mayor compromiso de la calidad de vida (DV) evaluada por el SF-36 comparados con pacientes con hepatitis C y pancreatitis crónica. *Rev Gastroenterol Mex* 2000;65(Suppl 1):50.

57  Schmulson M. El escrutinio diagnóstico limitado puede disminuir el impacto económico directo del síndrome de intestino irritable (SII). *Rev Med Chil* 2008;136:1398–1405.

58  Casiday RE, Hungin APS, Cornford CS *et al*. GPs' explanatory models for irritable bowel syndrome: a mismatch for patient model? *Fam Pract* 2009;26:34–39.

59  Zhao Y, Zou D, Wang R *et al*. Dyspepsia and irritable bowel syndrome in China: a population-based endoscopy study of prevalence and impact. *Aliment Pharmacol Ther* 2010;32:562–572.

60  Hori K, Matsumoto T and Miwa H. Analysis of the gastrointestinal symptoms of uninvestigated dyspepsia and irritable bowel syndrome. *Gut Liver* 2009;3:192–196.

61  Hu WH, Wong WM, Lam CL *et al*. Anxiety but not depression determines health care-seeking behaviour in Chinese patients with dyspepsia and irritable bowel syndrome: a population-based study. *Aliment Pharmacol Ther* 2002;16:2081–2088.

62  Kumano H, Kaiya H, Yoshiuchi K *et al*. Comorbidity of irritable bowel syndrome, panic disorder, and agoraphobia in a Japanese representative sample. *Am J Gastroenterol* 2004;99:370–376.

63  Kanazawa M, Endo Y, Whitehead WE *et al*. Patients and nonconsulters with irritable bowel syndrome reporting a parental history of bowel problems have more impaired psychological distress. *Dig Dis Sci* 2004;49:1046–1053.

64  Reséndiz-Figueroa FE, Ortiz-Garrido OM, Pulido D *et al*. Impacto de los rasgos de ansiedad y depresión sobre aspectos clínicos y calidad de vida en pacientes con síndrome de intestino irritable. *Rev Gastroenterol Mex* 2008;73:3–10.

65  Lee SY, Lee KL, Kim SJ and Cho SW. Prevalence and risk factors for overlaps between gastroesophageal reflux disease, dyspepsia and irritable bowel syndrome: a population-based study. *Digestion* 2009;79:196–201.

66  Wanj AJ, Liao XH, Xiong LS *et al*. The clinical overlap between functional dyspepsia and irritable bowel syndrome based on Rome III criteria. *BMC Gastroenterolgy* 2008;8:43.

67  Yarandi SS, Nasseri-Moghaddam S, Mostajabi P and Malekzadeh R. Overlapping gastroesophageal reflux disease and irritable bowel syndrome: increased dysfunctional symptoms. *World J Gastroenterol* 2010;16:1232–1238.

68  Spiegel BM, Gralnek IM, Bolus R *et al*. Clinical determinants of health-related quality of life in patients with irritable bowel syndrome. *Arch Intern Med* 2004;164:1773–170.

69  Rey E, García-Alonso MO, Moreno-Ortega M *et al*. Determinants of quality of life in irritable bowel syndrome. *J Clin Gastroenterol* 2008;42:1003–1009.

70  Gwee K-A, Lu C-L and Ghoshal UC. Epidemiology of irritable bowel syndrome in Asia: something old, something new, something borrowed. *J Gastroenterol Hepatol* 2009;24:1601–1607.

71  Gwee KA. Irritable bowel syndrome in developing countries – a disorder of civilization or colonization? *Neurogastroenterol Motil* 2005;17:317–324.

72 Dapoigny M, Bellanger J, Bonaz B *et al*. Irritable bowel syndrome in France: a common, debilitating and costly disorder. *Eur J Gastroenterol Hepatol* 2004;16:995–1001.

73 Quigley EMM, Bergmann J-F, Bytzer P *et al*. An evidence-based approach to the management of irritable bowel syndrome in Europe. *Eur J Gastroenterol Hepatol* 2007;19(Suppl 1):S1–S37.

74 Gwee K-A, Bak Y-T, Ghoshal UC *et al*. Asian consensus on irritable bowel syndrome. *J Gastroenterol Hepatol* 2010;25:1189–1205.

75 Chang F-Y and Lu C-L. Irritable bowel syndrome in the 21st century: Perspectives from Asia or South-east Asia. *J Gastroenterol Hepatol* 2007;22:4–12.

76 Hammer J, Eslick GD, Howell SC *et al*. Diagnostic yield of alarm features in irritable bowel syndrome and functional dyspepsia. *Gut* 2004;53:666–6672.

77 Ford AC, Marwaha A, Lim A and Moayyedi P. Systematic review and meta-analysis of irritable bowel syndrome in individuals with dyspepsia. *Clin Gastroenterol Hepatol* 2010;8:401–409.

78 Kang JY. Systematic review: the influence of geography and ethnicity in irritable bowel syndrome. *Aliment Pharmacol Ther* 2005; 21: 663–676.

79 Desmond AN, McWilliams S, Maher MM, Shanahan F, Quigley EM. Radiation exposure from diagnostic imaging among patients with gastrointestinal disorders. *Clin Gastroenterol Hepatol* 2012;10:886–892.

80 Gerson CD, Gerson MJ, Awad RA *et al*. Irritable bowel syndrome: an international study of symptoms in eight countries. *Eur J Gastroenterol Hepatol* 2008;20:659–667.

81 Cash BD, Rubenstein JH, Young PE *et al*. The prevalence of coeliac disease among patients with nonconstipated irritable bowel syndrome is similar to controls. *Gastroenterology* 2011;141:1187–1193.

82 Ford AC, Speigel BM, Talley NJ and Moayyedi P. Small intestinal bacterial overgrowth in irritable bowel syndrome: systematic review and meta-analysis. *Clin Gastroenterol Hepatol* 2009;7:1279–86

83 Wedlake L, A'hern R, Russell D *et al*. Systematic review: the prevalence of idiopathic bile acid malabsorption as diagnosed by SeHCAT scanning in patients with diarrhea-predominant irritable bowel syndrome. *Aliment Pharmacol Ther* 2009;30:707–717.

84 Carmona-Sánchez R and Tostado-Fernández FA. Prevalence of use of alternative and complementary medicine in patients with irritable bowel syndrome, functional dyspepsia, and gastroesophageal reflux disease. *Rev Gastroenterol Mex* 2005;70:393–398.

85 Hussein Z and Quigley EMM. Complementary and alternative medicine in the irritable bowel syndrome. *Aliment Pharmacol Ther* 2006;23:465–471.

86 Grunkeimer DM, Cassara JE, Dalton CB and Drossman DA. The narcotic bowel syndrome: clinical features, pathophsyiology and management. *Clin Gastroenterol Hepatol* 2007;5:1126–1139.

87 Gwee KA, Hwang JE, Ho KY *et al*. In-practice predictors of response to proton pump inhibitor therapy in primary care patients with dyspepsia in an Asian population. *J Clin Gastroenterol* 2008;42:134–138.

# Multiple Choice Questions

1 Which of the following factors has the greatest impact on quality of life (QOL) in IBS?
   A Patient age
   B The presence of extra-intestinal and/or psychological comorbidities
   C Patient ethnicity
   D An alternating (mixed) rather than constipation- or diarrhoea-predominant bowel pattern

Answer: B

2 Regarding the investigation of a patient presenting to your outpatient clinic for the first time with IBS-type symptoms, which of the following approaches is appropriate?
   A Tissue transglutaminase assay in serum from a 25-year-old Argentinian female with diarrhoea-predominant IBS.
   B Stool studies to detect *Entamoeba histolytica* in a 34-year-old Egyptian male.
   C Colonoscopy in an otherwise well 19-year-old female with constipation-predominant IBS and prominent bloating.
   D Lactose tolerance testing in a 23-year-old Indian male with alternating IBS.

Answer: A

3 Regarding the use of complementary and alternative medicine (CAM) practices in IBS, which of the following is true?
   A Those who use CAM will typically and reliably inform their doctor of this at their first consultation
   B The prevalence and patterns of CAM use are uniform world-wide
   C Dietary changes self-instituted on the basis of 'allergy tests' are commonly employed by IBS sufferers in Western Europe and North America
   D Use of CAM by IBS sufferers is rare in Latin America

Answer: C

**PART 2**

# Diagnosis of Irritable Bowel Syndrome

## CHAPTER 4

# What is the Best Way to Identify and Quantify Irritable Bowel Syndrome?

*Gururaj J. Kolar and G. Richard Locke, III*

Division of Gastroenterology and Hepatology, Mayo Clinic College of Medicine, Rochester, MN, USA

---

**Key points**

- Current diagnostic criteria allow clinicians to make a positive diagnosis of IBS.
- Better implementation of existing guidelines can decrease the number of diagnostic tests and minimize the cost.
- The proposed severity scale represents a great start towards a reproducible measure of IBS severity but needs to be evaluated in further studies.

---

Irritable Bowel Syndrome (IBS) has come from being a 'diagnosis of exclusion' to becoming a positive diagnosis. With the combination of positive diagnostic criteria and an absence of 'alarm symptoms', a diagnosis can be made without subjecting the patient to numerous diagnostic tests. However, a recent survey showed that community providers still believe IBS is a diagnosis of exclusion while the experts comply more closely with guidelines to diagnose IBS with minimal testing [1]. This goes to show that the implementation of guidelines needs improvement, so as to decrease variation and better provide cost-effective care.

## Best way to identify IBS

Since IBS lacks anatomic and physiologic markers, it is a diagnosis made on clinical grounds [2].

---

*Irritable Bowel Syndrome: Diagnosis and Clinical Management*, First Edition.
Edited by Anton Emmanuel and Eamonn M.M. Quigley.
© 2013 John Wiley & Sons, Ltd. Published 2013 by John Wiley & Sons, Ltd.

---

**Box 4.1  Alarm features in the diagnosis of IBS**

1. Weight loss, anaemia, and occult blood in the stool.
2. History of travel to locations with endemic parasitic diseases.
3. Night-time symptoms.
4. New onset after age 50.
5. Family history of colon cancer, inflammatory bowel disease, or coeliac disease.
6. Arthritis or skin findings on physical examination.
7. Signs or symptoms of malabsorption.
8. Signs or symptoms of thyroid dysfunction.

Adapted from Vanner *et al. Am J Gastroenterol* 1999;94:2912–2917, with permission from Macmillan Publishers Ltd.

---

## The role of history taking

In a clinical scenario, the key to diagnosing IBS is astute history taking. The history taking should focus on presence or absence of:

1 abdominal pain or discomfort
2 bloating
3 constipation, diarrhoea or an alternation between both.

Also, one must be sure to eliminate the presence of 'alarm features', which modifies the diagnosis in IBS patients. The 'alarm features' are summarized in Box 4.1.

The American College of Gastroenterology (ACG) undertook a review of studies of lower GI symptoms and reporting on the accuracy of rectal bleeding [3]. These studies found that rectal bleeding had a pooled sensitivity of 64% (95% CI=55–73%) and a pooled specificity of 52% (95% CI=42–63) for diagnosing colorectal cancer. Another review of seven studies reporting the accuracy of anaemia found that it had a pooled sensitivity of 19% (95% CI=5.5–33%) and a pooled specificity of 90% (95% CI=87–92%) for diagnosing colorectal cancer in patients with lower GI symptoms [3]. Weight loss studies found that there was a pooled sensitivity of 22% (95% CI=14–31%) and a pooled specificity of 89% (95% CI=81–95%) for colorectal cancer [3]. Two studies have also shown that nocturnal abdominal pain is not more likely in patients with organic diseases than it is in patients with IBS [4].

Thus, it can be concluded that rectal bleeding and nocturnal pain offer little discriminative value in separating patients with IBS from those with organic diseases. However, even though anaemia and weight loss have poor sensitivity for organic diseases, they do offer very good specificity. Presence of one of these alarm features makes it pertinent to undertake diagnostic testing for the relevant condition to rule out the cause of the presenting symptoms. But in cases where the 'alarm features' are absent,

> **Box 4.2  Rome III Criteria [35]: Diagnostic Criteria\* for Irritable Bowel Syndrome**
>
> Recurrent abdominal pain or discomfort\*\* at least three days per month in the last three months associated with *two or more* of the following:
> 1. Improvement with defecation.
> 2. Onset associated with a change in frequency of stool.
> 3. Onset associated with a change in form (appearance) of stool.
>
> \*Criteria fulfilled for the last three months with symptom onset at least six months prior to diagnosis.
> \*\*Discomfort means an uncomfortable sensation not described as pain. In pathophysiology research and clinical trials, a pain/discomfort frequency of at least two days a week during screening evaluation for subject eligibility.
> Reproduced from Longstreth GF, Thompson WG, Chey WD *et al.* Functional Bowel Disorders. *Gastroenterology* 2006;130:1480–1491.

the clinician can rest assured that a positive diagnosis of IBS with diagnostic criteria (which will be discussed subsequently) is correct.

## The role of diagnostic criteria

Functional diseases have been described more in terms of what they are not as opposed to what they are. While this may make scientific sense, it has not proven very useful for the sufferers of the disease for whom the problem is very real and not just the absence of other diseases. This diagnosis of exclusion approach ended up generating numerous tests and consultations for patients; this not only raised the cost of health care but also robbed the patients of the dignity of having a 'real' disease. The rationale for symptom-based diagnostic criteria arose from the presumption that there are symptom clusters that are found to be more coherent for clinical and population groups suffering from these disorders. The initial diagnostic criteria were the Manning criteria [5]. Then came the Rome criteria (1989 and 1990), Rome I criteria (1992) and Rome II criteria (1999). Box 4.2 shows the Rome III criteria, the present and latest available diagnostic criteria for IBS.

## The role of physical examination

The physical examination in patients with IBS is almost always unremarkable. Hence, physical examination is not the most important criteria to base one's diagnosis upon.

 Symptoms such as abdominal pain, loose or frequent stools associated with pain, incomplete evacuation, mucus per rectum and abdominal distension were thought to have less accuracy in diagnosing IBS. Lower abdominal pain had the highest sensitivity (90%) but very poor specificity (32%), whereas patient-reported visible abdominal distension had the highest specificity (77%) but low sensitivity (39%) [6]. The problem with this approach remains that Rome II and III criteria remain to be validated yet. No studies have been undertaken in this regard. Also, since the diagnosis of IBS cannot be confirmed by available diagnostic tests, the application of the term 'gold standard' to the Rome criteria remains a controversial issue.

## The role of diagnostic testing in patients with IBS symptoms

Multiple diagnostic testing should be avoided in patients as it is not only an expensive proposition but it also exposes patients to risk and discomfort and creates doubts in their minds as to the validity of the diagnosis.

When making decisions on using diagnostic tests, clinicians should consider the following two points:

1 If the pretest probability of the disease is small, the diagnostic test is unlikely to uncover the disease.
2 If the probability of the disease is high, consideration should also be given to the characteristics of the diagnostic tests with regards to sensitivity, specificity, positive and negative predictive values.

The 2009 ACG evidence-based position statement on the management of IBS [3] suggested that routine diagnostic testing with complete blood count, serum chemistries, thyroid function studies, stool for ova and parasites, and abdominal imaging was not recommended in patients with typical IBS symptoms and no alarm features because of a low likelihood of uncovering organic disease.

In patients presenting with a short duration of symptoms, exhibiting demographic features such as a more advanced age at the time of onset of symptoms, possessing a family history of organic gastrointestinal disease, or in whom there is a lack of concurrent psychosocial difficulties, a complete clinical history and physical examination followed by screening via a complete blood count (CBC) and faecal occult blood testing (FOBT) are recommended. Thereafter, the patient's individual symptom pattern, geographic location and relevant clinical features should direct the clinician towards whether or not to perform additional tests, such as erythrocyte sedimentation rate (ESR), serum chemistries and stool testing for ova and parasites (O&P).

In a study which evaluated the role of measuring thyroid-stimulating hormone (TSH) levels as part of the diagnostic evaluation of patients with suspected IBS, 67 patients (6%) among more than 1200 patients fulfilling the Rome criteria had thyroid function abnormalities [7]. These abnormalities were evenly distributed between hyper- and hypothyroidism. However, following correction of thyroid dysfunction, it was noted that there was no symptom response. This led to the conclusion that there is no clear role for thyroid gland dysfunction among individuals with IBS symptoms.

Routine serologic screening for coeliac sprue should be pursued in patients with IBS-D and IBS-A. Coeliac disease can present with a wide spectrum of insidious symptoms including diarrhoea, bloating and abdominal cramping [8].

However, patients with coeliac disease tend to have a diarrhoea-predominant illness with a relative absence of pain. Also, the presence of alarm symptoms such as weight loss, anaemia and other biochemical markers such anti-gliadin antibodies, anti-tissue transglutaminase and anti-endomysial antibodies are commonly present. Patients suspected of coeliac disease may undergo further testing including the above mentioned antibodies and upper endoscopy with small bowel biopsy. It is important to remember that the prevalence of coeliac disease in IBS patients is low; 2% in a recent study using Rome III criteria [9]. Another study by Locke *et al.* [10] reported that the prevalence of positive antibodies for anti-tissue transglutaminase IgA among patients with IBS in the general population was 4%, which was similar to a prevalence of 2% found in a control group. They also concluded that coeliac disease did not explain the symptoms of IBS in the vast majority of symptomatic subjects, but no comment was made on the relevance of coeliac disease screening in the population.

Lactose breath testing can be considered when lactose maldigestion remains a concern despite a lactose-free diet. The prevalence of lactose malabsorption has been reported to be approximately 25% in a Western population and almost 75% worldwide [11, 12]. However, a study which recommended an evaluation for lactose malabsorption being relevant in a subset of patients with functional bowel disorders [13] suffered from possible selection bias, and other studies have shown no difference in the prevalence of lactose intolerance between IBS and the general population [14]. Studies on diet in IBS are often difficult to interpret because of inadequate controls, poor methodology, heterogeneous populations and a large placebo effect. Nonetheless, IBS and lactose deficiency share a very similar set of symptoms and can exist simultaneously in the same patient. Hence, the lesson for clinical practice is that it is important to seek a history of lactose intolerance in patients who present with abdominal cramping, diarrhoea, bloating or other symptoms suspicious of IBS. Patients should be encouraged to keep a food diary to assess the relationship between symptoms and dairy intake, and if a consistent association is identified, consumption of milk, ice cream and soft cheeses should be avoided or at least minimized.

Currently, there are insufficient data to recommend breath testing for small intestinal bacterial overgrowth (SIBO) in IBS patients. Studies thus far, which have shown that a high percentage of patients diagnosed by Rome I criteria for IBS had test results consistent with SIBO, have suffered from several shortcomings, including potential selection bias, the absence of a gold standard for the diagnosis of SIBO, short study duration and incomplete follow-up data for the majority of enrolled patients; thus limiting the ability to draw firm conclusions [15].

There is a low pretest probability for Crohn's disease, ulcerative colitis and colonic neoplasia in the general population. Hence, routine colonic imaging

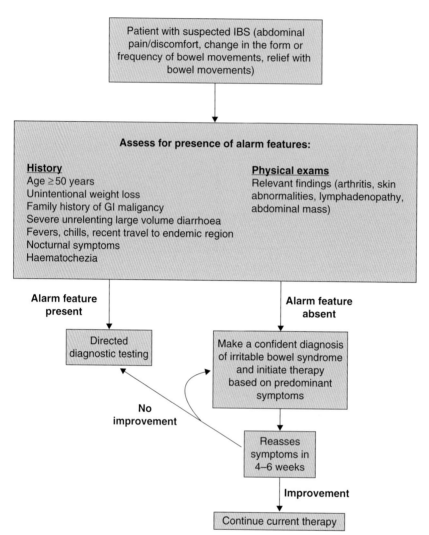

**Figure 4.1** Irritable bowel syndrome – an evidence-based approach to diagnosis. (Reproduced from Cash and Chey [17], with permission from John Wiley & Sons Ltd.)

is not recommended in patients younger than 50 years of age with typical IBS symptoms and no alarm features. Colonoscopic imaging should be performed in IBS patients with alarm features to rule out organic diseases and in those over the age of 50 years for the purpose of colorectal cancer screening. When colonoscopy is performed in patients with IBS-D, obtaining random biopsies should be considered to rule out microscopic/lymphocytic colitis.

The role of radiologic imaging in IBS was recently reviewed [16]. Despite the extensive use of imaging in the assessment of subjects presenting with IBS-type symptoms, good data on the optimal use of these diagnostic modalities are surprisingly scanty.

Despite the above recommendations, it must be conceded that there have been no studies performed to date that have prospectively assessed a diagnostic approach or approaches to IBS. Unlike many other diseases, there is not a single screening test that can be used for identifying IBS. Current evidence does not support the need for the performance of exhaustive tests to exclude the presence of organic diseases in the absence of alarm features in patients fulfilling symptom criteria for IBS. However, patients above the age of 50 years presenting with IBS should undergo colonoscopy (or other acceptable regimen) for age appropriate colorectal cancer screening. Lack of well-defined diagnostic tests that can be used to confirm the disease as opposed to eliminate the presence of other disorders further complicates the process. Suffice it to say that this requires further study [16].

A step-wise guide to the diagnosis of IBS [17] is shown in Figure 4.1; it summarizes the information provided thus far.

## Best way to quantify IBS

The challenge to assigning a degree of severity to an individual patient with IBS is compounded by a lack of a valid biomarker for the disorder. Hence, severity is typically determined based on an assessment of the patients' self-reported symptoms and behaviours. As a consequence, IBS and functional gastrointestinal diseases (FGIDs), in general, are best understood from the patient's personal experience of ill health. Patients' adherence to medications, adjustment of their lifestyles and pursuit of health care are based on their perception of severity of the disease. Clinicians may not always take this into consideration. They should weigh the patient's symptom reports and behaviours to make diagnostic and treatment decisions. Hence, there should be some way to understand and quantify the severity disease from the patient's perspective.

There is, as yet, no clear categorization of IBS patients into clinical subgroups of severity; there is only symptom categorization according to diagnostic criteria. The initial attempts at categorizing symptom severity into clinically meaningful subgroups were done many years ago [18, 19]. It proposed subcategorizing IBS into mild, moderate and severe based on certain clinical features. When severity is 'mild', patients have low-intensity, infrequent symptoms and good health-related quality of life (HRQOL) and may not seek health care; epidemiological studies of individuals with mild IBS indicate that many have never been to a physician. When severity is 'moderate', there are more persistent and discomforting symptoms with some impairment of HRQOL, reduced socializing and some work absenteeism. When IBS is 'severe', symptoms are more frequent, even persistent and of greater intensity, as well as being associated with marked functional impairment, psychosocial comorbidities and a high prevalence of health care referrals to specialists. However, these categorizations were based on the authors' clinical experience and not scientific data. As of now, there has been a lack of systematic categorization based on evidence. This leads to numerous problems, one of them being an inability to determine the natural history of symptom severity in IBS. Hence, there is a need for a standardized categorization which assesses severity and places patients into meaningful subgroups that can be validated and used to determine the prevalence and natural history of IBS. This will also lead to unambiguous separation of patients by severity, which can only enable better communication amongst clinicians and researchers alike, eventually resulting in better outcomes.

Two instruments have been used to assess severity in IBS. The first is the Functional Bowel Disorder Severity Index (FBDSI) [20] which assesses severity based on a patient's pain behaviours: the presence and intensity of pain and the number of health care visits. Predictions by physicians of the severity of patients' clinical features across different medical centres in the United States, Canada and the United Kingdom led to its development. Using regression analysis to assess the predictability of physician-rated severity identified only three significant variables: (i) the amount of pain present today, (ii) a diagnosis of functional abdominal pain syndrome (chronic or frequently recurring pain) and (iii) the number of physician visits in the previous six months. These three variables produced a numerical score for severity that was categorized into subgroups: a score of $\leq 36$ for mild illness, 37–110 for moderate illness and $\geq 111$ for severe symptoms. The FBDSI has construct validity, which means that a scale measures or correlates with a theorized psychological scientific construct that it purports to measure. It also demonstrates discriminant validity by differentiating non-IBS patients from IBS patients with and without fibromyalgia [21]. It shows, too, concurrent validity by its ability to correlate with psychological distress and illness behaviour. The FBDSI is used as well to assess other painful functional bowel conditions, such as functional abdominal pain syndrome, and has been used for the purpose of identifying or stratifying groups based on pain severity for clinical studies.

The second instrument is the IBS Severity Scoring System (IBS-SSS) [22]. This scale primarily evaluates the intensity of IBS symptoms over a 10-day period: abdominal pain, distension, stool frequency and consistency and interference with life in general. It calculates the sum of these five items each scored on a visual analogue scale from 0 to 100. Even though it may appear that the IBS-SSS uses patient-rated intensity of IBS symptoms, the determination of severity by the scoring system was originally anchored to a physician's assessment of patient severity. In one study of cognitive behavioural therapy, a 37-point reduction in the IBS-SSS score was seen over one year ($P=0.01$) [23]. In an acupuncture study, changes in the IBS-SSS scores were comparable with other commonly used measures of improvement in IBS trials [24]. Hence, it would be safe to say that the IBS-SSS is responsive to treatment. However, this is true only for studies which have evaluated behavioural interventions; its responsiveness in clinical trials using pharmacological agents has not been tested as yet. Nevertheless, the data suggest that the IBS-SSS could be used for selecting symptomatic patients for clinical trials and for measuring response to treatment [25]. Thus, the IBS-SSS can be considered to be a measure of the severity of IBS symptoms including abdominal pain and distension and bowel satisfaction.

In summary, there are two validated measures of IBS symptom severity based on physician ratings of severity – the FBDSI and the IBS-SSS. Their advantages are that they are relatively easy to use and have psychometric validity and reproducibility. The disadvantages are that they do not truly measure severity of the disease from the patients' perspective but rather from the clinician's perspective.

Many have tried to measure IBS severity based on patient perceptions [26–31]. However, all had limitations in terms of the value of the information provided. For example, one study reported that patient-derived IBS severity was predicted by abdominal pain, bloating, straining, urgency, myalgias and the belief that 'something serious is wrong with body' [26], but another reported that patients self-classify their symptoms as discomfort-like more than twice as often as abdominal pain [27]. Several quality of life measures have been developed, but that is a different concern. The impact of IBS on quality of life can be measured, but this is different from measuring IBS severity, including from a patient's perspective. A bird's-eye view of these studies shows that self-rated severity negatively correlates with health-related quality of life and positively with health care use and costs [28, 29]. There are insufficient data from studies of patient self-reported severity to come to meaningful conclusions and much more needs to be done.

## Relation of symptom severity to clinical response

There have been hardly any studies which can confirm our theoretical assumption that symptom severity can be reduced with an appropriate treatment and adherence thereto. As was mentioned before, the IBS-SSS has been shown to be responsive specifically to behavioural but not to pharmacological treatments. Drossman *et al.* conducted a multicentre randomized prospective trial involving 431 patients with moderate-to-severe functional bowel disorders (FBD) who received cognitive behavioural therapy vs an educational programme as control, or desipramine vs a placebo.

It found that those with moderate illness severity according to the FBDSI responded significantly better to either treatment than the severe group [32]. In a study of 30 patients with severe, refractory IBS undergoing hypnotherapy, those with intractable abdominal pain with little bloating or bowel habit disturbance had a poorer outcome than did patients with more 'classical' cases of IBS [33].

Aware of these inconsistent data, a Rome Foundation Working Committee which focused on measuring the severity of IBS suspended its activity for two years and instead awaited results from new studies by its committee members that were directed towards gaining more knowledge in the field of assessing severity in IBS. This led them to provide us with several empirical factors that can correlate the severity of IBS called the 'Proposed clinical profile for patient-rated severity in IBS' (Table 4.1).

This same committee had several other suggestions for the ideal patient-derived severity measure [34]:

1 Develop and validate a multicomponent rating scale:
   a that includes GI symptoms and other clinical domains (e.g., psychosocial factors, physiological dysfunction, disability) and which can be reduced to a single linear score or verbal description (e.g., mild, moderate, severe);
   b which is anchored to a patient self-rated scale of severity to establish clinical meaningfulness; and
   c aligns with the FDA Patient-Reported Outcomes Guidance document.
2 Using this multicomponent rating measure, validate and/or modify the proposed clinical profiles that attempt from existing data to characterize severity in a dimensional manner and categorically as mild, moderate and severe.
3 Perform multinational prospective epidemiological studies to assess the degree of variability and fluctuation of severity, and identify factors predictive of change in severity. Determine the degree to which the severity measure developed is responsive to change, as in clinical trials.
4 Determine whether differences in severity exist in other subgroups (e.g. based on gender, age, psychosocial difficulties, or symptoms such as stool subtype or diarrhoea).
5 Conduct research studies in other clinical settings (primary care, tertiary care) to further characterize severity.
6 Identify through multinational studies whether cross-cultural differences exist in severity and responsiveness to treatments.
7 Incorporate an assessment of severity in clinical trials as a measure of response to treatment and outcome.
8 Establish guidelines for severity assessment in clinical practice and research based on the newly acquired data.
9 Establish for clinicians a short version of a severity measure, as well as algorithms for diagnosis and treatment based on severity.

**Table 4.1** Proposed clinical profile for patient-rated severity in IBS*.

| Clinical Feature | Mild | Moderate | Severe |
|---|---|---|---|
| Estimated prevalence (%) | 40 | 35 | 25 |
| Psychometric correlate | FBDSI: <36 IBS-SSS: 75–175 | FBDSI: 36–109 IBS-SSS: 175–300 | FBDSI: >110 IBS-SSS: >300 |
| Physiological factors | Primarily bowel dysfunction | Bowel dysfunction and CNS pain dysregulation | Primary CNS pain dysregulation |
| Psychosocial difficulties | Non or mild psych distress | Moderate psych distress | Severe high psych distress |
| Gender | Men = Women | Women > Men | Women >> men |
| Age | Older > Younger | Older = Younger | Younger > Older |
| Abdominal pain | Mild/intermittent | Moderate/frequent | Severe/very frequent or constant |
| Number of other symptoms | Low (1–3) | Medium (4–6) | High (≥7) |
| Health-related quality of life | Good | Fair | Poor |
| Health care use | 0–1/year | 2–4/year | ≥5/year |
| Activity restriction | Occasional (0–15 days) | More often (15–50 days) | Frequent/constant (>50 days) |
| Work disability | <5% | 6–10% | ≥11% |

CNS, central nervous system; FBDSI, Functional Bowel Disorders Severity Index; IBS, irritable bowel syndrome
*This is based on existing data on severity in IBS and needs to be further tested and validated
Reproduced from Drossman *et al.* [34], with permission from Macmillan Publishers Ltd.

10  Develop responder and state-attainment criteria for clinical research and practice applications.
11  Consider the use of a multi-axial classification scheme that includes severity along with other parameters (diagnostic criteria, psychosocial distress, physiological dysfunction, disability / overall severity) for Rome IV [34].

## Conclusion

The current diagnostic criteria allow us to make a positive diagnosis in a great number of patients. Better implementation of existing guidelines can decrease the number of unnecessary diagnostic tests performed and, thereby, minimize cost. All of the data on severity leaves us with many possible leads to explore but no conclusive data. The proposed clinical profile for a patient-rated severity scale in IBS as shown in Table 4.1 is a great place to start to gain more data from further studies. In the end, progress is being made on the best way to identify and quantify IBS.

## References

1 Spiegel BMR, Farid M, Esrailian E, *et al.* Is irritable bowel syndrome a diagnosis of exclusion?: a survey of primary care providers, gastroenterologists, and IBS experts. *Am J Gastroenterol* 2010;105:848–858.

2 Olden KW. Irritable bowel syndrome: an overview of diagnosis and pharmacologic treatment. *Cleve Clin J Med* 2003;70:S3.

3 An evidence-based position statement on the management of irritable bowel syndrome. *Am J Gastroenterol* 2008;104:S1–S35.

4 Hammer J, Eslick GD, Howell SC *et al.* Diagnostic yield of alarm features in irritable bowel syndrome and functional dyspepsia. *Gut* 2004;53:666–672.

5 Manning AP, Thompson WG, Heaton KW *et al.* Towards positive diagnosis of the irritable bowel. *BMJ* 1978;2:653–654.

6 Ford AC, Talley NJ, Veldhuyzen van Zanten SJO *et al.* Will the history and physical examination help establish that irritable bowel syndrome is causing this patient's lower gastrointestinal tract symptoms? *JAMA* 2008;300:1793–1805.

7 Hamm LR, Sorrells SC, Harding JP *et al.* Additional investigations fail to alter the diagnosis of irritable bowel syndrome in subjects fulfilling the Rome criteria. *Am J Gastroenterol* 1999;94:1279–1282.

8 Green PHR, Stavropoulos SN, Panagi SG *et al.* Characteristics of adult coeliac disease in the USA: results of a national survey. *Am J Gastroenterol* 2001;96:126–131.

9 Korkut E, Bektas M, Oztas E *et al.* The prevalence of coeliac disease in patients fulfilling Rome III criteria for irritable bowel syndrome. *Eur J Intern Med* 2010; 21:389–392.

10 Locke GR, 3rd, Murray JA, Zinsmeister AR *et al.* Coeliac disease serology in irritable bowel syndrome and dyspepsia: a population-based case-control study. *Mayo Clin Proc* 2004;79:476–482.

11 Scrimshaw NS and Murray EB. The acceptability of milk and milk products in populations with a high prevalence of lactose intolerance. *Am J Clin Nutr* 1988; 48:1079–1159.

12 Bourlioux P, Pochart P. Nutritional and health properties of yogurt. *World Rev Nutr Diet* 1988;56:217–258.

13 Tolliver BA, Jackson MS, Jackson KL *et al.* Does lactose maldigestion really play a role in the irritable bowel? *J Clin Gastroenterol* 1996;23:15–17.

14 Farup PG, Monsbakken KW and Vandvik PO. Lactose malabsorption in a population with irritable bowel syndrome: prevalence and symptoms. A case-control study. *Scand J Gastroenterol* 2004;39:645–649.

15 Pimentel M, Chow EJ and Lin HC. Eradication of small intestinal bacterial overgrowth reduces symptoms of irritable bowel syndrome. *Am J Gastroenterol* 2000; 95:3503–3506.

16 O'Connor OJ, McSweeney SE, McWilliams S *et al.* Role of radiologic imaging in irritable bowel syndrome: evidence-based review. *Radiology* 2012;262:485–494.

17 Cash BD and Chey WD. Irritable bowel syndrome – an evidence-based approach to diagnosis. *Aliment Pharmacol Ther* 2004;19:1235–1245.

18 Drossman DA, Camilleri M, Mayer EA *et al.* AGA technical review on irritable bowel syndrome. *Gastroenterology* 2002;123:2108–2131.

19 Drossman DA and Thompson WG. The irritable bowel syndrome: a review and a graduated multicomponent treatment approach. *Ann Intern Med* 1992;116: 1009–1016.

20 Drossman DA, Li Z, Toner BB *et al.* Functional bowel disorders. *Dig Dis Sci* 1995;40: 986–995.

21 Sperber AD, Carmel S, Atzmon Y *et al.* Use of the Functional Bowel Disorder Severity Index (FBDSI) in a study of patients with the irritable bowel syndrome and fibromyalgia. *Am J Gastroenterol* 2000;95:995–998.

22 Francis CY, Morris J and Whorwell PJ. The irritable bowel severity scoring system: a simple method of monitoring irritable bowel syndrome and its progress. *Aliment Pharmacol Ther* 1997;11:395–402.

23 Kennedy T, Jones R, Darnley S *et al.* Cognitive behaviour therapy in addition to antispasmodic treatment for irritable bowel syndrome in primary care: randomised controlled trial. *BMJ* 2005;331:435.

24 Lembo AJ, Conboy L, Kelley JM *et al.* A Treatment Trial of Acupuncture in IBS Patients. *Am J Gastroenterol* 2009;104:1489–1497.

25 Lembo A, Ameen VZ and Drossman DA. Irritable bowel syndrome: toward an understanding of severity. *Clin Gastroenterol Hepatol* 2005;3:717–725.

26 Spiegel B, Strickland A, Naliboff BD *et al.* Predictors of patient-assessed illness severity in irritable bowel syndrome. *Am J Gastroenterol* 2008;103:2536–2543.

27 Sach J, Bolus R, Fitzgerald L *et al.* Is there a difference between abdominal pain and discomfort in moderate to severe IBS patients[quest]. *Am J Gastroenterol* 2002;97: 3131–3138.

28 Hahn BA, Kirchdoerfer LJ, Fullerton S, *et al.* Patient-perceived severity of irritable bowel syndrome in relation to symptoms, health resource utilization and quality of life. *Aliment Pharmacol Ther* 1997;11:553–559.

29 Longstreth GF, Wilson A, Knight K *et al.* Irritable bowel syndrome, health care use, and costs: a U.S. managed care perspective. *Am J Gastroenterol* 2003;98:600–607.

30 Hillilä MT and Färkkilä MA. Prevalence of irritable bowel syndrome according to different diagnostic criteria in a non-selected adult population. *Aliment Pharmacol Ther* 2004;20:339–345.

31 Tack J, Broekaert D, Fischler B *et al.* A controlled crossover study of the selective serotonin reuptake inhibitor citalopram in irritable bowel syndrome. *Gut* 2006; 55:1095–1103.

32 Drossman DA, Toner BB, Whitehead WE *et al.* Cognitive-behavioral therapy versus education and desipramine versus placebo for moderate to severe functional bowel disorders. *Gastroenterology* 2003;125:19–31.

33 Whorwell PJ, Prior A, Faragher EB. Controlled trial of hypnotherapy in the treatment of severe refractory irritable-bowel syndrome. *Lancet* 1984;324:1232–1234.

34 Drossman DA, Chang L, Bellamy N *et al.* Severity in irritable bowel syndrome: A Rome Foundation Working Team Report. *Am J Gastroenterol* 2011;106:1749–1759.

35 Longstreth GF, Thompson WG, Chey WD *et al.* Functional Bowel Disorders. *Gastroenterology* 2006;130:1480–1491.

# Multiple Choice Questions

1 What is the best way to identify IBS?
  A Perform an upper endoscopy, a colonoscopy, several blood tests and other testing as thought needed.
  B Use specific criteria such as the Rome criteria with attention to alarm symptoms.
  C Colonoscopy regardless of age followed by blood tests.
  D No evaluation needed regardless of symptoms.

Answer: B

2 What is the best way to quantify IBS?
  A Use an IBS quality of life scale such as the IBS-QoL.
  B Use a generic health status measure such as the SF-36.
  C Use a generic GI symptom measure such as the Gastrointestinal Symptom Rating Scale.
  D Use the Functional Bowel Disorder Severity Index (FBDSI) or the Irritable Bowel Syndrome Severity Scoring System (IBS-SSS).

Answer: D

3 IBS can be diagnosed on the basis of one week of symptoms in an emergency room:
  A True
  B False

Answer: B

4 The portion of the evaluation which provides the most evidence for IBS would be the:
  A History
  B Physical examination
  C Diagnostic testing

Answer: A

**5** Gastroenterologists are most likely to be involved in the care of
patients with what form of IBS:
  **A** Mild
  **B** Moderate
  **C** Severe

Answer: C

## CHAPTER 5

# Practical Approach to Clinical Assessment of Irritable Bowel Syndrome

*Robin Spiller and Ching Lam*

NIHR Nottingham Digestive Diseases Biomedical Research Unit, University of Nottingham, Nottingham UK

---

**Key points**

- IBS accounts for 40% of gastrointestinal outpatient referrals.
- Abdominal pain or discomfort is typically intermittent, related to bowel habit and often at least partially relieved by defaecation.
- Patients often complain of a sensation of bloating with or without visible distension.
- Over half the patients will be abnormally anxious.
- Multiple unexplained somatic symptoms are characteristic.
- Physical examination is usually normal.
- Alarm features include unintended weight loss, nocturnal symptoms, family history of colorectal cancer, age >50 years at first presentation, a short history, blood mixed with stool or abnormal physical examination.
- Multiple somatic symptoms predict frequent consultations and poor response to treatment.
- Those meeting diagnostic criteria who have no alarm features can be confidently diagnosed with IBS after a minimum of simple screening tests.

---

## Introduction

Irritable bowel syndrome (IBS) is important because it accounts for up to 40% of gastroenterology referrals from primary to secondary care [1] and, hence, has the potential to involve the use of a lot of medical resources. Managing it efficiently will also improve the management of patients with other diseases by freeing up investigations for those most likely to benefit from them. The symptoms of abdominal pain and altered bowel habit

This article presents independent research funded by the National Institute for Health Research (NIHR). The views expressed are those of the authors and not necessarily those of the NHS, the NIHR or the Department of Health.

---

*Irritable Bowel Syndrome: Diagnosis and Clinical Management*, First Edition.
Edited by Anton Emmanuel and Eamonn M.M. Quigley.
© 2013 John Wiley & Sons, Ltd. Published 2013 by John Wiley & Sons, Ltd.

may mimic many diseases, often leading to numerous expensive and unpleasant investigations which are a burden to both the patient and the healthcare system. The condition can markedly reduce the patient's quality of life and impair their performance at work and at home [2, 3].

As the condition is poorly understood, most physicians' training does not prepare them to effectively manage this group of patients. Physicians are often baffled by their multiple somatic problems and 'medically unexplained symptoms' which, in these days of marked specialization, often lead to multiple referrals to other specialists who focus on specific symptoms without recognizing the psychological distress which may be underlying some of the symptoms. As a result, patients often feel that their real concerns and symptoms are not listened to. The physician should have a flexible, yet systematic, approach to the assessment of such patients so that they feel understood and confident that the correct diagnosis has been made and are, hence, more likely to respond to management plans.

## Gathering information before the interview

Prior to patient consultation, it is useful to have an overview of the patient's previous illnesses and comorbidities. A good referral letter is vital and should list the most important concerns and prior consultations with their general practitioner or specialist clinic, especially for 'medically unexplained' symptoms. The typical IBS patient will have multiple previous consultations in the last five years. Absence of this feature should alert the physician to an alternative diagnosis. Looking through the medical notes or practice notes before meeting the patient will give insight as to how the patient has responded to other medical conditions or symptoms. The next most important features are patient's demographic details. Most IBS patients are young to middle aged females, although there are patients who develop IBS for the first time when they are older than 50 years of age. Other diagnoses, particularly colonic cancer and diverticular disease, become more common after this age, so new symptoms in this age group should raise concerns and prompt further investigations.

## Interview

The clinic consultation is usually the beginning of a patient–doctor relationship. There is increasing pressure to meet hospital targets and shorten interview time, which may compromise care of patients with functional GI disorders (FGIDs). They often have emotional problems that may take some time to elicit and, if not aired, may lead to a misdiagnosis and/or a feeling from the patient that 'they have not been listened to'.

A clinic consultation may vary from a doctor-dominated consultation to patient-dominated consultation, the latter being preferable with FGIDs. It is important to ensure that the patient feels at ease during the first few minutes of each consultation. This can be achieved by acknowledging the patient personally, positive gestures such as smiling, good eye contact and appearing 'unhurried' [4]. This might be a mundane task for a physician but from a patient's perspective meeting a 'specialist' may be of great importance in their patient journey.

Most medical diagnoses can be made from the initial consultation if done well and further tests add surprisingly little. During the consultation one should ask open-ended questions, so that patients are allowed to tell their story using their own words. By using open-ended questionnaires, one can elicit more information [5], especially about emotionally important factors and leave the patient satisfied that they have ' told the whole story', an unburdening which can have an important therapeutic benefit. Taking a full psychosocial history is worth the effort, as it has been shown to reduce return visits for IBS symptoms [6]. This would include questions about past or current anxiety, depression or panic attacks, quality of personal relationships as well as early family events like separation or family break up. As well as asking the patient about the potential role of psychosocial stressors it is also appropriate to ask about dietary precipitants and whether the symptoms began with an episode of gastroenteritis. Detailing the precise time course of onset and fluctuation in severity is often helpful here. Worsening of symptoms on Mondays and improvement on the weekend might suggest the role of work stress, while aggravation after eating out might suggest some dietary precipitant.

## Clinical features

IBS is a chronic condition whose key features are abdominal pain/discomfort together with an erratic bowel habit. Pain is sometimes, or often, relieved with defaecation and associated with increased stool frequency and looseness of stool form. Many patients find pain worsens soon after eating [7], which may also stimulate a bowel movement. Other associated symptoms are urgency, which may be severe enough to cause actual incontinence, straining and bloating. IBS patients often describe a feeling of incomplete evacuation and may return repeatedly to try to empty their bowels, often straining to do so, even if the stool is soft. They also describe bloating, an unpleasant sensation which may or may not be associated with visible abdominal distension and the need to loosen clothing. Those without visible distension demonstrate hypersensitivity to rectal distension such that they feel distended even though the bowel calibre is normal [8].

---

**Box 5.1  Rome III Diagnostic criteria for IBS\***

Recurrent abdominal pain or discomfort:
- ≥3 days per month in the last three months

- associated with two or more of the following

  ○ Improvement with defecation; *and/or*

  ○ Onset associated with a change in frequency of stool; *and/or*

  ○ Onset associated with a change in form (appearance) of stool.

\*Criteria fulfilled for the last 3 months with symptom onset ≥ 6 months prior to diagnosis

---

The Rome III diagnostic criteria for IBS (Box 5.1) [9], which were developed by an international consensus group, have been widely adopted as entry criteria for clinical trials of new IBS treatments and have reduced the heterogeneity of patients enrolled and improved consistency of findings. However, the criteria are somewhat insensitive and only 2/3 patients with IBS meet the criteria [10], which are not widely used in clinical practice. Most clinicians will make the diagnosis based on abdominal pain or discomfort with an erratic bowel habit in the absence of alarm features.

IBS symptoms typically wax and wane with symptoms occurring in clusters or 'attacks' and then subsiding [11]. These flares in symptoms typically last 2–3 days but may last for up to a week. Such a pattern is compatible with either dietary or emotional stressors aggravating symptoms as many patients recognize.

Since many conditions such as coeliac disease, diverticular disease and, very rarely, colorectal cancer can mimic IBS symptoms it is important to be alert to alarm symptoms which might suggest other diseases (Box 5.2). A key difference between IBS and other organic disease such as inflammatory bowel disease (IBD) is the erratic nature of the bowel disturbance. One study comparing IBD with IBS found that if patients agreed that '*Every day, my bowel pattern is different because I don't know if I will have a bowel movement and what it will look like. It varies every day*'; the sensitivity to diagnose IBS compared to IBD was 0.79 and specificity 0.7 [12] while the positive predictive value was 0.82. IBS patients have varied stool forms and using ≥3 stool forms/week as a diagnostic test for IBS, the sensitivity was 0.81, specificity 0.6 and positive predictive value of 0.77. IBD flares are typically more long lasting, usually weeks rather than days, and more consistent.

Commonly in clinical practice, pain and stool frequency and consistency are based on patient recall. In general, the accuracy of a patient's recall, especially for pain intensity, is poor and subject to overestimation, usually biased by the most recent events [13, 14]. This is probably also influenced by the current emotional state when recall occurs. The use of a diary

---

**Box 5.2  Alarm features**

- Age >50 years old at first presentation
- Unintended weight loss
- Short history of symptoms
- Nocturnal symptoms
- Blood mixed with stool
- Family history of colonic cancer
- Abnormally abdominal examination
- Anaemia
- Recent antibiotics.

---

provides a more reliable method of capturing details of pain/symptoms. At present, the standard is the Bristol Stool Chart scale incorporated in a one-week daily diary of stool frequency and consistency, severity of pain, bloating symptoms and overall general well-being (Figure 5.1). This gives a better understanding of the clustering of episodes of IBS symptoms and how they affect the patient's activities of daily living. The disadvantage of using paper diaries is that many patients forget to complete the diaries and do it all at once just before the clinic visit. More recently, electronic portable devices are being used which get round this problem.

It is worth asking about a family history of IBS, as there is a genetic tendency with increased prevalence of IBS in monozygotic (17%) compared to dizygotic twins (8%) [15]. There is also an important role for early learning, since having a mother with IBS increases the risk of having IBS even more than having a dizygotic twin with IBS.

## Somatization and comorbidities

One of the most difficult aspects of managing IBS patients is the high incidence of multiple comorbidities. These include psychological disorders such as somatization disorder and panic attacks, urinary symptoms such as dysuria, nocturia, frequency and urgency of micturition, gynaecological symptoms such as dyspareunia and chronic pelvic pain and other musculoskeletal problems, including chronic fatigue syndrome. Some may have undergone unnecessary investigations and treatments such as laparotomy, hysterectomy and cholecystectomy [16–18]. The rates of abdominal/pelvic surgery were reported to be twice as high as those of in the normal population and there is as high as a threefold increase in rates of gall bladder surgery in IBS patients [19].

Another comorbidity associated with between 30 and 60 % of IBS patients is fibromyalgia [20]. A study performed by Sperber *et al.* [21], in which

| Day | Date | Abdominal pain None = 0 Mild = 1 Moderate = 2 Severe = 3 | Urgency None = 0 Mild = 1 Moderate = 2 Severe = 3 | Bloating Yes/no | | Stool time and form | | | | | | | | | | |
|---|---|---|---|---|---|---|---|---|---|---|---|---|---|---|---|---|
| | | | | | | 1st | 2nd | 3rd | 4th | 5th | 6th | 7th | 8th | 9th | 10th | 11th |
| 1 | | | | | Form | | | | | | | | | | | |
| | | | | | Time | | | | | | | | | | | |
| 2 | | | | | Form | | | | | | | | | | | |
| | | | | | Time | | | | | | | | | | | |
| 3 | | | | | Form | | | | | | | | | | | |
| | | | | | Time | | | | | | | | | | | |
| 4 | | | | | Form | | | | | | | | | | | |
| | | | | | Time | | | | | | | | | | | |
| 5 | | | | | Form | | | | | | | | | | | |
| | | | | | Time | | | | | | | | | | | |
| 6 | | | | | Form | | | | | | | | | | | |
| | | | | | Time | | | | | | | | | | | |
| 7 | | | | | Form | | | | | | | | | | | |
| | | | | | Time | | | | | | | | | | | |

**Bristol Stool Form Score**

1 = Separate hard lumps, like nuts
2 = Sausage shaped but lumpy
3 = Like a sausage or snake, but with cracks on its surface
4 = Like a sausage or snake, smooth and soft
5 = Soft blobs with clear cut edges
6 = Fluffy pieces with ragged edges, a mushy stool
7 = Watery, no solid pieces

**Figure 5.1** The Bristol stool Chart scale.

approximately one-third of IBS patients had fibromyalgia and one-third of patients with fibromyalgia had IBS, showed that patients with both conditions had worse health-related quality of life and displayed more hypersensitivity to pain compared to those with IBS or fibromyalgia alone.

Somatization disorder (SD), a psychiatric disorder which features multiple medically unexplained symptoms, including psychiatric and neurological complaints, is rare, with an incidence of around 1 per 1000 but a much commoner problem is the 'physical symptom disorder',defined as one or more medically unexplained physical symptoms present for at least six months, which is found in as many as 1 in 10 of primary care consultees [22]. It may go unrecognized by physicians and general practitioners because training is focused on the identification and treatment of specific organic diseases [23]. Documenting the patient's complaints, comorbidities and previous attendances to hospitals is a helpful pointer towards the existence of SD. Patients with irritable bowel syndrome who manifest a degree of somatization often meet diagnostic criteria for other functional disorders [24]. It is important to recognize and identify these patients at the first interview. The evidence is that they are more difficult to manage, visit the emergency department more often, see more physicians, report worse global IBS symptomatology and have a poorer response to conventional IBS treatments [23].

The Patient Health Questionnaire 15 (PHQ-15) is a useful questionnaire that documents somatic symptoms from different parts of the body system and only takes 1–2 minutes to complete. The PHQ15 contains three gastrointestinal symptoms which, if deleted, leaves the PHQ12 Somatic Symptoms scale (PHQ12SS) as a useful measure of nongastrointestinal symptoms [25]. A PHQ12SS score >6 identifies patients with IBS with a sensitivity of 66.4% and specificity of 94.7% and a positive likelihood ratio of 13.2. A low score is unusual in IBS and should prompt a search for other diagnoses. Another tool that is useful is the 14 item Hospital Anxiety and Depression scale (HAD). This is a reliable tool to detect anxiety and depression [26]. It is important to recognize these since they contribute to the severity of disease and may warrant specific treatment.

## Precipitating events

IBS develops when a susceptible individual is exposed to external stressors; these include emotional stressors, gastrointestinal infection or a change in diet, factors which one should look out for during the consultation.

### Psychological stressors

It is important to take a full psychosocial history. Going through the response to the Hospital Anxiety and Depression scale is a useful way of reviewing anxieties and concerns. Creed *et al.* [27] demonstrated that severe adverse life events and chronic stressors are much commoner before the onset of IBS symptoms compared with other gastrointestinal disorders. Severe stressors include marital problems, enforced changes at work, bereavement, housing crises and court appearance with threat of imprisonment. Approximately 30% of patients with IBS have psychiatric illness and/or an anxiety provoking event that precede symptoms of functional abdominal symptoms [28]. Continuing chronic stressors are important to recognize, since they are one of the best predictors of success or otherwise of treatment [29].

## Gastroenteritis

A documented bout of infectious gastroenteritis is one of the strongest known risk factor for developing IBS in the subsequent year, with a relative risk of 11.9 [30]. After adjusting for age and gender the relative risk is similar to anxiety and greater than that for depression, sleep disorders, smoking, body mass index and alcohol excess [31]. Depending on the setting, between 6 and 17% of patients with IBS believe that their symptoms occurred following bacterial gastroenteritis [32] while 4–31% of documented bacterial infections are followed by IBS [33]. Post-infectious IBS has been defined by the development of IBS symptoms following an acute illness comprising two of the following symptoms: fever, vomiting, acute diarrhoea and positive stool culture [34]. Although a positive stool culture is desirable this is often not available, as many cases occur while travelling abroad when the patient may not have ready access to a public health laboratory.

Both psychological and intestinal factors predispose patients to develop post-infectious IBS, with bacterial factors and the local inflammatory response playing the dominant roles (Figure 5.2). Independent predictors for the development of post-infectious IBS are, in ascending order of importance: adverse life event in the preceding three months (relative risk (RR) = 2.0), depression (RR = 3.2), hypochondriasis (RR = 2.0) [35], female gender (RR = 3) [36], lymphocytosis and enterochromaffin cell hyperplasia in the colonic mucosa (each 1 Standard Deviation rise in cells counts increasing the risk 3.2 and 3.8 fold respectively) [34], smoking (RR = 4.8) [37], duration of initial illness >3 weeks (RR = 11.5) [36] and infection with a strain of *Campylobacter jejuni* which produces an elongating toxin (RR = 12.8) [38]. Age <60 years seem to be protective, RR = 0.36 [39]. It is important to take a patient's travel history, as 50% of patients with post-infectious IBS still have symptoms after five years [33]. It is worth noting that bile salt malabsorption can also present in this way with sudden onset after a bout of gastroenteritis but distinguishing features include severe nocturnal diarrhoea, with large volume watery stool. This can be tested for

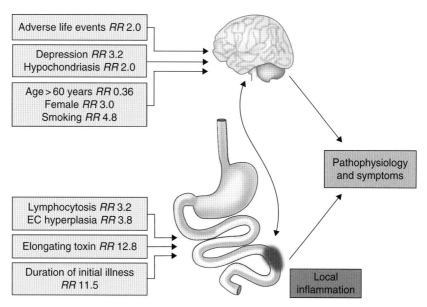

**Figure 5.2** Interaction between local inflammation and psychosocial factors in determining risk of developing post-infectious IBS. (Reproduced from Spiller and Garsed [39], with permission from Elsevier.)

using the SeCHAT test, which assesses the seven-day retention of Selenium [75] HomoCholic Acid Taurine. Bile salt malabsorption is diagnosed if retention is less than 10%. Intermediate degrees of malabsorption (10–15%) are less helpful but those with <10% show a good response to bile salt binding agents such as colestyramine [40].

## Diet

It is important to take a dietary history to assess intake of fruit and vegetables. Promoting a healthy diet, 'five a day', which includes dietary intake of five '80 g' portions of fruit and vegetables daily makes much sense from a public health perspective as it may well reduce the risk of cardiovascular disease, type-2 diabetes and obesity. However, many IBS patients are intolerant of the 'five a day' diet, since these foods typically have a high content of fibre, fructose, fructans and polyhydric alcohols. These are poorly absorbed even by a normal gut and the increased volume of chyme delivered to the colon along with the gas resulting from fermentation of unabsorbed carbohydrate can cause bloating, flatulence and pain in IBS patients who are hypersensitive to gut distension.

A dietary history should distinguish soluble from insoluble 'fibre', which is a misnomer since most 'fibre' is not fibrous. However, the term is widely used to describe nonstarch polysaccharide often found in plants, characteristically resistant to human digestive enzymes. Soluble 'fibre' consists of

> **Box 5.3  Common foods containing FODMAPs**
>
> • Lactose: dairy products from cow, goat and sheep milk.
>
> • Fructans: wheat, rye, onion, garlic, cruciferous vegetable and some fruit such as melon and peach.
>
> • Galactans: legumes such as kidney and baked beans, lentils and chickpeas.
>
> • Polyols (sorbitol, xylitol, mannitol and maltitol): apples, apricots, avocado, cherries and nectarines.

pectins, gums and mucilages, the best known being guar and psyllium which, characteristically, form viscous solutions with water and can be prescribed in pure form. Insoluble fibre consists of the harder structural components of plants, including celluloses, hemicelluloses and lignins. These are typically particulate and insoluble in water, for example as wheat bran. While soluble fibre can help IBS patients with constipation [41] insoluble fibre can adversely affect symptoms so intake should be assessed.

### Effect of bran

Patients who are symptomatic may modify their diet or increase their fibre intake prior to consulting their general practitioner. Increasing fibre intake such as bran may be beneficial in constipation but not diarrhoea. Randomized placebo controlled trials show that it aggravates abdominal distension, flatulence and diarrhoea in IBS patients [42, 43]. Anecdotally, about half (55%) of IBS patients believe it worsens their symptoms, while only a small proportion (10%) report any improvement [44].

### FODMAPs

FODMAPs consist of fructose, lactose, fructo- and galacto-oligosaccharides (fructans and galactans) and polyols (sorbitol, mannitol, sylitol and malti-tol) (Box 5.3). Recent randomized placebo controlled trials in Australia have shown that adding FODMAPs (Fermentable Oligo-Di and Mono-saccharides and Polyhydric alcohols) to the diet can trigger abdominal symptoms such as flatulence, bloating, abdominal discomfort and change in bowel habit [45, 46].

Fructose is a six-carbon monosaccharide found in many foods in three forms. Free fructose is found in fruit and honey. Fructose may also be present in the diet as a constituent of the disaccharide sucrose or as fructans, which are polymers of fructose with small amounts of glucose. Fructose absorption is less efficient than glucose so it is possible to exceed the absorptive capacity of the small bowel and excessive doses lead to malabsorbed fructose entering the colon. Here it is rapidly fermented by the microbiota, producing short fatty acids, carbon dioxide, hydrogen and methane [47, 48]. Hydrogen and methane so produced are expired through the breath or passed as flatus. When these osmotic changes and rapid gas production occur, symptoms such as flatus, bloating and abdominal discomfort are induced and gut motility altered [49, 50]. IBS patients do not appear to malabsorb more than normal but do seem to be more sensitive to the effects of these carbohydrates compared to healthy volunteers [51].

Assessing dietary intolerance to FODMAPs by history is difficult since the effect of each component depends on what else is consumed at the same time [49, 52]. Thus, if fructose and sorbitol are given in a mixture, they seem to cause more symptoms compared to when given separately [49], while if given with readily absorbed glucose, malabsorption is reduced [53], which may explain why sources of fructose with low glucose content like pears may be less well tolerated than sources with high glucose content such as grapes [54].

Some IBS patients respond to a low FODMAPs diet, though with such a complex diet, requiring intensive dietician input, placebo effects are likely also to be important [45]. One reason why this topic has generated a lot of interest is that over recent years there has been a marked increase in consumption of fructose and fructans, particularly in the United States, where high-fructose corn syrup is widely used as a sweetener in soft drinks, sugared fruit drinks, jams and baked goods [55, 56].

## Lactose intolerance

Lactose malabsorption affects up to 70% of adults worldwide but for most this causes no problem. Normally lactase levels fall post-weaning but a mutation which arose in North Western Europe prevents this, causing levels to remain high throughout adult life (lactase persistence) [57]. The prevalence of this mutation is maximal in Scotland and declines as one moves South and West [58]. Only about 1 in 3 are aware of their intolerance, and, in some, it can cause IBS-like symptoms [59]. Severity of the resulting symptoms is dose dependent and reduced if the lactose is taken with other food because this delays gastric emptying causing slower delivery to the small intestine [60]. Identifying lactose intolerance only helps if the patient's daily intake of lactose amounts more than is found in about half a pint of milk, something which applies to relatively few IBS patients.

## Drugs

A complete drug history is important since many drugs, including over the counter medications, can mimic IBS symptoms. Particular attention should be paid to opiates, which cause constipation [61], antibiotics which cause diarrhoea and proton pump inhibitors (PPIs) which can also cause diarrhoea due to microscopic colitis [62–66]. Probiotics are widely used and some have a laxative effect [67] so it is always worth specifically enquiring if they are being taken since many patients do not regard them as drugs.

Other rare causes of diarrhoea due to medications are cardiac medications; angiotensin converting enzyme inhibitors [68], beta-blockers, drugs affecting the central nervous system; lithium and carbamazepine [69, 70] and weight control medication; lipase inhibitors [71, 72].

## Physical examination

The general examination of IBS patients will usually be normal. You should look for signs of systemic diseases such as anaemia (pallor, koilo-nychias), clubbing, as well as features of hyperthyroidism and Addison's disease. IBS does not cause weight loss so cachexia or signs of malnutrition are alarm features which should lead to further investigations.

   Examination gives one the chance to observe where a patient places his/her hands on their abdomen when asked to show where the pain is felt. Visceral pain is typically diffuse and will be shown by placing the hand across the abdomen. If pain is localized by pointing with one finger this suggests a somatic origin. Pain originating in the abdominal wall can be demonstrated by asking the supine patient to raise their head and shoulders off the couch by tensing their abdominal muscles. Applying local pressure to the 'tender' area allows one to distinguish between intra-abdominal pain, which decreases, and abdominal wall pain, which increases with this manoeuver. This increase in pain on tensing the abdominal muscles is called a positive Carnett's sign. A recent study in Japan [73] has shown the reproducibility and utility of Carnett's test. The final diagnosis of patients with a positive Carnett's sign included idiopathic myofascial syndrome, radiculopathy, epidemic pleurodynia, peripheral nerve entrapment and cellulitis. Carnett's test has been reported to have a sensitivity of 81% and specificity of 88% [74]. Its main value is in preventing extensive negative examinations of the gut.

   Painful rib syndrome is another nongastrointestinal cause of abdominal pain which accounts for 3% of referrals to general medical/gastroenterology clinics [75] and can cause difficulty to the inexperienced practitioner. Patients complain of pain in the lower chest or upper abdomen with local tender spot(s) on the lower costal margin where local pressure can reproduce the pain. It is important to recognize this condition in order to avoid numerous unnecessary and unhelpful gastrointestinal investigations. Patients should be reassured that this is benign and for some that is all that they require. Some patients respond well to local anaesthetic injections to which steroid can be added if symptoms persist. Resection of the anterior end of the rib has been used in severe cases [76].

   Abdominal examination is usually unremarkable apart from vague tenderness, without guarding. Occasionally, one can feel a tender sigmoid colon in the left iliac fossa. Perineal inspection and rectal examination are useful to exclude any induration or local tenderness which might suggest Crohn's disease or an anal fissure. Assessment of voluntary squeeze is useful in assessing patients with urgency to see if there is any sphincter defect. It is also useful if constipation is a problem to ask the patient to bear down as if attempting defecation. This may identify inadequate propulsive effort or inappropriate puborectalis contraction which should prompt further investigation for disordered defecation [77]. Sigmoidoscopy and air insufflations may also be useful both to exclude colitis and to see if it reproduces the patient's pain. Typically, IBS patients experience the pain referred to the abdomen while, for most other patients, it is localized to the perineal region [78]. Direct visualization of stool form is also useful in objectively assessing bowel disturbance.

## Investigations and management

If the Rome criteria are met in the absence of alarm features (Figure 5.3) and physical examination is unremarkable, then the positive predictive value for the diagnosis of IBS is 98% [10]. At this stage it is important to state that you feel the diagnosis is IBS and that you think the limited screening tests will be normal. That way when the tests come back normal you do not then get pressure to do yet more tests as 'there must be something wrong'. The screening tests should vary according to the main bowel habit. All should have a full blood count and thyroid function tests if not already done but those with diarrhoea will warrant further tests, including tissue transglutaminase to exclude coeliac disease [79], C-reactive protein (CRP), calcium and albumin. Depending on the pattern of diarrhoea it may also be reasonable to do a colonoscopy to exclude microscopic colitis, particularly if the patient is >50 years of age and the diarrhoea is persistent or disturbs sleep. Colonoscopy is not necessary with constipation unless there are other indications like blood in the stool, age >50 years or a family history of colorectal cancer [80]. While faecal calprotectin has a 89% sensitivity to detect inflammatory bowel disease, it also gives quite a few false positives (21%) [81] and so is not widely used for diagnosis.

It is important to use time as a diagnostic test and to see the patient again after 6–8 weeks to ensure there has been no progression. Rare diseases like GIST tumours, pseudo-obstruction and not so rare diseases like Crohn's disease or ovarian cancer may present with vague IBS-like features but their symptoms progress and alarm features like weight loss, nocturnal diarrhoea and new symptoms should prompt a reconsideration of the diagnosis, especially in the over 50-year-old patient. The typical IBS patient's symptoms are intermittent and not progressive.

While subsequent chapters will deal with specific treatments it is worth saying here that it is important to ensure that the patient has realistic expectations of treatment. They should understand that symptoms are a balance of peripheral gut factors, which may respond to specific drugs or

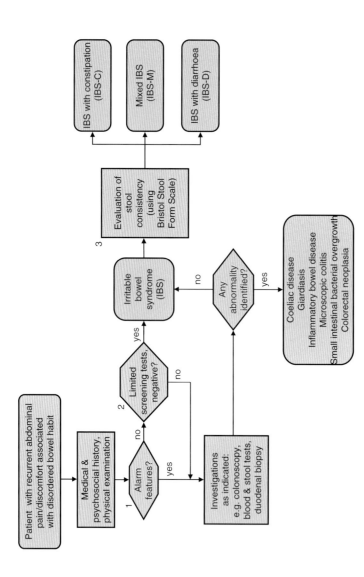

**Figure 5.3** Management algorithm for the assessment of patients with IBS. (Adapted from Spiller and Thompson [80], with permission from Macmillan Publishers Ltd.)

1. Alarm features include: Age >50 years old at first presentation, unintended weight loss, short history of symptoms, nocturnal symptoms, blood mixed with stool, family history of colonic cancer, abnormal abdominal examination, anaemia, recent antibiotics.

2. Screening tests include full blood count, thyroid function, tissue transglutaminase and, for those with diarrhoea, serum calcium albumin and C reactive protein (CRP).

3. Stool diary can be examined at the six-week visit to clarify bowel habit. Depending on whether diarrhoea or constipation predominates the patient can be recommended drugs to modify bowel habit, including low dose amitriptyline, loperamide, 5HT3 receptor antagonists or 5HT4 agonists (if available).

---

Content within the figure:

Patient with recurrent abdominal pain/discomfort associated with disordered bowel habit

Medical & psychosocial history, physical examination

1 — Alarm features?
- no
- yes

2 — Limited screening tests, negative?
- yes → Irritable bowel syndrome (IBS)
- no → Investigations as indicated: e.g. colonoscopy, blood & stool tests, duodenal biopsy

Investigations as indicated → Any abnormality identified?
- no → Irritable bowel syndrome (IBS)
- yes → Coeliac disease / Giardiasis / Inflammatory bowel disease / Microscopic colitis / Small intestinal bacterial overgrowth / Colorectal neoplasia

3 — Evaluation of stool consistency (using Bristol Stool Form Scale)
- IBS with constipation (IBS-C)
- Mixed IBS (IBS-M)
- IBS with diarrhoea (IBS-D)

treatments, and central psychological factors, which may be more difficult to change. The very anxious patient may respond to the mild tranquillizing effect of low dose amitriptyline, always assuming they can accept the side effects. Cognitive behavioural therapy or hypnotherapy may be successful in some patients but availability is very limited at present.

## Conclusion

Clinical assessment of IBS patients demands great attention to details. Adequate time needs to be allocated to hear the full story, particularly focusing on the emotional factors and events which have precipitated referral. A systematic approach in history taking, awareness of the patient's multiple medical and social problems and a thorough examination will lead to a more satisfactory consultation for both the physician and patient and ultimately a more accurate diagnosis with the minimum of investigations.

## Useful web links

- http://www.theibsnetwork.org
- http://www.aboutibs.org
- http://www.corecharity.org.uk/Irritable-Bowel-Syndrome.html
- http://www.romecriteria.org

---

**CASE STUDY 5.1**

A 28-year-old female lawyer presents with six years history of abdominal discomfort with erratic bowel habit. Symptoms have increased in severity and frequency over the last year. This has now prompted her general practitioner to refer her to a gastrointestinal outpatient clinic. She has experienced symptoms intermittently for the past six years. Each episode occurs every 3–4 weeks and lasts 1–4 days. Her abdominal discomfort is poorly localized, with a variable location, mainly central. When the pain begins her stools usually become softer and at times even watery. She opens her bowels up to five times per day, mostly in the morning. Once her bowels are opened, there is some relief of her abdominal discomfort. These episodes can last for days, following which she has no bowel movements for up to three days when her stool will be lumpy and hard to pass. She also complains of a sense of abdominal bloating and towards the end of the day notices her abdomen visibly swells and her clothing feels tight. Sometimes, she has to stay at home to rest during her bouts of pain and may lose 1–2 days off work. She feels that sometimes food aggravates her symptoms, especially when eating out, but cannot identify any specific food. She often turns down invitations to eat out because she fears it will bring on the pain. She has no upper gastrointestinal symptoms such as nausea, vomiting, reflux or dysphagia. There are no sinister symptoms, in particular, no weight loss, nocturnal symptoms, rectal bleeding or recent antibiotic usage. Her menstrual cycle is regular and menses last for four days.

She has had lower back pain for many years but no other significant past medical history. She does not smoke and drinks less than four units of alcohol per week. She is on paracetamol intermittently and an oral contraceptive pill. She eats a well-balanced diet with no obvious food intolerances. Her caffeine intake is minimal and, on further questioning of her dietary intake, it becomes clear that she does not take in excessive amounts of fibre, fructose or dairy products. She lives with her husband and works full time as a lawyer. She finds managing her job and two children, aged three and seven years, difficult and tiring. She thinks stress at work aggravates her symptoms. Twelve months ago, she had a miscarriage.

On examination there are no signs of anaemia. When asked to show where the pain would start she places her outstretched hand over her umbilical region and spreads both hands over her abdomen to show how the pain radiates all over her abdomen. The remainder of the examination, including perianal and rectal examination, is normal.

The gastroenterologist makes a confident diagnosis of IBS and explains to the patients that he will confirm this with a few simple tests which he expects to be normal. These include a complete blood count which is normal (haemoglobin 12.6 gm/dl, mean cell volume 88 fl), tissue transglutaminase is negative.

The gastroenterologist discusses the diagnosis of IBS to the patient at the first consultation and reassures her that it is very common and does not lead to more serious conditions. Further explanation regarding possible causes and how symptoms occur, including the idea of visceral hypersensitivity and hyper-reactivity of her bowel, was given. To further subtype her IBS, the patient is given the Bristol Stool Form Scale diary which she completes before attending for a follow-up appointment at six weeks to review the symptoms and results of the screening test. On review of her stool diary, she has stool consistency of various types, that is type 1 or 2 (hard or lumpy) to type 6 or 7 (mushy or watery). These occurred more than 25% of the time for each pattern. The patient was diagnosed as IBS of mixed type (IBS-M) (Figure 5.4).

She was prescribed mebeverine 135 mg before meals t.d.s and ispaghula husk 3.5 g b.d. Three months later symptoms were still present but she was coping better with them and was thinking of reducing her hours of work as she had come to the conclusion that stress at work was exacerbating her symptoms.

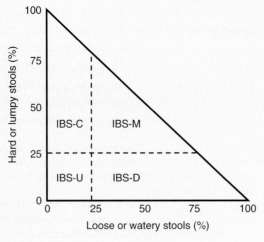

**Figure 5.4** IBS subtypes according to stool consistency.

# References

1  Thompson WG, Heaton KW, Smyth GT and Smyth C. Irritable bowel syndrome in general practice: prevalence, characteristics, and referral. *Gut* 2000;46(1):78–82.

2  Amouretti M, Le Pen C, Gaudin AF *et al*. Impact of irritable bowel syndrome (IBS) on health-related quality of life (HRQOL). *Gastroenterol Clin Biol* 2006;30(2):241–246.

3  Cain KC, Headstrom P, Jarrett ME *et al*. Abdominal pain impacts quality of life in women with irritable bowel syndrome. *Am J Gastroenterol* 2006;101(1):124–132.

4  Pandhi N, Bowers B and Chen FP. A comfortable relationship: a patient-derived dimension of ongoing care. *Fam Med* 2007;39(4):266–273.

5  Takemura Y, Sakurai Y, Yokoya S *et al*. Open-ended questions: are they really beneficial for gathering medical information from patients? *Tohoku J Exp Med* 2005; 206(2):151–154.

6  Owens DM, Nelson DK and Talley NJ. The irritable bowel syndrome: long-term prognosis and the physician-patient interaction. *Ann Intern Med* 1995;122(2):107–112.

7  Ragnarsson G and Bodemar G. Pain is temporally related to eating but not to defaecation in the irritable bowel syndrome (IBS). Patients' description of diarrhea, constipation and symptom variation during a prospective 6-week study. *Eur J Gastroenterol Hepatol* 1998;10(5):415–421.

8  Agrawal A, Houghton LA, Lea R *et al*. Bloating and distention in irritable bowel syndrome: the role of visceral sensation. *Gastroenterology* 2008;134(7):1882–1889.

9  Longstreth GF, Thompson WG, Chey WD *et al*. Functional bowel disorders. *Gastroenterology* 2006;130(5):1480–1491.

10  Vanner SJ, Depew WT, Paterson WG *et al*. Predictive value of the Rome criteria for diagnosing the irritable bowel syndrome. *Am J Gastroenterol* 1999;94(10):2912–2917.

11  Stevens JA, Wan CK and Blanchard EB. The short-term natural history of irritable bowel syndrome: a time-series analysis. *Behav Res Ther* 1997;35(4):319–326.

12  Pimentel M, Hwang L, Melmed GY *et al*. New clinical method for distinguishing D-IBS from other gastrointestinal conditions causing diarrhea: the LA/IBS diagnostic strategy. *Dig Dis Sci* 2010;55(1):145–149.

13  Jamison RN, Sbrocco T and Parris WC. The influence of physical and psychosocial factors on accuracy of memory for pain in chronic pain patients. *Pain* 1989;37(3): 289–294.

14  Gendreau M, Hufford MR and Stone AA. Measuring clinical pain in chronic widespread pain: selected methodological issues. *Best Pract Res Clin Rheumatol* 2003; 17(4):575–592.

15  Levy RL, Jones KR, Whitehead WE *et al*. Irritable bowel syndrome in twins: heredity and social learning both contribute to etiology. *Gastroenterology* 2001;121(4):799–804.

16  Francis CY, Duffy JN, Whorwell PJ and Morris J. High prevalence of irritable bowel syndrome in patients attending urological outpatient departments. *Dig Dis Sci* 1997;42(2):404–407.

17  Prior A, Wilson K, Whorwell PJ and Faragher EB. Irritable bowel syndrome in the gynecological clinic. Survey of 798 new referrals. *Dig Dis Sci* 1989;34(12):1820–1824.

18  Jones R, Latinovic R, Charlton J and Gulliford M. Physical and psychological comorbidity in irritable bowel syndrome: a matched cohort study using the General Practice Research Database. *Aliment Pharmacol Ther* 2006;24(5):879–886.

19  Cole JA, Yeaw JM, Cutone JA *et al*. The incidence of abdominal and pelvic surgery among patients with irritable bowel syndrome. *Dig Dis Sci* 2005;50(12):2268–2275.

20  Whitehead WE, Palsson O and Jones KR. Systematic review of the comorbidity of irritable bowel syndrome with other disorders: What are the causes and implications? *Gastroenterology* 2002;122(4):1140–1156.

21 Sperber AD, Atzmon Y, Neumann L *et al*. Fibromyalgia in the irritable bowel syndrome: studies of prevalence and clinical implications. *Am J Gastroenterol* 1999;94(12):3541–3546.

22 Kroenke K. Physical symptom disorder: a simpler diagnostic category for somatization-spectrum conditions. *J Psychosom Res* 2006;60(4):335–339.

23 North CS, Downs D, Clouse RE *et al*. The presentation of irritable bowel syndrome in the context of somatization disorder. *Clin Gastroenterol Hepatol* 2004;2(9):787–795.

24 Sperber AD and Dekel R. Irritable Bowel syndrome and co-morbid gastrointestinal and extra-gastrointestinal functional syndromes. *J Neurogastroenterol Motil* 2010; 16(2):113–119.

25 Spiller RC, Humes DJ, Campbell E *et al*. The Patient Health Questionnaire 12 Somatic Symptom scale as a predictor of symptom severity and consulting behaviour in patients with irritable bowel syndrome and symptomatic diverticular disease. *Aliment Pharmacol Ther* 2010;32(6):811–8120.

26 Zigmond AS and Snaith RP. The hospital anxiety and depression scale. *Acta Psychiatr Scand* 1983;67(6):361–370.

27 Creed F, Craig T and Farmer R. Functional abdominal pain, psychiatric illness, and life events. *Gut* 1988;29(2):235–242.

28 Ford MJ, Miller PM, Eastwood J and Eastwood MA. Life events, psychiatric illness and the irritable bowel syndrome. *Gut* 1987;28(2):160–165.

29 Bennett EJ, Tennant CC, Piesse C, Badcock CA and Kellow JE. Level of chronic life stress predicts clinical outcome in irritable bowel syndrome. *Gut* 1998;43(2):256–261.

30 Rodriguez LA and Ruigomez A. Increased risk of irritable bowel syndrome after bacterial gastroenteritis: cohort study. *BMJ* 1999;318(7183):565–566.

31 Ruigomez A, Garcia Rodriguez LA and Panes J. Risk of irritable bowel syndrome after an episode of bacterial gastroenteritis in general practice: influence of comorbidities. *Clin Gastroenterol Hepatol* 2007;5(4):465–469.

32 Longstreth GF, Hawkey CJ, Mayer EA *et al*. Characteristics of patients with irritable bowel syndrome recruited from three sources: implications for clinical trials. *Aliment Pharmacol Ther* 2001;15(7):959–964.

33 Spiller RC. Role of infection in irritable bowel syndrome. *J Gastroenterol* 2007;42(Suppl 17):41–47.

34 Dunlop SP, Jenkins D, Neal KR and Spiller RC. Relative importance of enterochromaffin cell hyperplasia, anxiety, and depression in postinfectious IBS. *Gastroenterology* 2003;125(6):1651–1659.

35 Gwee KA, Graham JC, McKendrick MW *et al*. Psychometric scores and persistence of irritable bowel after infectious diarrhoea. *Lancet* 1996;347(8995):150–153.

36 Neal KR, Hebden J and Spiller R. Prevalence of gastrointestinal symptoms six months after bacterial gastroenteritis and risk factors for development of the irritable bowel syndrome: postal survey of patients. *BMJ* 1997;314(7083):779–782.

37 Parry SD, Barton JR and Welfare MR. Factors associated with the development of post-infectious functional gastrointestinal diseases: does smoking play a role? *Eur J Gastroenterol Hepatol* 2005;17(10):1071–1075.

38 Thornley JP, Jenkins D, Neal K *et al*. Relationship of Campylobacter toxigenicity in vitro to the development of postinfectious irritable bowel syndrome. *J Infect Dis* 2001;184(5):606–609.

39 Spiller R and Garsed K. Postinfectious irritable bowel syndrome. *Gastroenterology* 2009;136(6):1979–1988.

40 Sinha L, Liston R, Testa HJ and Moriarty KJ. Idiopathic bile acid malabsorption: qualitative and quantitative clinical features and response to cholestyramine. *Aliment Pharmacol Ther* 1998;12(9):839–844.

41 Prior A and Whorwell PJ. Double blind study of ispaghula in irritable bowel syndrome. *Gut* 1987;28(11):1510–1513.

42 Cann PA, Read NW and Holdsworth CD. What is the benefit of coarse wheat bran in patients with irritable bowel syndrome? *Gut* 1984;25(2):168–173.

43 Snook J and Shepherd HA. Bran supplementation in the treatment of irritable bowel syndrome. *Aliment Pharmacol Ther* 1994;8(5):511–514.

44 Francis CY and Whorwell PJ. Bran and irritable bowel syndrome: time for reappraisal. *Lancet* 1994;344(8914):39–40.

45 Shepherd SJ, Parker FC, Muir JG and Gibson PR. Dietary triggers of abdominal symptoms in patients with irritable bowel syndrome: randomized placebo-controlled evidence. *Clin Gastroenterol Hepatol* 2008;6(7):765–771.

46 Ong DK, Mitchell SB, Barrett JS *et al*. Manipulation of dietary short chain carbohydrates alters the pattern of gas production and genesis of symptoms in irritable bowel syndrome. *J Gastroenterol Hepatol* 2010;25(8):1366–1373.

47 Shepherd SJ and Gibson PR. Fructose malabsorption and symptoms of irritable bowel syndrome: guidelines for effective dietary management. *J Am Diet Assoc* 2006;106(10):1631–1639.

48 Oku T and Nakamura S. Comparison of digestibility and breath hydrogen gas excretion of fructo-oligosaccharide, galactosyl-sucrose, and isomalto-oligosaccharide in healthy human subjects. *Eur J Clin Nutr* 2003;57(9):1150–1156.

49 Rumessen JJ and Gudmand-Hoyer E. Malabsorption of fructose-sorbitol mixtures. *Interactions causing abdominal distress. Scand J Gastroenterol* 1987;22(4):431–436.

50 Fernandez-Banares F, Esteve M and Viver JM. Fructose-sorbitol malabsorption. *Curr Gastroenterol Rep* 2009;11(5):368–374.

51 Symons P, Jones MP and Kellow JE. Symptom provocation in irritable bowel syndrome. Effects of differing doses of fructose-sorbitol. *Scand J Gastroenterol* 1992;27(11):940–944.

52 Goldstein R, Braverman D and Stankiewicz H. Carbohydrate malabsorption and the effect of dietary restriction on symptoms of irritable bowel syndrome and functional bowel complaints. *Isr Med Assoc J* 2000;2(8):583–587.

53 Truswell AS, Seach JM and Thorburn AW. Incomplete absorption of pure fructose in healthy subjects and the facilitating effect of glucose. *Am J Clin Nutr* 1988;48(6): 1424–1430.

54 Nobigrot T, Chasalow FI and Lifshitz F. Carbohydrate absorption from one serving of fruit juice in young children: age and carbohydrate composition effects. *J Am Coll Nutr* 1997;16(2):152–158.

55 Park YK and Yetley EA. Intakes and food sources of fructose in the United States. *Am J Clin Nutr* 1993;58(5 Suppl):737S–747S.

56 Hanover LM and White JS. Manufacturing, composition, and applications of fructose. *Am J Clin Nutr* 1993;58(5 Suppl):724S–732S.

57 Jarvela IE. Molecular genetics of adult-type hypolactasia. *Ann Med* 2005;37(3): 179–185.

58 Swallow DM. Genetics of lactase persistence and lactose intolerance. *Annu Rev Genet* 2003;37:197–219.

59 Lomer MC, Parkes GC and Sanderson JD. Review article: lactose intolerance in clinical practice–myths and realities. *Aliment Pharmacol Ther* 2008;27(2):93–103.

60 Ladas S, Papanikos J and Arapakis G. Lactose malabsorption in Greek adults: correlation of small bowel transit time with the severity of lactose intolerance. *Gut* 1982; 23(11):968–973.

61 Moore RA and McQuay HJ. Prevalence of opioid adverse events in chronic non-malignant pain: systematic review of randomised trials of oral opioids. *Arthritis Res Ther* 2005;7(5):R1046–1051.

62 Mukherjee S. Diarrhea associated with lansoprazole. *J Gastroenterol Hepatol* 2003; 18(5):602–603.

63 Rammer M, Kirchgatterer A, Hobling W and Knoflach P. Lansoprazole-associated collagenous colitis: a case report. *Z Gastroenterol* 2005;43(7):657–660.

64 Chande N and Driman DK. Microscopic colitis associated with lansoprazole: report of two cases and a review of the literature. *Scand J Gastroenterol* 2007;42(4):530–533.

65 Keszthelyi D, Jansen SV, Schouten GA, de Kort S, Scholtes B, Engels LG, *et al.* Proton pump inhibitor use is associated with an increased risk for microscopic colitis: a case-control study. *Aliment Pharmacol Ther* 2010;32(9):1124–1128.

66 Thomson RD, Lestina LS, Bensen SP *et al.* Lansoprazole-associated microscopic colitis: a case series. *Am J Gastroenterol* 2002;97(11):2908–2913.

67 Agrawal A, Houghton LA, Morris J *et al.* Clinical trial: the effects of a fermented milk product containing Bifidobacterium lactis DN-173 010 on abdominal distension and gastrointestinal transit in irritable bowel syndrome with constipation. *Alimentary Pharmacology & Therapeutics* 2009;29(1):104–114.

68 Simpson K and Jarvis B. Lisinopril: a review of its use in congestive heart failure. *Drugs* 2000;59(5):1149–1167.

69 Fosnes GS, Lydersen S and Farup PG. Constipation and diarrhoea – common adverse drug reactions? A cross sectional study in the general population. *BMC Clin Pharmacol* 2011;11:2.

70 Grandjean EM and Aubry JM. Lithium: updated human knowledge using an evidence-based approach: part III: clinical safety. *CNS Drugs* 2009;23(5):397–418.

71 Filippatos TD, Derdemezis CS, Gazi IF *et al.* Orlistat-associated adverse effects and drug interactions: a critical review. *Drug Saf* 2008;31(1):53–65.

72 Acharya NV, Wilton LV and Shakir SA. Safety profile of orlistat: results of a prescription-event monitoring study. *Int J Obes (Lond)* 2006;30(11):1645–1652.

73 Takada T, Ikusaka M, Ohira Y, Noda K and Tsukamoto T. Diagnostic usefulness of Carnett's test in psychogenic abdominal pain. *Intern Med* 2011;50(3):213–217.

74 Matsunaga S and Eguchi Y. Importance of a physical examination for efficient differential diagnosis of abdominal pain: diagnostic usefulness of Carnett's test in psychogenic abdominal pain. *Intern Med* 2011;50(3):177–178.

75 Scott EM and Scott BB. Painful rib syndrome – a review of 76 cases. *Gut* 1993; 34(7):1006–1008.

76 Gregory PL, Biswas AC and Batt ME. Musculoskeletal problems of the chest wall in athletes. *Sports Med* 2002;32(4):235–250.

77 Bharucha AE and Wald AM. Anorectal disorders. *Am J Gastroenterol* 2010;105(4): 786–794.

78 Mertz H, Naliboff B, Munakata J, Niazi N and Mayer EA. Altered rectal perception is a biological marker of patients with irritable bowel syndrome. *Gastroenterology* 1995;109(1):40–52.

79 Cash BD, Schoenfeld P and Chey WD. The utility of diagnostic tests in irritable bowel syndrome patients: a systematic review. *Am J Gastroenterol* 2002;97(11):2812–2819.

80 Spiller RC and Thompson WG. Bowel disorders. *Am J Gastroenterol* 2010;105(4): 775–785.

81 Tibble JA, Sigthorsson G, Foster R, Forgacs I and Bjarnason I. Use of surrogate markers of inflammation and Rome criteria to distinguish organic from nonorganic intestinal disease. *Gastroenterology* 2002;123(2):450–460.

82 Mylotte M, Egan-Mitchell B, McCarthy CF and McNicholl B. Incidence of coeliac disease in the West of Ireland. *BMJ* 1973;1(5855):703–705.

# Multiple Choice Questions

1 A 70-year-old man presented with acute onset of painless watery diarrhoea for the past 12 months. Frequently he is woken up in the middle of the night needing to open his bowels. He has no travel history and no exposure to antibiotics.
   **A** This is very unlikely due to microscopic colitis.
   **B** Part of investigation includes a bile salt malabsorption test SeHCAT test.
   **C** This is typical of functional diarrhoea.
   **D** IBS is the most likely diagnosis.

Answer: B

Microscopic colitis is a cause of chronic diarrhoea which occurs commonly in middle age and elderly patients, so is part of the differential diagnosis here. Functional diarrhoea does not cause nocturnal symptoms. IBS is by definition associated with abdominal pain or discomfort. Bile acid malabsorption normally causes acute onset of diarrhoea and also occurs nocturnally.

2 A 35-year-old Irish lady presented to the gastroenterology clinic with altered bowel habit. This has been going on for two years but has never been investigated before. She tells the doctor that she had a bout of gastroenteritis while on holiday in Malaysia and has had diarrhoea intermittently since. She gets bouts of severe abdominal pain and bloating associated with her diarrhoea. She has lost 10 kilograms in weight over the past year.
   **A** This lady likely has post-infectious irritable bowel syndrome.
   **B** The probable cause of her symptoms is due to intestinal carcinoid.
   **C** It is worth checking tissue transglutaminase antibodies for coeliac disease.

Answer: C

Although post-infectious IBS should be considered, weight loss is an alarm feature and warrants further investigation. Intestinal carcinoid does not cause malabsorption and is extremely rare compared with coeliac disease which is the most likely cause in this lady. Coeliac disease is prevalent in the USA and Western Europe especially in Ireland (1 in 300) [82]. Carcinoid syndrome has an annual incidence of around two per million patients and should only be considered when the much commoner causes have been excluded.

3 A 40-year-old anxious thin gentleman presents to the gastroenterology clinic complaining of worsening diarrhoea. On examination, he was very anxious, thin, tremulous and tachycardic. His abdominal examination and a rigid sigmoidoscopy were normal. What is the next step?
  A Check his thyroid function test.
  B Refer him to the psychiatrist.
  C Prescribe some loperamide to help with his diarrhoea.

Answer: A

It is important to remember that other systemic diseases can cause gastrointestinal symptoms. Endocrine problems such as hyperthyroidism could cause the above features. This emphasizes the importance of a thorough general examination. Hyperthyroidism should be promptly treated to avoid further complications such as heart failure. Prescribing antidiarrheal medication before a proper diagnosis is made could be dangerous if it delays a proper diagnosis.

4 An 80-year-old male presents with bloating and marked abdominal distension. He has lost weight. On examination, he looks pale and his abdomen is soft and nontender. His abdominal X-ray showed multiple fluid levels throughout the abdomen.
  A Request an urgent CT scan of his abdomen.
  B Refer the patient to the surgeon for consideration of laparotomy.
  C A glucose breath test would be helpful.

Answer: C

This is a typical presentation of jejunal diverticulosis. Dilated loops of bowel with fluid levels on plain abdominal X-ray normally indicate intestinal obstruction when associated with a tender abdomen. The fluid levels in this patient represent stagnant fluid within the diverticula which create a blind loop allowing bacterial overgrowth. A glucose breath test will detect around 70% of cases of small intestinal bacteria overgrowth.

**5** A GP refers a 43-year-old nurse to you. She has a long history of constipation with abdominal pain. She opens her bowels once to twice a week and the stool is hard and lumpy. There is no rectal bleeding. She is concerned about her chronic condition as her partner's bowel habit seems to be more regular than hers. What do you do?
   **A** Reassure and offer symptomatic treatment with ispaghula husk.
   **B** Organize a colonoscopy.
   **C** Refer her to a surgeon.

Answer: A

This patient has irritable bowel syndrome, predominantly constipation. She has no 'red flag' signs and symptoms and IBS is common in a patient of her age and gender. Her response to treatment should be assessed at six weeks when two out of three will show improvement.

# CHAPTER 6

# Interface between Primary Care and Secondary Care

*Nicholas S. Coleman[1] and Hazel Everitt[2]*

[1]Department of Gastroenterology, University Hospital Southampton, Southampton, UK
[2]Primary Medical Care, School of Medicine, University of Southampton, Southampton, UK

---

### Key points

- Many people with IBS symptoms remain undiagnosed and rely on self-care.
- GPs are the first point of contact for patients seeking medical advice and continue to provide long-term community-based care in the majority of cases.
- Only a minority of patients with IBS are referred to secondary care.
- Current guidelines encourage GPs to make a positive diagnosis based on symptoms in the absence of any 'red flags' or abnormalities on simple tests.
- Initial management in primary care is based on explanation, reassurance and treatment with lifestyle advice, diet and medications.
- Establishing an effective doctor–patient relationship is important.
- Patients with IBS would like doctors to spend more time providing information, listening, answering questions and giving support.
- Managing their symptoms and identifying trigger factors are more important to IBS patients than understanding aetiology.
- Primary and secondary care clinicians must work together to develop more integrated, comprehensive health services based in the community.
- GPs with a specialist interest can provide the expertise in primary care to manage the majority of patients with IBS in the community.

---

## Introduction

IBS is a common disorder worldwide although many people in the community remain undiagnosed and self-manage their symptoms. General Practitioners provide long-term care of IBS in the community and refer only a minority of patients to secondary care. The symptoms of IBS can impact greatly on quality of life and social functioning and lead to time off work. Therefore,

---

*Irritable Bowel Syndrome: Diagnosis and Clinical Management,* First Edition.
Edited by Anton Emmanuel and Eamonn M.M. Quigley.
© 2013 John Wiley & Sons, Ltd. Published 2013 by John Wiley & Sons, Ltd.

managing the burden of disease is important both for society and the health services.

In this chapter we look at what drives people to seek health care and at their journey once in the system. We discuss the core values of general practice and assess the key role of GPs in diagnosing and managing long-term conditions like IBS. The attitudes of doctors and patients towards IBS and the central role of the doctor–patient relationship are explored. We examine the interface between primary and secondary care and discuss how the re-organization of health systems and increasing specialization in primary care can provide a more comprehensive, integrated service to manage IBS more effectively in the community.

## IBS in primary care

The prevalence of IBS ranges worldwide from 3 to 25% depending on the diagnostic criteria used [1] (Figure 6.1). It is a complex, long-term condition and thus generates a substantial workload for health services. The true prevalence of IBS in the whole population is likely to be higher than esti-mated in health settings, as 33–90% of patients with IBS symptoms do not consult their general practitioner (GP) and self-manage their symptoms in the community [2]. Patients presenting with gastrointestinal symptoms account for 1 in 12 GP consultations in the United Kingdom [3] and approx-imately one quarter of these will have IBS. It has been estimated that, on average, a GP in full-time practice will see eight patients with IBS per week, of whom one will be presenting for the first time [4]. Although only 14–29% of patients who see their GP are referred to a specialist [5], patients with IBS account for 20–50% of all cases seen in gastroenterology clinics [1]. Some patients may seek alternative or complementary therapists in addi-tion, or as an alternative, to medical services.

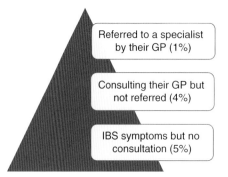

**Figure 6.1** Estimate of the percentage of the UK general population seeking medical advice in primary and secondary care for symptoms of IBS assuming a community prevalence of 10%. (Adapted from Williams *et al.* [1] and Spiller *et al.* [2].)

## Presentation to primary care

The majority of people manage significant gastrointestinal symptoms at home without seeking medical care and only when they decide to present to medical services is there the potential for diagnosis. Various factors influence the decision to consult or not and the impact of physical symptoms on the individual and their family's life, social circumstances and psychological factors all play a role. Worry about serious illness, advice or pressure from friends and relatives, life events and underlying health beliefs can all drive health-seeking behaviour. These factors also affect an individual's ability and willingness to self-manage their IBS symptoms. General Practitioners are usually the first point of contact and it is important that they explore why a person is presenting at a particular point in time; particularly when they may have had symptoms for many years. This will help to clarify their primary concerns and symptoms and can greatly assist the planning of appropriate education, reassurance, advice and management.

## Principles of primary care

Primary care services play a central role in the local community, providing comprehensive health care for all members of society with an emphasis on health promotion, disease prevention and the management of patients with a wide range of physical, mental and social health issues. There are significant differences between the practice of medicine in primary and secondary care. The traditional medical model – characterized by history taking, examination, investigation, diagnosis, treatment and follow-up – is still frequently followed in secondary care but does not recognize the complexity and diversity of the consultation in general practice, where undifferentiated disease, multiple comorbidities and hidden agendas need to be assessed in a short consultation.

In most healthcare systems GPs provide first contact care for patients in the community. Their role as clinical generalists combined with a close knowledge of the individual patient and their social circumstances dictates that they are uniquely placed to manage complex long-term conditions such as IBS. Because of the nature of general practice, GPs must adopt a problem-solving approach rather than the disease-based approach traditionally used in secondary care. Managing uncertainty, using time as a diagnostic tool and reduced reliance on investigations are all important aspects of this. General Practitioners have an important gatekeeping role and by identifying the minority of patients with significant gastrointestinal pathology they provide a safety net so that timely investigation and refer-ral can be arranged.

The delivery of person-centred care, whereby an individual patient's unique circumstances, expectations, preferences and beliefs are all taken into consideration, is an important goal of modern general practice [6]. When problems arise both the doctor and patient must take responsi-bility and difficult issues should be resolved by negotiation in order to maintain a good doctor–patient relationship. Empowerment of patients has given them a role in developing local services that meet their needs rather than those of the medical establishment. As a corollary to this, patients are expected to take a greater responsibility for their own management.

The ideal of being cared for from the cradle to the grave by a single prac-titioner has been eroded in recent times by increasing expectations and demands on primary care services. Nevertheless, there is evidence that such personal continuity of care is associated with greater patient satisfac-tion and more efficient use of resources. Patients find it frustrating to go over the same ground with a succession of different practitioners as this interrupts the smooth progression of care. Patients with IBS often receive care from many sources and they value their GPs central role in providing coordinated care across these different interfaces.

Primary care is said to be comprehensive in that a wide range of physi-cal, psychological and social problems must often be addressed in a single consultation. This can be challenging and, while patients must be given an opportunity to discuss the problems which are of most concern to them, effective management requires prioritization by the GP. Patients with IBS often find it difficult to understand how their multiple, seemingly unre-lated, problems can be attributed to a single disorder. The recognition that illnesses have both psychological and physical components, and that there is a dynamic relationship between them, has led to the holistic approach to patient care in general practice (Box 6.1).

---

**Box 6.1 Characteristics of general practice/family medicine**
- Comprehensive health care
- Problem-solving approach
- Person-centred care
- Holistic approach
- Good doctor–patient relationship
- Personal continuity of care
- Coordinated care

## Diagnostic criteria and guidelines – making a positive diagnosis

IBS is frequently viewed as a diagnosis of exclusion by GPs after investigations have eliminated organic diseases [7]. It is now proposed that a positive diagnosis can be made if the patient fulfils certain symptomatic criteria for IBS in the absence of any 'red flags' or abnormalities on simple laboratory investigation [8]. An early positive diagnosis benefits patients by giving them a clear diagnostic label, enabling early disease-specific education and advice on management. It also helps to reduce uncertainty, worry and time-consuming and costly investigations.

Over the last four decades diagnostic criteria for IBS have evolved from those originally devised by Manning through to the current Rome III criteria, although the latter were originally developed for research purposes and their applicability to primary care has not been established [9]. In isolation, diagnostic criteria cannot exclude the possibility of organic gastrointestinal disease but the pre-test probability of such diseases in the community is low [7]. In any case, only a minority of GPs are aware of these criteria and even fewer use them in clinical practice [10]. Distinguishing organic from functional GI disease was not thought to be particularly problematic in a survey of British GPs, who tended to weight other factors including unexplained or multiple symptoms, frequent consultation and female sex when considering a diagnosis of IBS [4]. Irritable bowel syndrome commonly presents between the ages of 30 and 50, although in many cases the symptoms have already been present for a number of years, a factor often used to support a diagnosis of IBS in primary care [4]. Current guidelines do not recommend that GPs should make a new diagnosis of IBS in a patient over 50 years of age without further investigation given the increased risk of cancer; nevertheless, IBS is a common diagnosis in the elderly and should be considered if investigations are normal. Although data in primary care are lacking, gastrointestinal symptoms in older people were more likely to be attributed to an organic or drug-related cause than a functional disorder in a study undertaken in elderly care clinics [11].

It should be noted that patients in primary care are less likely to be given a clear diagnosis of IBS in comparison with those seen in hospital clinics [12]. Evidence-based guidelines for the management of IBS have been produced by both the American College of Gastroenterology [13] and the British Society of Gastroenterology [2]. However, the first IBS guidelines specifically intended for use in primary care by GPs and patients were published by the UK National Institute of Clinical Excellence (NICE) in 2008 [14]. Although these have been criticized because of the lack of validation of the symptom-based approach in primary care [9], they have the potential to improve uniformity of care, patient engagement and cost effectiveness if widely taken up by GPs.

## Diagnosis of IBS based on symptoms

GPs should elicit the key symptoms of IBS in patients presenting with undifferentiated symptoms including abdominal pain, bloating or a change in bowel habit. If any of these are present, the NICE guidelines [14] recommend a formal assessment using specific diagnostic criteria for IBS. These require that the patient has abdominal pain or discomfort that is either relieved by defecation or associated with altered bowel frequency or stool form for at least three months. This should be accompanied by at least two of four additional symptoms: (i) altered stool passage, which may include straining, urgency or a sense of incomplete evacuation; (ii) abdominal bloating, visible distension, tension or hardness; (iii) symptoms made worse by eating; (iv) the passage of rectal mucus. Nongastrointestinal symptoms, such as lethargy, nausea, backache and bladder symptoms, are also frequent in patients with IBS and, although not diagnostic, their recognition as part of the IBS symptom complex is important to support the diagnosis, allay patient concerns and avoid unnecessary investigation and referral.

## Red flags

GPs should try to identify patients with organic pathology by enquiring about red flag symptoms, although there is no universal agreement about which red flags should be used and research shows them to have only modest predictive value [15]. The NICE guidelines consider unexplained weight loss, rectal bleeding, a family history of bowel or ovarian cancer and a persistent change in bowel habit in a person aged over 60 years of age to be important. Constant pain that has a fixed site and nocturnal symptoms is also considered significant.

Examination may also identify red flags such as anaemia and abdominal mass. Although benign rectal bleeding is common in IBS, digital rectal examination is recommended to exclude a mass. It should be noted, however, that rectal examinations are infrequently performed in primary care [16] and studies suggest that rectal examination is a poor predictor of palpable rectal tumour when performed by GPs [17]. Furthermore, it would appear that nonmedical factors, including a lack of time, absence of a chaperone or an expectation that the test will be performed by someone else, influence the decision to perform the examination [18]. Pelvic examination should also be considered if there is significant concern about ovarian cancer. A comparison of features of IBS and alternative diagnoses is shown in Table 6.1.

Patients should be told about red flag symptoms and advised to return for review if any of these occur. The emergence of any new red flags during longitudinal follow-up should prompt reassessment and referral for further investigation although, in practice, this is rare once a diagnosis of IBS has been made.

**Table 6.1** Shared and distinguishing features of IBS and alternative diagnoses in primary care.

| | Shared features | Distinguishing features | Typical age at diagnosis (years) | Sex distribution |
|---|---|---|---|---|
| Coeliac disease | diarrhoea, pain, bloating | malabsorption, including anaemia (iron and folate), weight loss and steatorrhoea; dermatitis herpetiformis | 20–40 | slightly more common in women |
| IBD | diarrhoea, pain | PR bleeding, frequent/nocturnal diarrhoea, weight loss, raised inflammatory markers, perianal disease, extra-GI features | 10–40 | equal |
| Colorectal cancer | altered bowel habit | rectal bleeding, iron deficiency anaemia, abdominal or rectal mass | over 50 | slightly more common in men |
| Ovarian cancer | pain, bloating, distension, | urinary frequency, PV bleeding, weight loss, abdominal mass | over 50 | all female |

## Investigating IBS in primary care

The low pre-test probability of serious gastrointestinal disease in primary care supports the concept of minimizing investigation when IBS is suspected [7]. As well as being more expensive, repeated investigation undermines confidence in the positive diagnostic approach, delays diagnosis and does not provide additional reassurance [19]. The NICE guidelines recommend that patients with suspected IBS require only a full blood count, ESR, C-reactive protein (CRP) and coeliac serology; more invasive tests such as colonoscopy are not recommended in the absence of any alarm symptoms. Although guidelines recommend checking both ESR and CRP, in practice, many GPs will only check one of these and given the low probability of finding abnormal inflammatory markers in a patient with typical IBS symptoms this is unlikely to make a significant difference.

It should be noted, however, that while the NICE guidelines recommend investigating lower GI symptoms in the absence of alarm symptoms only in patients over 60 years of age, guidelines from the United States are more cautious and suggest routine investigation after 50 years of age [13]. Ovarian cancer can present with nonspecific IBS-like symptoms such as fatigue and abdominal pain initially; persistent abdominal distension as opposed to the variable distension seen with IBS has a relatively high predictive value and should prompt further investigation [20]. A frequent diagnostic dilemma, particularly in younger adults, is distinguishing patients with mild presentations of inflammatory bowel disease from those with IBS. Faecal inflammatory markers such as calprotectin may be useful in determining which patients have intestinal inflammation [21] and, therefore, require lower GI endoscopy. Faecal calprotectin still has limited availability in primary care but it has recently been incorporated into local IBS management guidelines by several primary care trusts in the UK (NHS Brighton and Hove, NHS North of Tyne) and may well become more widely available over the next few years.

In some healthcare systems investigations such as colonoscopy and imaging studies have been accessible only to hospital specialists. This situation may change as GPs are given greater access to advanced diagnostic testing in primary care in a drive to reduce diagnostic waits, especially in patients with suspected cancer. In this situation, IBS guidelines may provide important guidance, preventing an increase in unnecessary colonoscopy in patients with IBS.

## Management of IBS in primary care

Making an early diagnosis is the essential first step in managing IBS and allows the GP to provide explanation, reassurance and effective treatment. Since the causes of IBS are unknown and treatments rarely provide complete symptom relief, management focuses on providing patients with information on the variable and chronic nature of IBS, so that they can understand their diagnosis, address lifestyle factors that exacerbate their symptoms and make informed choices regarding a trial of medication and/or psychological treatments. Concern that the symptoms may represent a serious underlying illness is a common reason for patients to see their GP. In one study in primary care, half of the patients questioned expected reassurance from their GP and a third of patients reported adequate relief of IBS symptoms following only reassurance and counselling [22]. Thus, reassurance can be an important aspect of the management of IBS. The aim of treatment is the relief of the predominant symptoms, a reduction in the impact on daily activities and an improvement in quality of life. However, no single treatment is likely to alleviate the multiple symptoms usually present, and thus a combination of treatments is often required. The NICE guidelines are very patient-centred in their approach to management, providing an algorithm (Figure 6.2) and other sources of information that help the patient to work together with their GP to achieve symptom relief.

Ensuring an understanding of the condition and working through the possible lifestyle changes and treatments can be a time-consuming task that requires long-term effort and dedication from the patient and GP;

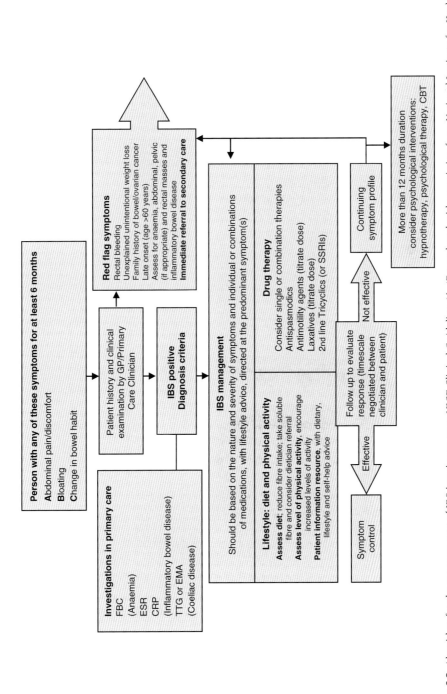

**Figure 6.2** Algorithm for the management of IBS in primary care: NICE Clinical Guideline 61. (Reproduced with permission from National Institute for Health and Clinical Excellence (2008) CG 61 Irritable bowel syndrome in adults: Diagnosis and management of irritable bowel syndrome in primary care. NICE, London. Available from www.nice.org.uk/guidance/CG61. This content was accurate at the time of going to press.)

a good doctor–patient relationship will help this process. Many patients find that education, reassurance and dietary and lifestyle advice are sufficient but a significant proportion will require further treatments at some stage. Pharmacological treatments widely used in general practice include antispasmodics, laxatives, antimotility agents and antidepressants. Behavioural and psychological therapies are recommended in severe cases although access to these is variable in primary care. A large number of patients rely on self-care including the use of over the counter medicines, self-help books and alternative or complimentary therapies. In a recent trial using sham acupuncture a positive interaction with the health practitioner accounted for the most significant component of the placebo effect in patients with IBS, suggesting that regular follow-up by a healthcare practitioner could be beneficial [23].

## Lifestyle advice

GPs are encouraged to educate patients and provide lifestyle advice with a particular emphasis on self-management. This should include information on general lifestyle, physical activity and diet. The pattern of daily activities may need to change to normalize physiology, for example by eating more regular meals, making plenty of time in the morning for defaecation or moving away from shift work. The NICE guidelines advise assessment of physical activity using the General Practice Physical Activity Questionnaire, which can be completed as an electronic template during the consultation and automatically generates a simple, four-level Physical Activity Index. Patients scoring 'less than active' should be encouraged to undertake a minimum of 30 minutes of moderate activity on five days of the week.

In one study a self-help guidebook reduced primary care consultations by 60% compared with controls with an associated reduction in healthcare costs [24]. Although global symptom scores were not reduced, patients perceived that their symptoms were improved, suggesting that the guidebook worked by helping them to manage their condition on a daily basis. Self-help resources are widely available, particularly on the internet, and GPs should be familiar with at least a few of the more popular websites. Information is also freely available from a variety of healthcare organizations, including the NHS, IBS charities and commercial interests. Notable online resources include 'The Irritable Bowel Syndrome Self Help and Support Group' and 'The IBS Network', a UK membership charity providing a helpline, fact sheets, a magazine and an interactive self-management programme for a yearly subscription. Self-help support groups and web-based chat rooms are an increasingly popular way of sharing information and experiences.

## Diet

Many patients with IBS do not like the idea of taking regular medications and consider dietary therapy to be a more 'natural' option. This is in keeping with the widely held belief of IBS patients that their condition is due to food allergy or intolerance. Although GPs and practice nurses are well placed to provide dietary advice, many feel that both a lack of nutritional training and time constraints prevent them from giving optimal advice [25]. However, as many patients with IBS believe that food exacerbates their symptoms, it is natural for them to see dietary modulation as a logical solution to their problem. It is important for the GP to acknowledge these concerns by helping the patient to identify specific food triggers, perhaps with the aid of a food diary, and by providing recommended dietary advice. Explaining that most food-related symptoms are due to food intolerance rather than allergy and highlighting the difference between these may help to dissuade patients from undertaking expensive and unproven commercially available treatments, such as exclusion diets based on the presence of IgG antibodies to food. Increasingly, patients who do not have coeliac disease are requesting gluten-free products from their GP, although they are not eligible to receive these on prescription. The majority will have IBS with wheat intolerance rather than true gluten sensitivity and it is, therefore, logical to try a wheat free diet before purchasing expensive gluten free products.

There is much conflicting advice regarding diet from both medical and lay sources and the role of dietary fibre, in particular, has been controversial. In the United Kingdom, access to a dietician in the community is variable and many patients are referred to secondary care for more specific advice. The NICE guidelines help to address some of these issues by providing detailed general advice within the treatment algorithm. In addition, a self-help diet sheet, produced in conjunction with the British Dietetic Association, provides more specific information depending on the predominant symptoms. Patients who do not respond to self-help dietary measures or advice in primary care may need to be referred to a hospital dietician, particularly if more complex dietary regimens are being considered. The NICE guidelines suggest that people wishing to try probiotics should give these a four-week trial but they can be surprisingly expensive if required on a long-term basis.

## Pharmacological therapy

Decisions about pharmacological management should be based on both patient choice and the nature and severity of symptoms. The use of single or combination medications is determined by the predominant symptoms, including pain and bloating (antispasmodics and antidepressants), constipation (laxatives) and diarrhoea (antimotility drugs). GPs should feel confident to discuss the use of these medications with patients and monitor and review response to treatment. A review of pharmacological therapies is covered in detail in other chapters of this book.

## Attitudes towards IBS

### The patient's perspective

Patients presenting with symptoms suggesting IBS often expect that investigations will be performed to rule out serious disease [22]. Failure to arrange these may be interpreted as a sign that the symptoms are not being taken seriously or that the doctor lacks appropriate knowledge. In this situation, an explanation of the diagnostic approach is necessary so that concerns about serious disease do not persist. In those patients who do undergo tests there is sometimes disappointment when they fail to show evidence of a disease that would validate the patient's symptoms and offer the prospect of a medical or even surgical cure. It is not uncommon for fears of serious disease to persist after consultation [4]; colorectal cancer and inflammatory bowel disease are the conditions that concern patients most [26].

In trying to understand IBS, the primary concern is more often with identifying trigger factors that provoke symptoms than understanding complex disease mechanisms. Patients consider food intolerance [22] to be one of the most frequent causes, although identifying specific food triggers can be a difficult and frustrating process. Stress is also recognized as an important factor [22] although, in contrast to the view held by their doctors, patients are more likely to see stress as an external factor over which they have little control [27].

The most important treatment goal from the patient's perspective is relief from their worst symptom, usually pain or bloating, rather than overall symptom relief [22]. Doctors need to be aware of the frustration that results from the long process of repeatedly trying treatments with little effect. Explaining the range of treatment options and encouraging patients to return if their treatment is not helping may help them to make sense of what is often a trial-and-error process.

In a large US study of IBS patients' expectations of their healthcare providers, the qualities most desired from their doctors included: giving comprehensive information, referring to sources of further information, listening, answering questions, giving support and a sense of hope and providing information about IBS studies and medications, although their previous experiences infrequently matched these ideals [28]. Despite the fact that patients often feel dissatisfied with the explanation and the lack of effective treatments provided by their GP, they more often attribute this to the paucity of current knowledge about IBS than poor consultation skills [27].

Many patients with IBS find that their condition impacts significantly on activities of daily living. The unpredictable onset of symptoms such as diarrhoea and urgency may lead to anxiety and social avoidance. A sense of isolation is common and patients often feel that family, friends and doctors do not understand their symptoms [29]. There may also be feelings of embarrassment, guilt or self-blame. Many patients feel a sense of frustration that their symptoms continue despite their best attempts to maintain a healthy lifestyle and follow medical advice.

Patients who do not seek health care tend to feel more in control of their symptoms and worry about them less [30]. They are also more likely to be able to talk to members of their extended family, many of whom will share similar symptoms. In one survey, the main reasons cited for avoiding medical care were either mild symptoms or having learned to live with them, being too busy or dislike of visiting the doctor [31].

## The general practitioner's perspective

Many GPs still consider IBS to be a diagnosis of exclusion [12]. The fear of missing serious illness is always a concern, although confidence should be taken from the comparative rarity of serious gastrointestinal diseases in primary care. In practice, missed diagnoses are uncommon and the majority of GPs are confident in excluding more serious conditions by using red flags and longitudinal observation.

Since the pathophysiology of IBS is poorly understood a chief concern for many GPs is providing a convincing explanatory model that will be accepted by the patient, since failure to do so drives patient anxiety and further consultation [32]. Engagement is more likely if a patient has confidence in their doctor's knowledge and willingness to listen to their concerns. Evidence suggests that GPs lack knowledge and have inconsistent views about the causes and treatment of IBS [33]. In particular, they are divided in their belief as to whether IBS is fundamentally a psychological disturbance or a primary gastrointestinal disease [34]. However, although many lack detailed knowledge of the putative causes of IBS, most GPs are aware of the importance of trigger factors. Stress is commonly cited, with many GPs believing that it triggers disordered bowel activity in susceptible individuals. A lack of dietary fibre is also considered important [22]. There appear to be national differences in opinion so that while UK practitioners, in one study, named infection, food and travel as being major trigger factors, their Dutch counterparts saw smoking, caffeine, diet, 'hasty lifestyle' and lack of exercise as being important [32].

The treatment of IBS is often viewed by GPs as a trial-and-error process and is frequently guided by the patient's personal health beliefs and views on trigger factors. Although the majority of patients in primary care are straightforward to manage, it is the most difficult patients that tend to formulate opinion about IBS, in general. In these patients, symptom resolution is rare and developing a long-term therapeutic partnership requires significant personal investment from the GP. There is evidence that GPs feel more negative towards this group of patients, particularly those who are anxious or attend frequently [32]. They often blame such patients for their own negative attitudes and behaviour and lack of personal responsibility, although the extent to which health-related quality of life is affected is frequently underestimated.

It is clear that if GPs are to take on a greater responsibility for the management of IBS there is a need for further training focused not only on diagnosis and management but also on dealing with patient concerns and expectations.

## The gastroenterologist's perspective

Although IBS is one of the disorders seen most frequently in gastroenterology clinics, little has been published on the attitude of gastroenterologists towards this condition. Nevertheless, it is clear that hospital specialists are far less likely to consider IBS as diagnosis of exclusion and more likely to make a diagnosis using symptomatic criteria with only minimal investigation [12]. In one survey, gastroenterologists viewed patients with IBS as being less sick but requiring more time per consultation than their colleagues in primary care [35]. In the same study, specialists were more likely to consider prior gastroenteritis and a history of abuse as being important causes of IBS. It seems a reasonable assumption that many specialists would be happy for 'routine' IBS cases to be managed in primary care if it gives them more time and resources to manage complex cases.

## Developing a positive doctor–patient relationship

Establishing a supportive doctor–patient relationship is a key aspect of caring for patients with IBS [36]. It requires a commitment to engage in a long-term therapeutic partnership with active involvement and responsibility by both parties. Developing good consultation skills based on empathy, active listening, open ended questioning and appropriate body language are all skills that GPs learn during their training (Box 6.2).

In primary care, a typical consultation lasts for only 10 minutes. In patients with complex presentations it may, therefore, be helpful to arrange an extended consultation or plan several consultations to give the patient sufficient time to express their concerns and to explore symptoms and psychosocial factors. It is important to show support and empathy by validating the symptoms, indicating that they are familiar to the doctor and that others share similar experiences. It may be difficult to give a clear diagnosis and explanation in one session and information leaflets and referral

> **Box 6.2  Developing a good doctor–patient relationship**
>
> - Validate symptoms
> - Listen to patient concerns
> - Refer to other sources of information
> - Negotiate a management plan
> - Encourage self-management
> - Explain the care versus cure approach
> - Maintain continuity of care
> - Follow-up at regular, fixed intervals
> - Set specific goals for each session
> - Offer practical advice and support

to other sources of information are important with an opportunity for further discussion at a later date.

At the end of the assessment a problem list can be agreed from which a management plan can be negotiated. The positive role that patients can play in managing their symptoms should be emphasized, helping them to take back control of their condition. Self-help through groups, organizations and web interactions should also be encouraged.

Patients should be told that complete symptom resolution is unlikely, although this needs to be presented in a positive way. Instead, patients need to know that the treatment goal is to improve symptoms, quality of life and coping skills; the so-called care versus cure approach. It is preferable to identify one doctor as a patient's principal point of contact, although, with a clear management plan, other professionals can be involved without setting back the progression of care. By arranging follow-up at regular, fixed intervals, setting specific goals for each session and discouraging consultation outside these times the number of interactions can be reduced and patients encouraged to become more self-reliant.

IBS is a long-term condition and management requires patience and commitment by both the patient and the doctor. Patients are likely to raise concerns about their condition at each consultation and it may require repeated discussions in which the same issues are reviewed more than once. Patients may question the practitioner's approach if there are inconsistencies or questions remain unanswered but this can be helped by clear documentation. Treatments should be tried one at a time in a stepwise fashion giving adequate time to assess the therapeutic response before making any changes; patients should be counselled that improvements are likely to occur slowly over time. Helping the patient to overcome problems with their daily activities by offering practical advice and support is an important aspect of the partnership; involving a relative or friend as a therapeutic ally can lend further support. Practical solutions may include counselling for marital or family conflicts, helping the patient to return to work by using a graded activity program and providing medical reports for employers or benefits agencies.

## Referral to secondary care

GPs may refer patients with IBS for a number of reasons. Many patients will have significant alarm symptoms while others will have typical IBS symptoms in association with minor features that create diagnostic uncertainty, such as rectal bleeding due to piles or mildly elevated inflammatory markers. Other patients will clearly have IBS according to diagnostic criteria but are referred because of treatment failure, request for a second opinion or because fears of serious disease persist despite reassurance [10]. In a study from UK general practice, major predictors for referral to a specialist included: denial of a role for stress, long history (>6 months) and increased stool frequency [4]. In another study, male sex, greater duration of time since diagnosis, frequent bowel motions, absence of dyspepsia in the previous three months and increased use of medication and alternative therapies predicted specialist consultation [37]. Multiple nongastrointestinal symptoms associated with IBS can initiate referral to inappropriate specialists if not recognized as part of the IBS symptom complex.

## The role of secondary care

Secondary care clinics should provide specialist assessment and management for patients who require services beyond the scope of primary care. Their role is to facilitate the management of IBS in the community rather than to undertake long-term care. The qualities of secondary care that make it more suited to managing complex disease include specialist expertise, a multidisciplinary approach and access to the full range of diagnostic tests. Additionally, there is access to a range of specialist practitioners who may not be universally available in the community, including dieticians, psychologists, pain specialists and IBS nurses. In tertiary referral centres, these practitioners may work directly alongside gastroenterologists in specialist IBS clinics.

## Primary/secondary care communication

As workloads have increased the opportunity for face-to-face or telephone interactions between GPs and hospital specialists have lessened and the majority of communication occurs indirectly. This is a shame, as direct doctor–doctor interactions are an effective way of building trust, cooperation and a sense of shared responsibility. Effective and timely communication between primary and secondary care is essential for the development of an efficient, integrated system of care but this requires education and effort by all parties. The use of explicit guidelines and care pathways can help this process.

A GP referral letter that provides all of the required information can save time and aid appropriate decision making by the specialist. The reason for referral should be stated clearly to ensure that the correct problem is addressed. Essential details include the main symptoms, a list of previous diagnoses and current medications, as patients frequently forget these. Psychosocial issues, hidden agendas and health-related concerns are particularly important as they may not readily be revealed in the hospital setting to an unfamiliar doctor. Ensuring that the results of any tests recommended by the guidelines are available can aid clinical decision making prior to the specialist consultation and facilitate a seamless patient journey. It is also important to document the results of tests undertaken in other healthcare facilities.

Hospital specialists should aim to provide the GP with a detailed care plan that will help them to manage the patient in the community and reduce the need for secondary care intervention. There should be a clear statement of the diagnosis with any associated comorbidities. It is helpful to record the explanatory models used and any information given to the patient so that the GP can continue to deliver a consistent message. Planned investigations and the rationale for these should be recorded. The management plan can be documented as a bulleted list so that treatment can be delivered in a stepwise fashion if initial treatments fail. Finally, further follow-up or the indications for re-referral should be stated. It is good practice to send a copy of the clinic letter to the patient to affirm the diagnosis, avoid misunderstandings and give the patient a sense of involvement in their care.

## Multidisciplinary management of complex IBS

A minority of patients with IBS have chronic symptoms that respond poorly to standard treatment. Psychological factors are more likely to be relevant in these patients and there may also be medically unexplained symptoms on a background of multiple referrals and investigations. Although few in number these patients may be regarded as 'heartsink' cases who demand a disproportionate amount of medical time and resources. The patient may be told that they have to 'learn to live' with their symptoms when the doctor reaches the limit of their medical expertise. In reality, these complex patients require a long-term management strategy delivered primarily by their GP but often with additional input from hospital specialists or a wider multidisciplinary team including pain specialists and psychologists.

There may be many volumes of hospital case notes containing potentially useful clues as to the underlying cause. Although time consuming, review of the notes by an experienced specialist is useful, not only to establish a definitive diagnosis and ensure that no significant clinical findings have been overlooked but also to prevent needless repetition of tests or treatment. Important details to document include current symptoms, a chronological list of investigations, previous treatments, confirmed medical diagnoses and operations, current medications and psychosocial history with information about the patients' personal and family circumstances. This summary can form the basis of a problem-based management plan. It is helpful if other members of the multidisciplinary team can validate the plan, preferably following discussion at a joint meeting which may be attended by the patient. Discussion with the GP can be particularly enlightening and may reveal many hitherto undisclosed psychosocial factors known as a result of their long-term knowledge of the patient. Copies of the plan should be given to the patient and should also be available in emergency departments and medical and surgical admissions units so that unnecessary admission can be avoided.

## Managing IBS in the community: future developments

Health services across the world are re-configuring to meet the challenges of rising healthcare expenditure and the provision of care for people with long-term disease. One of the key strategies will be to shift the focus of chronic disease management from hospitals into the community [6]. GPs, hospital specialists and patients will have to work together if genuinely integrated and comprehensive health services are to result. For an important condition like IBS, which accounts for up to half of the referrals seen in gastroenterology outpatient clinics, it will be necessary to re-develop both primary and secondary care gastroenterology services so that IBS can be managed more effectively in the community.

### Increasing specialization in primary care

There is a need for specialist leadership and knowledge in primary care if high quality gastroenterology services are to be delivered in the community. This could be provided by general practitioners with a specialist interest (GPwSIs) who have undertaken a period of training and accreditation under the supervision of a hospital specialist [38]. Community care could also be delivered by hospital specialists contracted to spend some of their time working in primary care clinics. Community-based specialists would work with a team of primary care nurses, dieticians, psychologists and physiotherapists, complementing rather than duplicating secondary care

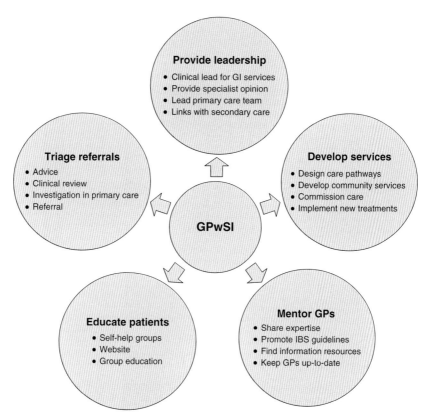

**Figure 6.3** The multiple roles a general practitioner with a special interest (GPwSI) in gastroenterology could play in improving the management of irritable bowel syndrome in primary care.

services. One of their main roles would be to triage referrals from local GPs by giving advice, reviewing patients in community clinics, arranging investigations in primary care or referring for specialist opinion. A reduction in waiting times, decreased hospital referrals and reduced costs would be key outcome measures (Figure 6.3).

It is important for GPwSIs to maintain a good working relationship with colleagues in secondary care to aid service coordination and the joint development of care pathways. As clinical leaders for their specialty, GPwSIs would take a leading role in developing community GI services based on the principles of general rather than hospital practice and commissioning care for GI disorders. They would also be expected to assess new treatments for IBS, implementing these if proven effective.

Most GPwSIs continue in their main role as a general practitioner, which limits the time they can devote to seeing specialty patients. An effective alternative use of their time may be to share their expertise with local GPs to improve standards, promote good clinical practice and encourage the

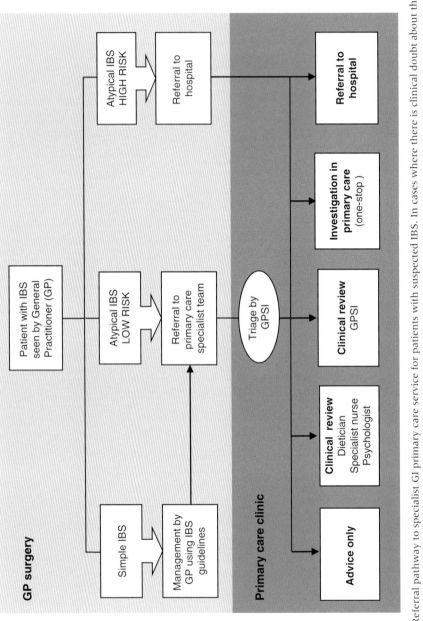

**Figure 6.4** Referral pathway to specialist GI primary care service for patients with suspected IBS. In cases where there is clinical doubt about the diagnosis of IBS but a low risk of serious GI pathology patients are referred to a primary healthcare team led by a GPwSI working in a community healthcare clinic. One-stop investigations including flexible sigmoidoscopy or faecal calprotection could be performed.

use of IBS guidelines. Patient education and self-care play an important role in IBS management but often GPs find it difficult to keep up to date with the latest developments. GPwSIs could assist their colleagues by providing regular updates and highlighting popular patient information resources. They could also play a direct role in patient education by running web sites and coordinating self-help groups. Educational sessions delivered to large groups of IBS patients by GPwSIs or other primary healthcare professionals could be more cost effective than following them up on an individual basis (Figure 6.4).

## Changing practice in secondary care

The shift of care into the community will also require hospital specialists to change their working practices. They will need to become more accessible, providing appropriate support and advice to both primary care clinicians and patients. A reduction in the number of IBS referrals to secondary care should improve waiting times for hospital clinics while allowing specialists to spend a greater proportion of their time managing complex cases. Intelligent booking systems will enable GPs to book an appointment with a chosen specialist at the convenience of the patient. The use of different modes of communication including e-mail, telephone and audio/video teleconferencing will allow specialists not only to provide timely advice but also to hold joint consultations without requiring patients to attend hospital. The development of more integrated IT systems will be necessary to share test results and patient information between GP surgeries, primary healthcare clinics, and hospitals.

## Conclusion

Effective management of patients with IBS depends on a well-integrated healthcare system with effective communication and clear pathways of care. Recent guidelines aimed at encouraging an early positive diagnosis and the development of increasing specialization based in primary care have the potential to improve the care of patients with IBS in the community.

## Useful web links

- http://guidance.nice.org.uk
- http://www.rcgp.org.uk
- http://globalfamilydoctor.com
- http://www.theibsnetwork.org

## References

1  Williams JG, Roberts SE, Ali MF *et al*. Gastroenterology services in the UK. The burden of disease, and the organisation and delivery of services for gastrointestinal and liver disorders: a review of the evidence. *Gut* 2007;56:1–113.

2  R Spiller, Q Aziz, F Creed *et al*. Guidelines on the irritable bowel syndrome: mechanisms and practical management. *Gut* 2007;56:1770–1798.

3  Royal College of General Practitioners, OPCS and DHSS. *Morbidity statistics from general practice 1991–1992. Fourth National Study*, Studies on Medical and Population Subjects. 1995; HMSO, London.

4  Thompson WG, Heaton KW, Smyth GT and Smyth C. Irritable bowel syndrome in general practice: prevalence characteristics and referral. *Gut* 2000;46:78–82.

5  Jones R. IBS: prime problem in primary care. *Gut* 2000; 46(1):7–8.

6  Royal College of General Practitioners. *The Future Direction of General Practice: A Roadmap*. 2007, Royal College of General Practitioners (RCGP), London. http://www.rcgp.org.uk/policy/rcgp-policy-areas/~/media/Files/Policy/A-Z%20policy/the_future_direction_rcgp_roadmap.ashx (accessed 10 October 2012).

7  Jellema P, van der Windt DA, Schellevis FG and van der Horst HE. Systematic review: accuracy of symptom based criteria for diagnosis of irritable bowel syndrome in primary care. *Aliment Pharmacol Ther* 2009;30(7):695–706.

8  Longstreth GF, Thompson WG, Chey WD *et al*. Functional bowel disorders. *Gastroenterology* 2006;130:1480–1491.

9  Talley NJ. Commentary; Controversies in NICE guidance on irritable bowel syndrome. *BMJ* 2008;336:558–559.

10  Thompson WG, Heaton KW, Smyth GT *et al*. Irritable bowel syndrome: the view from general practice. *Eur J Gastroenterol Hepatol* 1997;9:689–692.

11  Agrawal A, Khan MH and Whorwell PJ. Irritable bowel syndrome in the elderly: An overlooked problem? *Dig Liver Dis* 2009;41(10):721–724.

12  Spiegel BM, Farid M, Esrailian E, Talley J and Chang L. Is irritable bowel syndrome a diagnosis of exclusion?: a survey of primary care providers, gastroenterologists, and IBS experts. *Am J Gastroenterol* 2010;105(4):848–858.

13  Brandt LJ, Chey WD, Foxx-Orenstein AE *et al*. (American College of Gastroenterology Task Force on IBS). An evidence-based systematic review on the management of irritable bowel syndrome. *Am J Gastroenterol* 2009;104: S1–S35 (supplement 1).

14  National Institute for Health and Clinical Excellence. Irritable bowel syndrome in adults. Diagnosis and management of irritable bowel syndrome in primary care. 2008, National Institute for Health and Clinical Excellence (NICE), London. www.nice.org.uk/CG061 (accessed 10 October 2010).

15  Whitehead WE, Palsson OS, Feld AD *et al*. Utility of red flag symptom exclusions in the diagnosis of irritable bowel syndrome. *Aliment Pharm Ther* 2006;24;137–146.

16  Barwick TW, Scott SB and Ambrose NS. The 2 week referral for colorectal cancer: a retrospective analysis. *Colorectal Dis* 2004;6(2):85–91.

17  Ang CW, Dawson R and Farmer M. The diagnostic value of digital rectal examination in primary care for palpable rectal tumour. *Colorectal Dis* 2008;10(8):789–792.

18  Hennigan TW, Franks PJ, Hocken DB and Allen-Mersh TG. Rectal examination in general practice. *BMJ* 1990;8(30):478–480.

19  McDonald IG, Daly J, Jelinek JM *et al*. Opening Pandora's box: the unpredictability of reassurance by a normal test result. *BMJ* 1996; 313:329–332.

20  Hamilton W. Cancer diagnosis in primary care. *Br J Gen Pract* 2010;60(571): 121–128.

21 Jellema P, van Tulder MW, van der Horst HE *et al.* Inflammatory bowel disease: a systematic review on the value of diagnostic testing in primary care. *Colorectal Dis* 2011;13(3):239–254.

22 Bijkerk CJ, de Wit NJ, Stalman WA *et al.* Irritable bowel syndrome in primary care: the patients' and doctors' views on symptoms, etiology and management. *Can J Gastroenterol* 2003;17(6):363–368.

23 Kaptchuk TJ, Kelley JM, Conboy LA *et al.* Components of placebo effect: randomised controlled trial in patients with irritable bowel syndrome. *BMJ* 2008;336(7651):999–1003.

24 Robinson A, Lee V, Kennedy A *et al.* A randomized controlled trial of self-help interventions in patients with a primary care diagnosis of irritable bowel syndrome. *Gut* 2006;55(5):643–648.

25 Buttriss JL. Food and nutrition: attitudes, beliefs and knowledge in the United Kingdom. *Am J Clin Nutr* 1997;65(suppl):1985s–1995s.

26 Lacy BE, Weiser K, Noddin L *et al.* Irritable bowel syndrome: patients' attitudes, concerns and level of knowledge. *Aliment Pharmacol Ther* 2007;25(11):1329–1341.

27 Casiday RE, Hungin APS, Cornford CS, de Wit NJ and Blell MT. Patients' explanatory models for irritable bowel syndrome: symptoms and treatment more important than explaining aetiology. *Family Practice* 2009;26:40–47.

28 Halpert A, Dalton CB, Palsson O *et al.* Irritable bowel syndrome patients' ideal expectations and recent experiences with healthcare providers: a national survey. *Dig Dis Sci* 2010;55:375–383.

29 Drossman DA, Chang L, Schneck S *et al.* A focus group assessment of patient perspectives on irritable bowel syndrome and illness severity. *Dig Dis Sci* 2009;54(7):1532–1541.

30 Ringstrom G, Abrahamsson H, Strid H and Simren M. Why do subjects with irritable bowel syndrome seek healthcare for their symptoms. *Scand J Gastroenterol* 2007;42; 1194–1203.

31 Hungin AP, Whorwell PJ, Tack J and Mearin F. The prevalence, patterns and impact of irritable bowel syndrome: an international survey of 40 000 subjects. *Aliment Pharmacol Ther* 2003;17:643–650.

32 Casiday RE, Hungin APS, Cornford CS, de Wit NJ and Blell MT. GPs' explanatory models for irritable bowel syndrome: a mismatch with patient models? *Family Practice* 2009;26:34–39.

33 Longstreth GF and Burchette RJ. Family practitioners' attitudes and knowledge about irritable bowel syndrome. Effect of a trial of physician education. *Family Practice* 2003;20:670–674.

34 Gladman LA and Gorard DA. General practitioner and hospital specialist attitudes to functional gastrointestinal disorders. *Aliment Pharmacol Ther* 2003;17:651–654.

35 Lacy BE, Rosemore J, Robertson D *et al.* Physicians' attitudes and practices in the evaluation and treatment of irritable bowel syndrome. *Scand J Gastroenterol* 2006;41(8): 892–902.

36 Conboy LA, Macklin E, Kelley J *et al.* Which patients improve: characteristics increasing sensitivity to a supportive patient-practitioner relationship. *Soc Sci Med* 2010;70(3): 479–484.

37 Smith GD, Steinke DT, Kinnear M *et al.* A comparison of irritable bowel syndrome patients managed in primary and secondary care: the Episode IBS study. *British Journal of General Practice* 2004;54:503–507.

38 Royal College of General Practitioners. Guidance and competencies for the provision of services using practitioners with special interests (PwSIs): Adult endoscopy (upper and lower GI). 2006, Royal College of General Practitioners (RCGP), London. http://www.rcgp.org.uk/clinical-and-research/clinical-resources/~/media/62F4C7F1 49D04156BB33A4F21A35B7CA.ashx (accessed 5 November 2012).

# Multiple Choice Questions

1 A 35-year-old man with longstanding IBS has requested an appointment with you after one of the senior GP partners told him that that IBS is not a real condition and that he should learn to live with his symptoms. Which ONE of the following approaches would be most helpful during your consultation?

   A Arrange further investigations to allay his fears.

   B Keep the appointment short but provide information leaflets.

   C Agree with your partner to maintain a consistent medical approach.

   D Listen to the patient and validate his symptoms.

   E Refer him to a self-help web site to that he can self-manage his symptoms.

Answer: D

2 Which ONE of the following statements about General Practitioners with a specialist interest (GPwSI) is true?

   A The primary role of a GPwSI is that of a specialist.

   B GPwSI-led clinics are associated with reduced costs.

   C GPwSI-led clinics are associated reduced waiting times.

   D GPwSIs will usually work independently of secondary care.

   E Accreditation is not required.

Answer: C

3 Which ONE of the following is a defining feature of General Practice?

   A Doctor-centred care.

   B The traditional medical model.

   C Using time as a diagnostic feature.

   D Diagnosis of exclusion.

   E Problem-solving approach.

Answer: E

**4** Which ONE of the following is an appropriate indication for referral to secondary care in a patient with suspected IBS?

  **A** Patient fulfils the NICE diagnostic criteria for IBS.

  **B** Patient does not wish to take regular medication.

  **C** Poor response to antispasmodics.

  **D** Patient has nocturnal diarrhoea.

  **E** Patient wishes to have investigation for candida infection.

Answer: D

**5** Which ONE of the following is not appropriate lifestyle advice for a patient with IBS?

  **A** Avoid travel to tropical countries.

  **B** Have regular meals and take time to eat.

  **C** If activity levels are low 30 minutes exercise five days a week.

  **D** Encourage time for leisure and relaxation.

  **E** Drink at least eight cups of fluid per day.

Answer: A

# PART 3

# Symptom-specific Treatment of Irritable Bowel Syndrome

# CHAPTER 7

# Self-Management Strategies for Irritable Bowel Syndrome

*Monica E. Jarrett, Pamela Barney and Margaret M. Heitkemper*

Department of Biobehavioral Nursing and Health Systems, University of Washington, Seattle, WA, USA

---

**Key points**

- As the number of chronically ill patients in the United States has grown, the self-management model has become increasingly useful with the patient serving as the principle caregiver and the healthcare professionals serving as consultants in a supportive role.
- For self-management of IBS to be effective patients need to be able to monitor and manage their symptoms. This requires that they have an understanding of IBS, have effective strategies to manage the symptoms and know when to put them into practice.
- Self-management strategies for IBS might include medications, dietary management, relaxation skills, cognitive skills, leisure time, physical activity and adequate sleep.
- Self-management of IBS is patient specific and problem oriented. The patient defines the problem and identifies the most effective way for it to be managed.
- Self-management interventions can be integrated to primary and specialty care settings.

---

Irritable Bowel Syndrome (IBS) is a functional gastrointestinal (GI) disorder that often becomes a chronic condition [1, 2]. The symptoms of IBS affect physical functioning, emotional well-being and social and work activities. Similar to a number of other chronic disorders, self-management approaches are often recommended as the first step in controlling symptoms [3, 4]. Most self-management interventions for IBS fall on a continuum from using self-help books (e.g., IBS for Dummies [5]) to cognitive behavioural therapy or psychotherapy guided by specialist and medications prescribed by healthcare providers [6, 7]. In this chapter we will define self-management, describe specific elements of self-management therapies, review recommendations for self-management approaches from current guidelines, present case studies and factors that are associated with successful self-management.

---

*Irritable Bowel Syndrome: Diagnosis and Clinical Management*, First Edition.
Edited by Anton Emmanuel and Eamonn M.M. Quigley.
© 2013 John Wiley & Sons, Ltd. Published 2013 by John Wiley & Sons, Ltd.

Self-management, which is synonymous with self-care, is defined as a therapeutic approach where patients perform 'activities or tasks tradition-ally performed by professional healthcare providers' by the US National Library of Medicine [8]. This focus on the individual differs from the 2003 Institute of Medicine definition that focused on the role of providers, 'edu-cation and supportive interventions by healthcare staff to increase patients' skills and confidence in managing their health problems, including regular assessment of progress and problems, goal setting, and problem-solving support [9].' For self-management to be effective patients need to monitor and manage: knowledge of their disease and treatments, medications, dis-ease related symptoms, effects of the disease on functioning in their daily life, prevention strategies and risk reduction in collaboration with their healthcare provider(s) [3].

Traditionally healthcare providers have owned the knowledge and skill to restore health. Patients have been viewed as the passive recipients of care. With a growing number of chronically ill patients in the United States, a new paradigm has emerged where chronically ill patients are no longer the passive receivers of health care, instead they have become the principal caregivers, with healthcare professionals serving as consultants and supporting them in this role [10–12]. With this shift there is a growing need for a self-management model that prepares patients to effectively assume this role. Self-management education differs from traditional patient education in several ways. It is patient specific and problem ori-ented. Instead of providing disease-specific information with a focus on skills the provider deems important, a self-management approach allows the patient to take the lead, identifying problems of concern. The informa-tion and skills taught are specific to managing the patient's identified problems. Traditional patient education focuses on theory and disease spe-cific information with the belief that this will change health behaviours. Self-management education is based on the theory that better clinical outcomes are achieved when patients have increased confidence in their capacity to make life improving changes. Rather than striving for patient compliance, the overall goal of self-management education is increased patient self-efficacy [13].

## Self-efficacy

Self-efficacy refers to a person's belief in their ability to organize or execute a course of action to produce a desired outcome. The belief that a patient has the skill and ability to carry out an effective plan of action is associated with improved health status in patients involved in self-management programs [14]. Self-efficacy is influenced by four sources. These include:

- Skills mastery
- Modelling
- Interpretation of symptoms
- Social persuasion.

Mastering a skill and knowing when to put it into action are essential ingredients in effective symptom management of IBS. Goal setting, action plans, skill building and monitoring all contribute to this process. Modelling for IBS patients can be accomplished through a relationship with a health-care provider, other IBS patients, books, articles, classes and web sites. This process is most effective when patients can identify with the model and believe that the information will be of personal use. Interpretation of symptoms allows the patient to identify problematic symptoms and recognize their impact. For example, a patient who experiences abdominal pain following a distressing interaction with a teenager might interpret this as an inability to cope with the stressors of raising children. A reinterpretation of this might be recognizing that abdominal pain is a common physiologic response of a person that has IBS unrelated to one's ability to raise children or cope with the stressors involved. This reinterpretation does not serve to undermine a patient's confidence in their ability to manage their symptoms. Social persuasion can come in the form of instruction, advice, opinions and behaviours. Words of encouragement often increase self-efficacy and words of discouragement often decrease it.

## Five core self-management skills

A report from the Center for the Advancement of Health identified five core self-management skills: problem solving, decision making, resource use, forming an alliance with healthcare providers and taking action [9]. As an alternative to providing patients with the answers to their current problems, these skills will allow IBS patients to manage current and future problems, preparing them for the role of primary caregiver in a self-management model (Table 7.1).

As the primary care giver the IBS patient takes a problem-based, solution-focused approach. A systematic approach to problem solving builds confidence that a variety of problems can be solved using these skills. As IBS patients learn to specifically define the problem, generate possible solutions, implement solutions and evaluate results [15] they gain confidence and the ability to manage current and future problems effectively.

The skill of decision making requires knowing or having access to adequate appropriate information on which to base a decision [4]. This information, along with effective resources and a relationship with a healthcare provider, equips the IBS patient to make take effective steps in symptom management.

**Table 7.1** Roles of patients and healthcare provider in self-management. (Reproduced from Kennedy and Rogers [63].)

| Roles | Traditional health care | Self-management |
|---|---|---|
| Healthcare provider | Principle Caregiver, The Expert<br>• Diagnosis<br>• Medications<br>• Provider of disease specific information<br>• Identify problems and direct treatment options<br>• Provide emotional support | Health Consultant, The Collaborator<br>• Diagnosis<br>• Medications – if desired by patient<br>• Healthcare consultant – providing needed/desired information for problems identified by the patient |
| Patient | Care Receiver, The Recipient<br>• Seeker of diagnosis and treatment<br>• Receiver of health care | Principle Caregiver, The Director<br>• Seek diagnosis and desired information<br>• Skill building<br>• Problem solving<br>• Decision making<br>• Resource use<br>• Forming partnership with healthcare provider<br>• Taking action |

## Patient–clinician communication

In a self-management setting the establishment of a collaborative relationship between the patient and provider is essential. This therapeutic relationship has a patient-centred focus with the patient's perspective and symptoms addressed simultaneously [16]. A nonjudgmental, empathetic patient-focused communication effects patient satisfaction, motivation, trust and self-efficacy. These, in turn, influence adherence, self-management skills and social support, each of which is associated with improved health [17].

Learning to ask questions that elicit more information than the symptoms a patient experiences will serve to identify and describe illness experience and the coping mechanisms of the patient. Kennedy *et al.* [14] created a list of questions for their focus group meetings that invited patients to talk about many aspects of their IBS (Box 7.1). This type of questioning allows the patient to describe the impact that IBS has on their lives and the unique set of problems that result. Identifying and addressing the issues specific to each patient plays a significant role in helping a patient learn to manage their symptoms effectively. This sort of patient-centred care helps establish an environment for problem solving and collaborative decision making [14]. With an understanding of the patient's

---

**Box 7.1  Questions to elicit patient's symptoms and experiences with IBS(63)**

Assessment questions

Do you recall anything that triggered your first episode of IBS?

What was your initial response to your IBS diagnosis?

Do you have any strategies that help you manage your symptoms?

What do you know about IBS? What else would you like to know?

What are the biggest challenges that you face with IBS?

Do you have any fears about your diagnosis?

Is there anything about your IBS that you monitor or keep track of on a regular basis?

Who else knows about your IBS, and what have you told them?

---

perspective and symptoms the clinician can begin to identify and teach the information and skills needed by the patient to effectively manage the impact of IBS.

## Clinician/facilitator's role

The role of the clinician or the facilitator of a self-management programme requires a combination of medical knowledge and psychosocial skills. Functioning as an educator, coach and, in many cases, a consultant, the person in this role needs to be experienced in motivating, persuading, supporting, reinforcing, building confidence, problem solving and working collaboratively. With a complete understanding of IBS and the guidelines for management, the clinician must understand how to present information in a manner specific to the patient needs. General information is not sufficient to motivate patients to manage their symptoms effectively [14]. An understanding of self-management and the tasks associated with it provide the structure for assisting patients to effectively manage the condition. Information presented may include disease-specific information, strategies to manage symptoms, resources available and general self-management skills, such as problem solving, action plans, goal setting, dealing with difficult emotions, communication and collaboration with healthcare providers [9].

Because no therapeutic modality benefits all patients it can be a challenging and time consuming process to identify an effective treatment plan for each patient. Drossman *et al.* [18] have proposed a graduated multicomponent treatment approach based on symptom severity. Individualization is determined by symptom pattern, severity and psychosocial factors that exacerbate symptoms. Treatment for patients with mild symptoms is focused on education, reassurance and dietary recommendations. Patients with a moderate symptoms profile, experiencing intermittent disruption of activity, psychological distress and some insight into factors that exacerbate symptoms, may require additional options. These patients may benefit from symptom monitoring and modification, pharmacotherapy that targets specific intermittent symptoms, behavioural treatments including relaxation training, or hypnosis, or psychotherapy such as cognitive behavioural therapy, insight-oriented therapy, group or family counselling. Patients with severe or intractable IBS symptoms are often unresponsive to traditional psychotherapy or medications. These patients may benefit from improved patient–physician interaction thus avoiding maladaptive illness behaviour. Useful behavioural-based techniques for this population may include diagnostic and treatment measures based on objective findings rather than patient demands, realistic goal setting, shifting responsibility of treatment decisions to the patient by providing therapeutic options and demonstrating a commitment to the patient's well-being instead of commitment to treatment of the disease [18, 19].

## Patient barriers to success

Using a multicomponent self-management approach is a means of optimizing a patient's ability to manage the chronic and unpredictable condition of IBS. In spite of this fact it is often challenging to identify which patients will respond positively to this approach [15]. Patients must be able to participate in the self-management programme, learn new skills and strategies, set goals and make decisions and lifestyle changes to manage their symptoms. Lake and Straiger [17] identified several factors that clinicians felt limited the ability of some patients to succeed in a self-management programme. These included cognitive impairment, complex conditions, dysfunctional family situations and cultural differences.

IBS patients with severe psychological and GI symptoms may be less likely to complete a self-management programme [17]. Those with severe pain uncorrelated to meals, psychological disturbances (severe anxiety, depression or somatization), chronically impaired daily functioning and the inability to recognize psychological factors as contributors to their illness are often unresponsive to most treatment approaches [18]. In contrast, those that experience mild to moderate symptoms by which they are notably distressed, are open to the concept that psychological factors play a role in their condition and are willing to participate in this therapeutic approach, may be most appropriate for a self-management programmes [19].

## Self-management integrated into health care

Self-management can be integrated into usual health care and coordinated by the healthcare provider, nurse or other trained healthcare professionals. Most healthcare organizations, however, lack the structure to support self-care management [20]. In many cases, self-management programmes are conducted outside of the primary care setting. Healthcare providers may refer their patients to psychologists [21, 22], nurses [23], or advanced practice psychiatric nurses [24, 25] with an understanding of IBS and skill in self-management strategies. Treatment may include individual face-to-face sessions or combination face-to-face and telephone interventions. In a classroom setting a variety of disciplines, such as a nurse, dietician, physical therapist, psychologist and gastroenterologist, can combine their expertise to present an effective multicomponent self-management programme [26–28]. Patient-led support groups are another possible option [29, 30]. When the above options are unavailable, healthcare providers may suggest a self-management book for patients to read on their own [31].

## Self-management recommendations in current guidelines and systematic reviews

Over the last decade, a number of guidelines have been developed to identify treatment approaches for IBS by professional organizations and expert panels: American College of Gastroenterology Task Force on Irritable Bowel Syndrome [32], World Gastroenterology Organization [33], National Collaborating Centre for Nursing and Supportive Care [34], Rome Foundation report [35], Asian Consensus on Irritable Bowel Syndrome [36] and American College of Gastroenterology Functional Gastrointestinal Disorders Task Force [37]. Self-management approaches that are addressed jointly by patients and healthcare providers include elements such as education and reassurance, dietary modifications, physical activity, psychological approaches and complementary and alternative approaches.

### Education and reassurance

Education and reassurance is usually the first step [36, 38]. This involves confirming the diagnoses of IBS, explaining possible causes for the patients symptoms, the risk of other diagnoses (e.g., colorectal [39] or ovarian cancer [40], coeliac disease [41], inflammatory bowel disease [42]) and treatment options. If partnership between the patient and healthcare provider is going to occur then providers need to be willing to listen to the patient's concerns, accept the concerns as real, and appreciate the impact they have on the patient's life [43].

## Diet management

Many patients believe that what they eat affects their symptoms, so adjusting their diet is one way to manage IBS symptoms [44–47]. Over the last 10 years, the recommendations in guidelines have expanded from fibre and food allergies to include behavioural strategies [32–37, 43]. A patient's perception of the relationship of diet to symptoms has been explored in two ways: qualitative synthesis of interviews with IBS patients and surveys. As part of a larger study, women between 18 and 45 years of age were interviewed to explore the relationship between diet, eating behaviours and symptoms. Overall, women tried to adjust their diet so that their symptoms were manageable through a process of trial and error. If they could identify trigger foods then they excluded the food or created rules for when and how the food was eaten in an effort to maintain a healthy diet (e.g., for an accountant it was no ice cream during tax season and after a meal the rest of the year). Women who failed to find a relationship between diet and symptoms during the trial-and-error process either felt frustrated by the uncertainty or, for a few women, decided that the process was not worth the bother [44]. Additional themes were identified in a study of women with IBS and inflammatory bowel disease, including seeking dietary information from other than physicians, timing and awareness of surroundings when eating and giving in to temptations [48].

In a regional US survey, 1242 patients with IBS responded that their IBS symptoms were caused or triggered by eating too much food (67%), drinking coffee (57%), eating fatty foods (56%), dairy (52%), carbohydrates (36%), meat (31%), and drinking alcohol (17%), or food allergies (30%) along with other factors (85%). Over 40% said they used or could use such strategies as eating small frequent meals, eating low fat or carbohydrates and high fibre food while avoiding high protein, fatty foods, milk products, carbohydrates or caffeine [47]. A survey was conducted in the United Kingdom on the acceptability of treatment options by patients with IBS [49]. Of the 645 respondents, over 75% rated drugs, diet change and yoga as acceptable treatments. Moreover, for those who disliked drugs, nonmedical treatments (e.g., dietary, psychosocial) were seen as the preferred first approach to treatment. Thus, most patients with IBS believe that there is a relationship between what they eat, when they eat and how they eat and their gastrointestinal symptoms and have tried to change their diet to minimize symptoms. A few intervention trials have included modules on dietary approaches to manage symptoms [24, 25, 50].

---

### CASE STUDY 7.1 — Woman with diarrhoea-predominant IBS

Deborah, a 27-year-old woman has had IBS-like symptoms since she was a child, recently began a new job as a physical therapist. Long hours, a brisk pace and a steep learning curve contributed to an increase in abdominal pain, urgency and diarrhoea. Deborah had trouble falling asleep at night because of her concerns. She awoke worrying about the impact that her IBS would have on her work day and by the time she arrived at work she was experiencing moderate-to-severe abdominal pain. The stress of the situation felt like it was too much and Deborah was considering quitting her job.

At her healthcare provider's suggestion Debra made an appointment with a nurse practitioner trained in the treatment of IBS. After several weeks she was able to develop a plan that helped her manage her symptoms and allowed her to continue her job. Her plan contained the following strategies:

- Eat small meals every 3–4 hours.
- Avoid coffee on work days.
- Take a break for lunch and get out of the department.
- Practice one minute of abdominal breathing before each patient.
- Attend yoga class on Tuesday and Thursday evening.
- Get 7–8 hours of sleep on work nights.
- Continue to work on decreasing catastrophic thinking.

---

## Physical activity

Recommendations regarding physical activity are limited in the guidelines for IBS patients. It is frequently suggested/recommended that healthcare providers assess and encourage leisure, relaxation and physical activity time [33, 34]. However, 'there is no adequate proof' [33] that exercise helps. In a recent study, Daley *et al.* [51] tested the feasibility and efficacy of a twelve-week exercise intervention to usual care in 56 adults with IBS. The intervention goal was 30 minutes of moderate intensity exercise on five of seven days per week. The approach was chosen for its efficacy in other populations [52, 53] and its self-management characteristics (i.e., two consultant visits to facilitate exercises success [week 1] and to prevent relapse [week 4]). Of the primary outcomes only constipation symptoms improved in the exercise group compared to the usual care group.

Two researcher teams used yoga for the treatment of IBS. One in India found no difference in the outcomes (autonomic symptom score, bowel symptom score, state anxiety, or physical flexibility) in 22 men with diarrhoea-predominant IBS compared to conventional treatment controls (loperamide 2–6 mg/day) [54]. Researchers in the United States compared results in 25 adolescents, in which one group followed a daily home yoga practice with a video and the other group was placed on a wait-list for four weeks prior to receiving the intervention [55]. The yoga group reported less functional disability and use of emotion-focused avoidance, and less anxiety (criteria, p <0.10) than the wait-list control group after four weeks. The findings from these studies did include IBS symptoms and used relatively small samples; thus, further testing is needed to determine the efficacy of physical activity for IBS symptoms.

## Psychological therapies

Overall, cognitive behavioural therapy (CBT), assertion training, contingency management, psychotherapy and hypnotherapy have been shown to be more effective than usual care in treating symptoms of IBS. Relaxation therapy may not be generally effective, but may help patients to deal with moderate anxiety symptoms [33, 43]. In one guideline it was noted that in primary care settings 'talking' counselling by healthcare providers may be helpful, but patients in tertiary care often need psychological therapies by specialist for comorbid conditions such as anxiety or depression [43]. Some adverse events have occurred in psychological therapies such as suicidal ideation but no hospitalizations or deaths have been reported [24, 56]. Also, patient's preferences are not considered in randomized controlled trials (RCTs) but could be by healthcare providers [43]. One of the challenges for patients and providers is that well-trained therapists who are experienced with IBS patients may not be available [36].

Two recent meta-analyses and a symptomatic review found that psychological interventions are more effective than usual care or waiting-list control groups [56–58]. In one meta-analysis of 25 studies, psychological interventions were not more effective when the control group include some type of placebo (i.e., psycho-educational support, pseudo-meditation, biofeedback alpha-suppression, education, visualization, Tenso-stop, or self-help support group) [57]. This finding is worth considering, since it argues that some intervention may be better than usual care even if it is a placebo-type intervention. However, the post intervention follow-up period for many studies is at the end of the intervention (2 and 3 months) with only a few studies extending their follow-up assessments to test the sustainability of the findings (e.g., 6, 9 or 12 months).

Researchers are also testing the efficacy of less clinical-intensive CBT interventions. One researcher's approach was to decrease the number of CBT sessions to four (minimal contact) and compare it to a typical 10-session CBT intervention, and compare both to a wait-list control [59]. At the end of 12 weeks, 72% of subjects in the CBT-minimal contact and 61% of those in the CBT-10 sessions reported adequate relief of their IBS symptoms compared to 7% in the waiting list control group. Instead of decreasing the number of sessions, researchers in Sweden tested the efficacy of a 10-week CBT intervention delivered through the Internet with limited clinician support for 86 subjects with IBS. The control group was a waiting list control [60]. This CBT intervention was focused on mindfulness and exposure to fears. Each week the CBT group completed self-management exercises, posted their homework to the web site, had access to a discussion board and e-mailed their clinician weekly. The wait-list control group also had access to a discussion board and could contact their clinician for general support. The CBT group significantly decreased their IBS symptoms compared to the wait-list controls (Cohen's d=0.83; 95% confidence interval [CI], 0.36–1.29) as well as the secondary outcomes. In the next study the researchers compared their exposure-based CBT intervention to a stress management control group that included nonspecific therapeutics factors but not the unique elements of the exposure-based CBT intervention [61]. The exposure-based CBT intervention group reported a significant decrease in GI symptoms compared to the stress management control group at both the end-of-treatment and six-month follow-up assessments. These studies provided further support for exposure-based CBT, but also highlighted the efficacy of an intervention delivered through the Internet with limited therapist support and a low dropout rate (<15%).

In some clinical settings, hypnosis is used to relieve symptoms of IBS. A systematic review of four RCT of 147 patients who had failed prior medical treatment was used to determine the efficacy of hypnotherapy for IBS [62]. The control groups received psychotherapy, usual care or were wait-listed. Primary outcomes were summary scores for IBS symptoms (i.e., abdominal pain, diarrhoea or constipation and bloating). In three studies IBS symptoms decreased significantly at approximately three months follow-up but the effect was not seen at twelve months in the only study with long term follow-up. No adverse events were reported.

---

### CASE STUDY 7.2 — Woman with constipation-predominant IBS

Amelia, a 35-year-old airline attendant, was diagnosed with IBS 12 years ago. The symptoms intensified six years ago, however, when she began flying. The pain, constipation and bloating were almost unbearable when she travelled, with the pain and bloating beginning as soon as she boarded the plane. The constipation increased with each day of travel.

Amelia was afraid to try medication for constipation when she was travelling, as she did not feel that she could risk the possibility of diarrhoea or increased pain. Feeling stuck, and hoping for some additional strategies to help her manage her symptoms, Amelia attended a class on IBS Symptom Management recommended by her primary

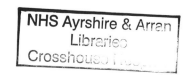

care provider. She developed the following plan that allowed her to travel with minimal symptoms:

- Increase fibre intake to 25–30 gm/day.
- Carry high fibre snacks when travelling.
- Drink 64 ounces of non-caffeinated liquid a day.
- Exercise 30 minutes a day – do not omit when traveling.
- Do Passive Progressive Muscle Relaxation exercise before boarding the plane.
- Prior to each flight, remain focused on increased ability to manage IBS symptoms.

One of the concerns of healthcare providers is how well findings from well controlled RCTs translate to clinical practice. One example is a study of 149 IBS patients recruited from 10 primary care practices in England to participate in an efficacy trial of CBT (six sessions) and mebeverine (anticholinergic) versus mebeverine only [50]. The intervention was delivered by trained nurses, not specialists. The CBT and mebeverine group significantly improved outcome measures (i.e., symptom severity, anxiety, work and social adjustment, coping behaviours related to IBS and illness-related negative cognitions) compared to the mebeverine group at 1.5 and three months follow-up. However, only 61% of the patients in the treatment group completed the intervention compared to 9% of controls. Similarly, researchers in Australia recruited 64 patients from primary care and randomized to a self-management or usual care [22]. The intervention was a self-help manual used for 7–8 weeks plus an initial in-person session with a health psychologist and two one-hour telephone sessions. Symptom relief across two, three and six month post intervention follow-up favoured the self-management group over the controls (odds ratio [OR] = 12.2 [95% CI, 3.72–40.1]). IBS symptom severity scores did not differ at three months follow-up, but improved at six months follow-up (OR 5.3 [95% CI, 1.64–17.26]). This suggests that motivated patients can benefit from a self-management approach that requires limited professional support. (See Chapters 8 and 14 for complementary and alternative medicine therapies)

## Summary

As the number of chronically ill patients in the United States has grown, the self-management model has become increasingly useful, with the patient serving the principle caregiver and the healthcare professionals serving as consultants in a supportive role. Researchers have demonstrated that for patients with IBS self-management interventions work significantly better than standard care and, even when nonspecific therapeutics factors are controlled, fewer sessions are used or minimal therapist support is provided. Translation of these effective interventions to primary and specialty care settings needs further exploration, as does the use of the Internet.

## Useful web links

- International Foundation for Functional Gastrointestinal Disorders (IFFGD) http://www.iffgd.org/
- The National Digestive Diseases Information Clearinghouse http://digestive.niddk.nih.gov/ddiseases/pubs/ibs/

## Self-help books for IBS patients

Barney P, Weisman P, Jarrett M, Levy RL and Heitkemper M. *Master Your IBS: An 8-Week Plan Proven to Control the Symptoms of Irritable Bowel Syndrome*. 2010, AGA Press, Bethesda, MD.
Written in a workbook format this step-by-step, multicomponent approach walks patients through the process of learning a variety of strategies to manage IBS symptoms. The book provides forms for monitoring symptoms, tracking diet, problem solving, cognitive restructuring, and tracking sleep.

Burstall D, Vallis M and Turnbull GK. *IBS Relief: A Complete Approach to Managing Irritable Bowel Syndrome*. 2006, John Wiley & Sons, Inc., Hoboken, NJ.
Written by a doctor, dietician and psychologist this book provides a multidisciplinary approach to managing IBS. This book provides an overview of IBS and covers topics such as diet, relaxation, stress management, pain control.

Davis M, Eschelman ER and Mckay M. T*he Relaxation and Stress Reduction Workbook*, 6th edn. 2008, New Harbinger Publications, Oakland, CA.
A self-help book focused on the understanding and management of stress. This book teaches a variety of relaxation skills including breathing, progressive relaxation, meditation, visualization, self-hypnosis and autogenics. Cognitive strategies and topics such as time management, nutrition and exercise are also addressed.

Guillory G. *IBS: A Doctor's Plan for Chronic Digestive Troubles: The Definitive Guide to Prevention and Relief*. 2001, Hartley & Marks Publishers Inc., Point Roberts, WA.

This informative approach to preventing and relieving IBS symptoms includes an explanation of IBS, the brain–gut connection, diet, exercise, stress management, medications and complimentary approaches.

Lackner J. *Controlling IBS The Drug Free Way.* 2007, Stewart, Tabori and Chang, New York.
A systematic approach with a focus on cognitive strategies that provides the reader with a description of IBS, tools for symptoms monitoring and opportunities to develop strategies for symptom management. Dr Lackner's extensive IBS research provides the foundation for this well written book.

## References

1 Drossman D, Corazziari E, Delvaux M *et al. Rome III: The Functional Gastrointestinal Disorders*, 3rd edn. 2006, Degnon Associates, Inc., MacLean, VA.

2 Neal KR, Barker L and Spiller RC. Prognosis in post-infective irritable bowel syndrome: a six year follow up study. *Gut* 2002;51(3):410–413.

3 Battersby M, Von Korff M, Schaefer J *et al.* Twelve evidence-based principles for implementing self-management support in primary care. *Jt Comm J Qual Patient Saf* 2010;36:561–570.

4 Lorig KR and Holman H. Self-management education: history, definition, outcomes, and mechanisms. *Ann Behav Med* 2003;26(1):1–7.

5 Dea CW and L. Christine. *IBS for Dummies.* 2005, John Wiley & Sons, Inc., Hoboken, NJ.

6 Longstreth GF. Teaching irritable bowel syndrome patients to care for themselves. *Am J Gastroenterol* 1998;93(6):860–861.

7 van der Horst HE, Schellevis FG, van Eijk JT and Bleijenberg G. Managing patients with irritable bowel syndrome in general practice. How to promote and reinforce self-care activities. *Patient Educ Couns* 1998;35(2):149–156.

8 Self Care [database on the Internet]. US National Library of Medicine, Medical Subject Headings (MeSH). 2011 [cited May 30, 2011]. http://www.ncbi.nlm.nih.gov/mesh/68012648 (accessed 10 October 2012).

9 Pearson ML, Mattke S, Shaw R, Ridgely MS and Wiseman SH. Patient Self-Management Support Programs: An Evaluation. 2007, Agency for Healthcare Research and Quality, Rockville, MD.

10 Holman H and Lorig K. Patients as partners in managing chronic disease. *BMJ* 2000;320(7234):526–527.

11 Von Korff M, Gruman J, Schaefer J, Curry SJ and Wagner EH. Collaborative management of chronic illness. *Ann Inter Med* 1997;127(12):1097–1102.

12 Lawn S and Schoo A. Supporting self-management of chronic health conditions: Common approaches. *Patient Educ Couns* 2009;80(2):205–211.

13 Bodenheimer T, Lorig K, Holman H and Grumbach K. Patient self-management of chronic disease in primary care. *JAMA* 2002;288(19):2469–2475.

14 Kennedy A, Robinson A and Rogers A. Incorporating patients' views and experiences of life with IBS in the development of an evidence based self-help guidebook. *Patient Educ Couns* 2003;50(3):303–310.

15 Adeyemo MA, Spiegel BM and Chang L. Meta-analysis: do irritable bowel syndrome symptoms vary between men and women? *Aliment Pharmacol Ther* 2010;32(6):738–755.

16  Lake AJ and Staiger PK. Seeking the views of health professionals on translating chronic disease self-management models into practice. *Patient Educ Couns* 2010;79(1):62–68.

17  Sanders K, Blanchard E and Sykes M. Preliminary study of a self-administered treatment for irritable bowel syndrome: comparison to a wait list control group. *Appl Psychophysiol Biofeedback* 2007;32(2):111–119.

18  Drossman DA and Thompson WG. The irritable bowel syndrome: a review and a graduated multicomponent treatment approach. *Ann Intern Med* 1992;116(12):1009–1016.

19  Hutton JM. Issues to consider in cognitive-behavioural therapy for irritable bowel syndrome. *Eur J Gastroenterol Hepatol* 2008;20(4):249–251.

20  Ladabaum U, Sharabidze A, Levin TR et al. Citalopram provides little or no benefit in nondepressed patients with irritable bowel syndrome. *Clin Gastroenterol Hepatol* 2010;8(1):42–48.e1.

21  Lackner JM, Jaccard J, Krasner SS *et al.* How does cognitive behavior therapy for irritable bowel syndrome work? A mediational analysis of a randomized clinical trial. *Gastroenterology* 2007;133(2):433–444.

22  Moss-Morris R, McAlpine L, Didsbury LP and Spence MJ. A randomized controlled trial of a cognitive behavioural therapy-based self-management intervention for irritable bowel syndrome in primary care. *Psychol Med* 2009;40(1):85–94.

23  Everitt HA, Moss-Morris RE, Sibelli A *et al.* Management of irritable bowel syndrome in primary care: feasibility randomised controlled trial of mebeverine, methylcellulose, placebo and a patient self-management cognitive behavioural therapy website. *BMC Gastroenterol* 2010;10(136). doi:10.1186/471-230X-10-136.

24  Jarrett ME, Cain KC, Burr RL *et al.* Comprehensive self-management for irritable bowel syndrome: randomized trial of in-person vs. combined in-person and telephone sessions. *Am J Gastroenterol* 2009;104(12):3004–3014.

25  Heitkemper MM, Jarrett ME, Levy RL *et al.* Self-management for women with irritable bowel syndrome. *Clin Gastroenterol Hepatol* 2004;2(7):585–596.

26  Saito YA, Rey E, Almazar-Elder AE *et al.* A randomized, double-blind, placebo-controlled trial of St John's wort for treating irritable bowel syndrome. *Am J Gastroenterol* 2010;105(1):170–177.

27  Saito YA, Prather CM, Van Dyke CT *et al.* Effects of multidisciplinary education on outcomes in patients with irritable bowel syndrome. *Clin Gastroenterol Hepatol* 2004;2(7):576–584.

28  Ringstrom G, Storsrud S, Lundqvist S, Westman B and Simren M. Development of an educational intervention for patients with Irritable Bowel Syndrome (IBS): a pilot study. *BMC Gastroenterol* 2009;9:10.

29  Von Korff M, Moore JE, Lorig K *et al.* A randomized trial of a lay person-led self-management group intervention for back pain patients in primary care. *Spine (Phila Pa 1976)* 1998;23(23):2608–2615.

30  Druss BG, Zhao L, von Esenwein SA *et al.* The Health and Recovery Peer (HARP) Program: A peer-led intervention to improve medical self-management for persons with serious mental illness. *Schizophr Res* 2010;118(1–3):264–270.

31  Robinson A, Lee V, Kennedy A *et al.* A randomised controlled trial of self-help interventions in patients with a primary care diagnosis of irritable bowel syndrome. *Gut* 2006;55(5):643–648.

32  American College of Gastroenterology Task Force on Irritable Bowel Syndrome, Brandt L, Chey W, Foxx-Orenstein A *et al.* An evidence-based position statement on the management of irritable bowel syndrome. *Am J Gastroenterol* 2009;104 (Suppl 1):S1–S35.

33 World Gastroenterology Organisation Global Guideline: irritable bowel syndrome: a global perspective [database on the Internet] 2009 [cited May 20, 2011]. http://www.ngc.gov/content.aspx?id=15232&search=world+gastroenterology+organisation+global+guideline%3a (accessed 10 October 2010).

34 NCCNSC. Irritable bowel syndrome in adults. Diagnosis and management of irritable bowel syndrome in primary care. National Collaborating Centre for Nursing and Supportive Care (NCCNSC) commissioned by National Institute for Health and Clinical Excellence (NICE) 2008 (updated 2012). http://guidance.nice.org.uk/CG61/Guidance/pdf/English (accessed 23 October 2012).

35 Spiegel B, Camilleri M, Bolus R *et al*. Psychometric evaluation of patient-reported outcomes in irritable bowel syndrome randomized controlled trials: a Rome Foundation report. *Gastroenterology* 2009;137(6):1944–1953.e1–3.

36 Gwee K-A, Bak Y-T, Ghoshal UC *et al*. Asian consensus on irritable bowel syndrome. *J Gastroenterol Hepatol* 2010;25:1189–1205.

37 American College of Gastroenterology Functional Gastrointestinal Disorders Task Force. Evidence-based position statement on the management of irritable bowel syndrome in North America. *Am J Gastroenterol* 2002;97(11 Suppl):S1–S5.

38 American Gastroenterological Association medical position statement: Irritable bowel syndrome. *Gastroenterology* 2002;123(6):2105–2107.

39 Norgaard M, Farkas DK, Pedersen L *et al*. Irritable bowel syndrome and risk of colorectal cancer: a Danish nationwide cohort study. *Br J Cancer* 2011;104(7):1202–1206.

40 Hamilton W, Peters T, Bankhead C and Sharp D. Risk of ovarian cancer in women with symptoms in primary care: population based case-control study. *BMJ* 2009;339:b2998.

41 Korkut E, Bektas M, Oztas E *et al*. The prevalence of coeliac disease in patients fulfilling Rome III criteria for irritable bowel syndrome. *Eur J Intern Med* 2010;21(5):389–392.

42 García Rodríguez LA, Ruigómez A, Wallander MA, Johansson S and Olbe L. Detection of colorectal tumor and inflammatory bowel disease during follow-up of patients with initial diagnosis of irritable bowel syndrome. *Scand J Gastroenterol* 2000;35:306–311.

43 Spiller R, Aziz Q, Creed F *et al*. Guidelines on the irritable bowel syndrome: mechanisms and practical management. *Gut* 2007;56(12):1770–1798.

44 Jarrett M, Visser R and Heitkemper M. Diet triggers symptoms in women with irritable bowel syndrome. The patient's perspective. *Gastroenterol Nurs* 2001;24(5):246–252.

45 Casiday RE, Hungin APS, Cornford CS, de Wit NJ and Blell MT. Patients' explanatory models for irritable bowel syndrome: symptoms and treatment more important than explaining aetiology. *Fam Pract* 2009;26(1):40–47.

46 Fletcher PC, Jamieson AE, Schneider MA and Harry RJ. 'I know this is bad for me, but…': a qualitative investigation of women with irritable bowel syndrome and inflammatory bowel disease: part II. *Clin Nurse Spec* 2008;22(4):184–191.

47 Halpert A, Dalton CB, Palsson O *et al*. What patients know about irritable bowel syndrome (IBS) and what they would like to know. national survey on patient educational needs in IBS and development and validation of the Patient Educational Needs Questionnaire (PEQ). *Am J Gastroenterol* 2007;102(9):1972–1982.

48 Jamieson AE, Fletcher PC and Schneider MA. Seeking control through the determination of diet: a qualitative investigation of women with irritable bowel syndrome and inflammatory bowel disease. *Clin Nurse Spec* 2007;21(3):152–160.

49 Harris LR and Roberts L. Treatments for irritable bowel syndrome: patients' attitudes and acceptability. *BMC Complement Altern Med* 2008;8:65.

50  Kennedy T, Jones R, Darnley S *et al.* Cognitive behaviour therapy in addition to antispasmodic treatment for irritable bowel syndrome in primary care: randomised controlled trial. *BMJ* 2005;331(7514):435–437.

51  Daley AJ, Grimmett C, Roberts L *et al.* The effects of exercise upon symptoms and quality of life in patients diagnosed with irritable bowel syndrome: a randomised controlled trial. *Int J Sports Med* 2008;29(9):778–782.

52  Lowther M, Mutrie N and Scott EM. Promoting physical activity in a socially and economically deprived community: a 12 month randomized control trial of fitness assessment and exercise consultation. *J Sports Sci* 2002;20(7):577–588.

53  Kirk A, Mutrie N, MacIntyre P and Fisher M. Increasing Physical Activity in People With Type 2 Diabetes. *Diabetes Care* 2003;26(4):1186–1192.

54  Taneja I, Deepak KK, Poojary G *et al.* Yogic versus conventional treatment in diarrhea-predominant irritable bowel syndrome: a randomized control study. *Appl Psychophysiol Biofeedback* 2004;29(1):19–33.

55  Kuttner L, Chambers C, Hardial J *et al.* A randomized trial of yoga for adolescents with irritable bowel syndrome. *Pain Res Manag* 2006;11(4):217–223.

56  Lackner JM, Mesmer C, Morley S, Dowzer C and Hamilton S. Psychological treatments for irritable bowel syndrome: a systematic review and meta-analysis. *J Consult Clin Psychol* 2004;72(6):1100–1113.

57  Zijdenbos IL, de Wit NJ, van der Heijden GJ, Rubin G and Quartero AO. Psychological treatments for the management of irritable bowel syndrome. *Cochrane Database Syst Rev* 2009;CD006442.

58  Dorn SD. Systematic review: self-management support interventions for irritable bowel syndrome. *Aliment Pharmacol Ther* 2010;32(4):513–521.

59  Lackner JM, Jaccard J, Krasner SS *et al.* Self-administered cognitive behavior therapy for moderate to severe irritable bowel syndrome: clinical efficacy, tolerability, feasibility. *Clin Gastroenterol Hepatol* 2008;6(8):899–906.

60  Ljótsson B, Falk L, Vesterlund AW *et al.* Internet-delivered exposure and mindfulness based therapy for irritable bowel syndrome – A randomized controlled trial. *Behav Res Ther* 2010;48(6):531–539.

61  Ljotsson B, Hedman E, Andersson E *et al.* Internet-delivered exposure-based treatment vs. stress management for irritable bowel syndrome: a randomized trial. *Am J Gastroenterol* 2011;106(8):1481–1491.

62  Webb AN, Kukuruzovic R, Catto-Smith AG and Sawyer SM. Hypnotherapy for treatment of irritable bowel syndrome. *Cochrane Database Syst Rev* 2007;CD005110.

63  Kennedy AP and Rogers AE. Improving patient involvement in chronic disease management: the views of patients, GPs and specialists on a guidebook for ulcerative colitis. *Patient Educ Couns* 2002;47(3):257–263.

# Multiple Choice Questions

1 Self-management is a collaborative approach with _____ in the lead.
   A the patient
   B the primary health care provider
   C the gastroenterologist
   D all of the above

Answer: A

The focus in self-management support is on the patient, with healthcare providers serving in supportive roles as educators, coaches and consultants.

2 A man who has experienced 10 years of constipation-predominant IBS asked if you have any 'tricks' for treating his constipation, bloating and abdominal pain. After asking about his current self-management strategies you discover that he is using commercial fibre supplements and eating bran cereal for breakfast every morning. What would you suggest?
   A Increase the Metamucil that he has been taking.
   B Begin including more fresh fruit and fluid in his diet.
   C Stop eating bran cereal for breakfast and begin eating oatmeal.
   D B and C

Answer: C

For a balanced, nutritious diet it is helpful to get fibre from your diet instead of commercial fibre supplements. It is often recommended that fresh fruit be limited in an IBS patient's diet. Switching from bran cereal (an insoluble fibre) to oatmeal (a soluble fibre) might help to decrease bloating and constipation.

3 After making several effective dietary changes a 35-year-old woman with abdominal pain and diarrhoea reports that her symptoms have improved but she continues to miss one to two days of work each month. She wants help to manage her symptoms more effectively but not with a drug. Which choice would most likely NOT be helpful to for her?

  **A** Planning regular leisure time into each week.
  **B** Beginning a yoga class.
  **C** Moderate exercise five days a week.
  **D** Cognitive behavioural therapy.

Answer: C

There is no adequate proof that exercise is an effective strategy in managing abdominal pain or diarrhoea. There is some evidence that it may be helpful in the management of constipation.

**4** A middle-aged woman came to see you because she was tired of her IBS symptoms ruling her life. Her symptoms began as a child but have increased to the point that she no longer participates in activities she once enjoyed. She is still able to work but feels too anxious to have dinner out with friends, attend movies or go hiking, biking or travel. She asks you for recommendation to a specialist. Which of the following would you recommend?
  **A** Psychologist.
  **B** Nurse trained in self-management strategies.
  **C** Dietician.
  **D** Hypnotist.

Answer: A

It is likely that this woman's symptoms are influenced by anxiety based on beliefs from her past. A psychologist is the best trained professional to identify and treat thoughts and beliefs that influence her anxiety and her IBS symptoms.

**5** Which of the following is not a core self-management skill?
  **A** Resource use.
  **B** Decision making.
  **C** Forming a patient/provider partnership.
  **D** Effective communication.

Answer: D

The five core self-management skills include: problem solving, decision making, resource use, forming a patient/provider partnership and taking action. Effective communication plays a significant role in the patient/provider relationship but it is not identified as a core self-management skill.

# CHAPTER 8

# Food-related Symptoms of Irritable Bowel Syndrome

*Michel Dapoigny*

Médecine Digestive, CHU Estaing, CHU Clermont-Ferrand, Clermont-Ferrand, France

---

**Key points**

- Strong relationship between the meals and the occurrence of IBS symptoms.
- Food intolerance is hard to prove.
- Elimination diets are popular but not very effective.
- FODMAP-free and gluten-free diets are to be evaluated more.
- Demonstration of the efficacy of probiotics in IBS is needed.

---

Irritable bowel syndrome (IBS) is the most common of the functional gastrointestinal disorders. The multiplicity of symptoms of IBS precludes developing a simple and reliable hypothesis regarding physiopathology. Many factors are potentially implicated in IBS physiopathology, but the presence of symptoms in single patient can remain unexplained. This is emphasized by the relative failure of conventional and /or alternative therapies; the management of IBS patients remains a difficult challenge for doctors. Most IBS patients try to modify their diet either as primary self-therapy or following some medical, paramedical or friendly advice. A majority of IBS patients seek dietary counselling from their GPs or the gastroenterologist. They often strongly believe that a (usually) restrictive diet will improve the IBS symptoms. Despite the potential deleterious effect of some foods, such as lactose, fermentable foods, coffee or even some fibre, on abdominal symptoms, it is very difficult to give general dietary advice to IBS patients. It was stated a few years ago [1] that food by itself is not responsible for IBS symptoms but that targeted dietary advice to individual patients could be helpful. Recently it has been proposed that Fermentable Oligo-, Di- and Monosaccharides and Polyols (under the acronym FODMAP) could trigger symptoms of IBS [2], especially bloating; as such a low FODMAP diet has been proposed in the management of IBS. Additionally,

---

*Irritable Bowel Syndrome: Diagnosis and Clinical Management*, First Edition.
Edited by Anton Emmanuel and Eamonn M.M. Quigley.
© 2013 John Wiley & Sons, Ltd. Published 2013 by John Wiley & Sons, Ltd.

changes in gut microflora have been increasingly described in IBS patients [3, 4], and it has been proposed that symptoms of IBS could originate from these changes. Thus, it is suggested that altering the microbiota could modulate IBS symptoms, in a facilitatory or inhibitory way. Altering the diet may influence the gut microflora and the addition of probiotics in alimentation could improve IBS symptoms [5]. How food and/or dietary interventions can modify symptoms in IBS patients is discussed in this chapter.

## Importance of the relationship between food and IBS

The first issue is to address whether we have enough scientific background to believe that foodstuffs can interact with symptoms of IBS. The personal feeling of most IBS patients is that food is important in inducing symptoms. It is usual to hear from patients that they cannot eat anymore or that every kind of food is bad for them. But the last definition of IBS (Rome III criteria) [6] does not take into account any point regarding food intake or alimentation. When searching the PubMed database using very simple criteria such as 'diet and IBS' 231 papers are proposed, but when using Google, like many IBS patient can do, with the same key words one can obtain up to 9 300 000 results. It seems that there is a big gap between science and popular feelings as expressed on Internet sites and in different kinds of forum. Nevertheless, ten years ago, Horwitz, in a review article published in the *New England Journal of Medicine* [7] underlined that change in diet should be the first line treatment in the three classical IBS subtypes. This was in accordance with a paper showing that about 66% of IBS patients perceived their symptoms to be diet related [8]. This could suggest that IBS patients and the normal population have different kinds of diet. But studies performed in different groups have shown that the IBS subpopulation has an adequate and balanced dietary intake when compared with other populations [9, 10]. So this discrepancy is not explained satisfactorily.

There is a well-recognized colonic motor response to eating [11, 12] although a colonic motility disorder is not thought to be the dominant pathophysiology in IBS [13–16]. The mechanisms of the colonic response to the meal were thought to be reflex mediated from the autonomic nervous system and/or hormonal via cholecystokinin, gastrin and other digestive hormones [17–19]. Lipids were described as the most potent stimulating factor of the colonic response to the meal [20, 21]. More recently, visceral (especially colonic) hypersensitivity has become prime in the aetiopathogenesis of IBS symptoms, and has even been claimed to be a biomarker of IBS [22]. More recently still, lipids intakes have also been shown to increase visceral sensitivity [23]. This correlates with the clinical report by IBS patients that they do not tolerate fatty diets.

An additional factor for some IBS patients is the question of a 'food allergy' or food intolerance, with some individuals grossly restricting their diets. In contrast with the high prevalence rate of IBS in the general population, the prevalence of food allergies is estimated between 0.6% (peanuts) and 2.6% (seafood) of the general population [24], and the estimated prevalence of food intolerance in United Kingdom was measured between 1.4 and 1.8% of the general population [25].

Avoidance of specific dietary components is much more frequent than supplementation, except for fibre and probiotics. In fact, for many years fibre has been argued to have a beneficial effect on IBS symptoms. The subject of dietary fibre, particularly wheat bran, became a popular one following Burkitt's work [26] on the possible role in preventing diverticular disease and colonic cancer, followed by Painter's subsequent letter in the *BMJ*: 'I believe that these symptoms (i.e. IBS-like symptoms) are often caused by an intestine that is struggling with our modern fibre-deficient diet' [27]. Despite no clear-cut advantages being demonstrated, bran continued to be used for IBS patients, probably because it was felt that at least it would not do any harm. A recent meta-analysis [28] stated that treatment benefit for fibre was not evident, and when there is a positive effect it might be through an improvement in gut transit. On the other hand, nondigestible carbohydrates, mostly derived from fibre, are fermented in the colon. This metabolism produces short chain fatty acids (butyrate, acetate and propionate) and gas [29]. The butyrate is supposed to have positive effect on the colon [30] and may increase colonic sensitivity in rats [31]. This last point could contribute to the variable effects of fibre in IBS patients.

Probiotic supplementation is a popular alternative to conventional treatment for many patients. Probiotics were defined by the Food and Agriculture Organization as live microorganisms which, when administered in adequate amounts, confer a health benefit to the host [32]. They may act to improve intestinal motility and sensitivity, and decrease the (even already low) level of mucosal inflammatory [33]. Some probiotics are already available as daily foodstuffs such as yogurt and some are sold as nutritional supports not needing medical prescription to be used by patients.

So whilst there may be a link between alimentation and IBS symptoms, the lack of evidence of scientifically demonstrated effect leaves the clinician unable to reliably make recommendations, and the IBS patient frustrated. So, examined now is the evidence on elimination and supplementation diets.

## Elimination diets

It has been proposed to eliminate a wide variety of foodstuffs from the diet of IBS patients who claim that they have a food allergy or food intolerance. One of the main points to discuss before advising an IBS patient to avoid a specific food component is the difference between *food intolerance* and *food allergy*. The latter is defined as an adverse health effect arising from a specific immune response that occurs reproducibly on exposure to a given food. It can result in anaphylaxis, which is a very severe condition, but it remains quite rare in the general population. In contrast, when foods elicit reproducible adverse reactions without immunologic mechanisms this is termed food intolerance [24].

The best example to illustrate this difference is probably the difference between lactose intolerance and the allergy to cow's milk proteins. Lactose intolerance is a much more frequent condition than allergy, but the condition is not so severe because the response is not immune based. There are four types of food allergy: IgE-mediated, non-IgE-mediated, mixed IgE- and non-IgE-mediated and, sometimes, cell-mediated. This can explain, at least in part, why food allergy has such a wide spectrum of expression, ranging from death due to severe anaphylaxis to mild abdominal bloating.

With regard to IBS symptoms, food allergy may need to be considered when a patient presents with any combination of symptoms listed in Table 8.1 that occur within minutes to hours of ingesting food, especially if

**Table 8.1** Food-induced allergic reactions.

| System | Immediate reactions | Delayed reactions |
|---|---|---|
| Gastrointestinal tract | Oral pruritus | Gastro-oesophageal reflux |
| | Tongue swelling | Nausea/Vomiting |
| | Nausea/vomiting | Abdominal pain |
| | Abdominal pain | Haematochezia |
| Respiratory | Cough/dyspnoea | Cough/dyspnoea |
| | Wheezing | Wheezing |
| | Chest tightness | – |
| Otolaryngology | Nasal congestion/pruritus | – |
| | Rhinorrhoea | – |
| | Sneezing | – |
| | Laryngeal edema | – |
| Ophthalmology | Pruritus | Pruritus |
| | Conjunctival erythema | Conjunctival erythema |
| | Tearing | Tearing |
| Cutaneous | Erythema | Erythema |
| | Pruritus | Pruritus |
| | Urticaria | Flushing |

these symptoms have followed the ingestion of specific food on more than one occasion [24]. The diagnosis of food allergy is always difficult, because it could take a long time to understand the patient's full history and to explore factors which could be implicated in the occurrence of the symptoms, such as physical exercise, alcohol consumption, and use of aspirin or nonsteroidal anti-inflammatory drugs [34]. The most recent guidelines from the USA [24] concluded that only few tests are useful (Table 8.2) and some nonvalidated tests such as endoscopic allergen provocation should be avoided [35]. In fact, the gold standard to identify the offending food is still the double blind placebo controlled food challenge [36], even if it may provoke some morbidity. However, a single blind or an open-food challenge may have some diagnostic value when objective symptoms (elicited by challenge) correlate with medical history and are supported by laboratory tests [24]. An open test with a strict avoidance of the suspected food during 2–8 weeks can be performed before initiating the single or double blind challenge [37]. But a very important question remains: is an IBS patient diagnosed with a real food allergy still an IBS patient? This author would suggest not, because the 'official' definition of IBS reports that symptoms are representative of IBS if there is any structural or metabolic abnormality.

True food allergy is quite rare (about 3% prevalence) whilst, in contrast, more than 20% of the population complains of food intolerance [38]. Food intolerances are nontoxic and nonimmune-mediated adverse reactions to food [39, 40]. So far, we can eliminate poisoning foods which elicit symptoms in an acute condition; this is not compatible with the chronic condition

**Table 8.2** Diagnostic testing for food allergy.

| Test | Potential usefulness | Diagnostic |
|---|---|---|
| Skin prick test | Identification of food | Not alone |
| Intradermal tests | Suggestive for carbohydrate-induced IgE-mediated allergy | Not to be done |
| Total serum IgE | Sensitivity and specificity too low | Not to be done |
| Allergen-specific serum IgE | Identification of food | Not alone |
| Atopy patch test | Evaluation of atopic dermatitis and eosinophilic esophagitis | Not to be done |
| Combination tests: | Identification of food | |
| Skin prick tests, serum IgE and atopy patch tests | Increasing positive and negative predictive values | Not to be done |
| Foods elimination diets | Identification of food | No consensus |
| Oral food challenge | Identification of food | Gold standard |

of IBS. Four different types of intolerance can be described but from a clinical point of view it is always difficult to differentiate between them in a single IBS patient. The usual symptoms of food intolerance are bloating, abdominal pain and diarrhoea, whatever the mechanism is, and this is very close of the symptoms of diarrhoea-predominant IBS.

First of all coeliac disease has to be discussed, because this represents an interface between food allergy and food intolerance. It was once referred to as gluten intolerance in some textbooks, before precise immune mechanisms were described. It is well known that symptoms of coeliac disease can mimic those of IBS, and it has been suggest that coeliac disease has to be ruled out before confirming IBS diagnosis [41–43]. But some IBS patients in whom coeliac disease has been excluded claim that they are improved with a gluten-free diet, although the objective evidence supporting this approach is poor. Wahnschaffe *et al.* suggested that the gluten-free diet could improve diarrhoea-predominant IBS patients but this was non-randomized study [44]. More recently, Biesiekierski *et al.* [45] published a randomized and controlled study demonstrating that a gluten-free diet can improve symptomatic IBS patients. Even if the conclusion was that 'non-coeliac gluten intolerance' may exist, the underlying mechanisms remain unknown. It is interesting to note that it may be that another component of gluten than gliadin (i.e. fructans) was responsible for the symptomatic effect. It has been shown recently that fructans are present even in gluten-free bread [46], but the analysis of the ingested gluten in the Biesiekierski's study demonstrated that it was also fructans-free. Those patients in this last study were IBS patients who responded to a gluten-free diet before inclusion; nevertheless, this suggests that there is a potential overlap between IBS and coeliac disease; but more studies are needed before concluding that a gluten-free diet could be useful in some selected IBS patients. Because the gluten-free diet is complicated to follow, and because it is still quite expensive, it is especially important to identify strong predictors of a positive response to the gluten-free diet.

The second very frequent problem to deal with in a patient presenting with IBS is lactose intolerance. To be absorbed, lactose needs the presence of lactase within the intestinal wall. This kind of food intolerance can be defined in three different ways [1, 47, 48]: biochemical malabsorption as measured by classical or simplified hydrogen breath test [49] after ingestion of 50 g of lactose; or the reproduction of symptoms after lactose challenge; or even the disappearance of symptoms on a lactose-free diet. But the lactase deficiency does not lead to IBS-like symptoms in all subjects, only those patients suffering from, abdominal pain, bloating and/or diarrhoea are said to have lactose intolerance [50]. On the other hand, a lot of patients who believe that lactose triggers their symptoms have no objective evidence of lactose malabsorption [51]. If we consider that lactose malabsorption can induce more symptoms in IBS patients than in normal subjects, it is not surprising to find that the prevalence of lactase deficiency is higher in the IBS group [52]. But the efficacy of the lactose-free or reduced diet is still controversial, not only in IBS patients [53].

---

### CASE STUDY 8.1

A 23-year-old Caucasian, male patient was presenting with abdominal pain, bloating and diarrhoea for at least five years. The physical examination, including rectal examination, was normal and the history reported that abdominal pain and bloating had occurred every day after the meals for three years, and diarrhoea was intermittent. He had at least two bowel movements per day and the stools were never hard. The patient was diagnosed with IBS a few years ago because he did not lose weight, the standard biology was normal every time it was done. Different treatments were proposed including low fibre diet, enriched fibre diet, antispasmodics, loperamide and even, recently, probiotics.

All these treatments were reported as nonefficient by the patient. At this point, the patient started a very restrictive diet because of the post prandial occurrence of the symptoms. He said that he was more comfortable when he did not eat anything at lunch, so he could carry out his work in better conditions. A few weeks later he was complaining of a weight loss of 3 kg. Then a gastroenterologist performed a total colonoscopy by hypothesizing Crohn's disease, or a microscopic or lymphocytic colitis. The multiple ileal and colonic biopsies did not find any abnormalities. The blood tests did not show any abnormality, including the antitransglutaminase antibodies and thyroid testing. The diagnosis of diarrhoea-predominant IBS was confirmed and a treatment with loperamide and probiotics was proposed again. The improvement was quite small and the patient again complained with a very low quality of life and a persistent weight loss. Then, the patient was given an antidepressant (amitriptyline 40 mg per day), but adverse events were significant (dryness of the mouth and poor sleep) and the patient stopped the treatment.

Because lactose intolerance was not suspected before, a breath test with lactose was performed. During the test (50 g of lactose in 250 ml water) the patient experienced important abdominal pain, nausea and bloating, and diarrhoea appeared 60 minutes after lactose ingestion. The rate of expired hydrogen was significantly higher than the basal rate from 30 minutes after ingestion to the end of the procedure (240 minutes). The correlation between breath test and symptoms after lactose ingestion demonstrated a lactose intolerance and the dietician proposed a strict lactose-free diet for the patient.

A few months later the patient had taken all the usual meals, including lunch, without problem. He had a weight gain by 4 kg. He did not complain of diarrhoea anymore, and he told us that the bloating was intermittent and acceptable. He noted that bloating was associated with abdominal pain but that these intermittent pain attacks were easily improved by antispasmodics.

In conclusion: lactose intolerance is quite rare in the Caucasian population and it is not very common in the primary care system to propose this diagnosis in a patient so young. In this case, the diagnosis of lactose intolerance was supported by a good correlation between breath test, symptoms and response to lactose-free diet. But, the patient was still suffering from IBS with abdominal discomfort and bloating occurring more than three days a month for years.

Fructose, which is another frequently incriminated sugar in IBS symptoms, is found in a lot of natural products, such as honey and fruits, and also in many diet drinks or prepared foods, in which it is used as a sweetener. Because the human intestine does not have a specific enzyme to digest the fructose, we can associate the natural fructose malabsorption with that of the lactose. The main difference is that the fructose is passively absorbed in presence of glucose. So far, fructose can initiate IBS-like symptoms when it is ingested in large amounts as compared with the ingested rate of glucose. The absorption of fructose is facilitated by glucose transporters (GLUT5 and GLUT2) which can be deficient or not activated enough [54]. If not absorbed, the fructose can have an osmotic effect when entering the distal small intestine and the proximal colon; it can also be fermented by the colonic microbiota. In both cases patients can suffer from IBS-like symptoms such as diarrhoea and bloating. Some authorities diagnose fructose malabsorption by breath testing, but this method and its clinical implication remain controversial because the breath testing with fructose alone (without glucose) may overestimate the malabsorption [55]. A recent publication showed that up to 67% of IBS patients with a positive breath test can improve over a long-term period with a diet low in or free of fructose, sorbitol and/or lactose [56]. Despite the fact that the literature remains too equivocal to definitively support the efficacy of this kind of elimination diet, the concept of carbohydrate malabsorption warrants further exploration.

## The FODMAPs diet

The FODMAPs concept arose from these last studies about short chain carbohydrates. Fructose and the lactose, respectively mono- and disaccharide, are included within the FODMAPs group, but have been discussed already. The remaining FODMAPs are fructans, polyols and galactooligosaccharides [57].

Fructans are linear or branched fructose (oligo) polymers which are either beta-2,1-linked inulins or beta-2,6-linked levans. Inulin is mainly of plant origin whereas fungi or bacteria are producers of levans [58]. It is recognized that three inulin-containing plants are used by the food industry (agave, Jerusalem artichoke and chicory) to produce short or long chain fructans. Usually, short chains of fructose (less than ten) are called fructo-oligo- saccharides (FOS) and long chain fructose (more than ten) are called inulins. Fructans are manufactured to be incorporated within a lot of different kinds of food products as sweetener, fat replacers, texturing agent, or stabilizer [59]. But inulin-type fructans are also found in significant amounts in a lot of fruits and vegetables (wheat, onions, bananas, garlic and leek). This kind of fructans has been classified as nondigestible oligosaccharides because the human intestine does not have the correct hydrolase to break the beta-2,1 bond. This effect has putative health benefits in humans [60] and the mean amount of daily ingested fructan is increasing in western countries [61].

Polyols are relatively underexplored despite their wide use, especially as sugar alternatives. Xylitol, sorbitol, mannitol, maltitol, lactitol, isomalt, erythritol, D-tagatose, isomaltulose, sucralose and polydextrose can be found in almost all foods. Their claimed effects are to improve dental health and decrease post prandial glycaemic response, but their labelling should include that an excessive consumption can lead to diarrhoea [62]. This is a well-known effect because sorbitol and lactitol are marketed as laxatives in many countries. One could explain that large ingestion of this kind of foodstuffs induces diarrhoea, bloating and abdominal pain as well in predisposed IBS patients.

The main dietary forms of galactooligosaccharides are raffinose (one fructose, one glucose and one galactose) and stachyose (one fructose, one glucose and two galactose) [57]. These nonabsorbed oligosaccharides are found in significant quantity in pulses such as beans, peas and lentils [63].

All these FODMAPs have three common properties: they are poorly absorbed, they are osmotically active and they are rapidly fermented by the microbiota [2]. This means that the transit time could be decreased and the intra luminal gas production could be increased. The arrival of FODMAP in the distal ileum and the proximal colon is a normal feature, but it may induce symptoms in some IBS patients because of an impaired visceral sensitivity or a dysmotility [2]. Thus, strict avoidance of FODMAPs in the diet to improve IBS patients has been proposed. But there is a confounding issue: many foodstuffs in the daily meals of citizens in western countries contain FODMAPs. To date there is only one Australian study [2] about FODMAPs-containing foods, and it remains impossible to give reliable advice to our IBS patients regarding this kind of elimination diet.

## Elimination and supplementation diet

This section only discusses the role of fibre in IBS. Increasing the amount of ingested dietary fibre in IBS patients has been a standard recommendation for a long time. The most recent meta-analysis [28] on the effect of dietary fibre in IBS included 12 trials with a total of almost 600 IBS patients. Many studies included constipation-predominant IBS, and in this case one can suppose that the improvement of transit can also improve the global evaluation of the symptoms. Moreover, there was a very small difference between the high fibre diet and the placebo or low fibre diet (52% vs 57%, respectively, have no improvement). This poor effect of fibre in IBS was previously reported by other studies [64, 65] in which the detrimental effect of fibre was even suggested. But in the same meta-analysis it was suggested that soluble fibre could have a positive effect on IBS symptoms, contrasting with the effect of insoluble bran. This point is highlighted by a systematic review and a randomized controlled study [66, 67] showing that soluble fibres such as ispaghula or psyllium are more effective that bran in IBS. All these data suggest that despite strong recommendations to use fibre in IBS it is important to take into account the symptom subtype of IBS patients and, if fibre is recommended, it seems more effective to use soluble rather than insoluble fibre.

## Supplementation diets

The microbiota of the normal human intestine represents a complex mostly anaerobic ecosystem that plays a key role in maintenance of health and physiological functions of the host. This microbiota acts as a barrier against pathogens, stimulates the host immune system and produces a great variety of compounds from the metabolism of dietary and endoge-nous substrates that could affect the host. Some microbial alteration may also be involved in the onset and maintenance of IBS. Disturbances in the composition and stability of the gut microbiota were reported in IBS indi-viduals compared to healthy ones [4, 68, 69]. These alterations of colonic microflora could explain, at least in part, excess gas production secondary to food ingestion and could make the link with food-related symptoms and disturbances of the microbiota. Probiotics are likely to have a variety of roles: enhance the intestinal barrier function, be immune modulators and improve the competitive adherence to the mucus and epithelium. A strong case can, therefore, be made to use probiotics in IBS patients [70]. Probiotics are commonly incorporated into our daily food but it is not clear how effective probiotics can be as nutritional supplementation in IBS patients. The last published meta-analysis concluded that probiotics could be effica-cious in symptomatic IBS patients, but also that the species, strains and dose of probiotics remain to determined, as well as the role of single and multiple strains [71]. A recent study showed that multiple strain probiotic mixtures could have a greater beneficial effect than single strain products in most forms of gut pathology except IBS where the results were more variable [72]. When comparing recently published papers (in 2011) the results remain controversial [73–75]. Nevertheless, probiotics treatment in IBS could be a promising approach, However, selection and characteriza-tion of potentially active strains should be done before testing dose and possible synergies.

   If one could accept that probiotics are useful in treating or improving IBS symptoms, it could also be worthwhile to consider prebiotics. Their definition has been recently revisited and stated as a selectively fermented ingredient that allows specific changes, both in the composition and/or activity in the gastrointestinal microflora, that confer benefits upon host well-being and health [76]. However, very few studies have addressed the effects of prebiotics in IBS patients. One study was performed in subjects with minor functional disorders and showed that short chain FOS could improve digestive comfort and quality of life [77]. There is only one randomized controlled trial showing that galactooligosaccharides act as a prebiotic and have an effect in alleviating IBS symptoms [78].

There is a degree of contradiction between FODMAP and prebiotic, which sometimes are the same product, such as galactooligosaccharides, inulin or oligo fructans. In reality, these should be considered as prebiotics [79]. Thus, it is difficult to separate the deleterious effects of FODMAPs (and propose a FODMAP-free diet) and the beneficial effects of prebiotics (and propose supplementation of the diet with prebiotics) in the IBS patients.

## Conclusions

Despite the high prevalence of IBS in the population and the very popular tendency to modify the diet in those patients, little evidence-based advice can be drawn from the literature (Table 8.3). True food allergy is rare and food intolerance is not so easy to prove. The most popular recommendation is for elimination diets, but the evidence base is especially weak here. The supplementation of the diet with bran or insoluble fibre is not to be recommended anymore. Some new concepts are emerging but remain, at least in

**Table 8.3** Possible diets to propose for IBS patients.

| Elimination diets | Supplementation diets |
| --- | --- |
| Lactose | Prebiotics: |
| Fructose | Galacto-oligosaccharides |
| Gluten | Short chain fructo-oligocaccharides |
| Fibre | Probiotics |
| FODMAPs: | Fibre |
| Galacto-oligosaccharides | |
| Fructans | |
| Polyols | |
| Specific foodstuffs related to proven food intolerance or allergy | |

part, controversial. It is suggested that in some IBS patients a gluten-free diet would be helpful. Probiotics may be efficient but we do not know which ones, which association and which dosage. Finally, there is the conflicting approach of prebiotics and FODMAPs. While it is certain that there is a clear relationship between meal ingestion and IBS symptoms, most dietary approaches currently employed by IBS sufferers are not supervised by their doctors and are not based on science. This underlines the need for the evaluation of new hypotheses regarding interactions between food, diet and IBS, and for the performance of relevant high quality trials.

## Useful web links

- http://www.eatright.org/
- http://www.iffgd.org
- http://www.apssii.org
- http://pharmabiotic-ri.org

## References

1 Dapoigny M, Stockbrügger RW, Azpiroz F *et al*. Role of alimentation in irritable bowel syndrome. *Digestion* 2003;67:225–233.
2 Gibson PR and Shepherd SJ. Evidence-based dietary management of functional gastrointestinal symptoms: The FODMAP approach. *J Gastroenterol Hepatol* 2010;25:252–258.
3 Malinen E, Rinttila T, Kajander K *et al*. Analysis of the fecal microbiota of irritable bowel syndrome patients and healthy controls with real time PCR. *Am J Gastroenterol* 2005;100:373–382.
4 Kassinen A, Krogius-Kurikka L, Makivuokko H *et al*. The fecal microbiota of irritable bowel syndrome patients differs significantly from that of healthy subjects. *Gastroenterology* 2007;133:24–33.
5 Hoveyda N, Heneghan C, Mahtani KR *et al*. A systematic review and meta-analysis: probiotics in the treatment in irritable bowel syndrome. *BMC Gastroenterology* 2009;9:15.
6 Longstreth CF, Thompson WG, Chey WD *et al*. Functional bowel disorders. *Gastroenterology* 2006;130:1480–1491.
7 Horwitz BJ and Fisher RS. The irritable bowel syndrome. *N Engl J Med* 2001;344: 1846–1850.
8 Simren M, Mansson A, Langkilde AM *et al*. Food-related gastrointestinal symptoms in the irritable bowel syndrome. *Digestion* 2001;63:108–115.
9 Saito YA, Locke GR3rd, Weaver AL *et al*. Diet abd functional gastrointestinal disorders: a population-based case control study. *Am J Gastroenterol* 2005;100:2743–2748.
10 Williams EA, Nai X and Corfe BM. Dietary intakes in people with irritable bowel syndrome. *BMC Gastroenterology* 2011;11:9.
11 Frexinos J, Bueno L and Fioramonti J. Diurnal changes in myoelectric spiking activity of the human colon. *Gastroenterology* 1985;88:1104–1110.

12 Rao SS, Sadeghi P, Beaty J, Kavlock R and Ackerson K. Ambulatory 24-h colonic manometry in healthy humans. *Am J Physiol Gastrointest Liver Physiol* 2001;280: G629–G639.

13 Deiteren A, Camilleri M, Burton D *et al*. Effect of meal ingestion on ileocolonic and colonic transit in health and irritable bowel syndrome. *Dig Dis Sci* 2010;55:384–391.

14 Bueno L, Fioramonti J, Ruckebusch Y, Frexinos J and Coulom P. Evaluation of colonic myoelectrical activity in health and functional disorders. *Gut* 1980;21: 480–485.

15 Sullivan MA, Cohen S and Snape WJ, Jr. Colonic myoelectrical activity in irritable-bowel syndrome. Effect of eating and anticholinergics. *N Engl J Med* 1978;298: 878–883.

16 Lee OY. Asian motility studies in irritable bowel syndrome. *J Neurogastroenterol Motil* 2010;16:120–130.

17 Snape WJ, Jr., Wright SH, Battle WM *et al*. The gastrocolic response: evidence for a neural mechanism. *Gastroenterology* 1979;77:1235–1240.

18 Niederau C, Faber S and Karaus M. Cholecystokinin's role in regulation of colonic motility in health and in irritable bowel syndrome. *Gastroenterology* 1992;102: 1889–1898.

19 Snape WJ, Jr., Matarazzo SA and Cohen S. Effect of eating and gastrointestinal hormones on human colonic myoelectrical and motor activity. *Gastroenterology* 1978;75:373–378.

20 Rao SS, Kavelock R, Beaty J *et al*. Effects of fat and carbohydrate meals on colonic motor response. *Gut* 2000;46:205–211.

21 Spiller RC, Brown ML and Phillips SF. Decreased fluid tolerance, accelerated transit, and abnormal motility of the human colon induced by oleic acid. *Gastroenterology* 1986;91:100–107.

22 Mertz H, Naliboff B, Munakata J *et al*. Altered rectal perception is a biological marker of patients with irritable bowel syndrome. *Gastroenterology* 1995;109:40–52.

23 Simren M, Abrahamsson H and Björnsson ES. Lipid-induced colonic hypersensitivity in the irritable bowel syndrome: the role of bowel habit, sex, and psychologic factors. *Clin Gastroenterol Hepatol* 2007;5:201–208.

24 Boyce JA, Assa'ad A,Burks WA *et al*. Guidelines for the diagnosis and management of food allergy in the United States: Summary of the NIAID-sponsored expert panel report. *J Allergy Clin Immuno.* 2010;126:1105–1118.

25 Young E, Stoneham MD, Petruckevitch A et al. A population study of food intolerance. *Lancet* 1994;343:1127–1130.

26 Painter NS and Burkitt DP. Diverticular disease of the colon: A deficiency disease of Western civilization. *BMJ* 197l;ii:450–454.

27 Painter NS. Irritable or irritated bowel? BMJ I 972;ii:46.

28 Ford AC, Talley NJ, Spiegel BM *et al*. Effect of fibre, antispasmodics, and peppermint oil, in the treatment of irritable bowel syndrome: systematic review and meta-analysis *BMJ* 2008; 337: a2313.

29 Bernallier-Donadille A. Fermantative metabolism by gut microbiota. *Gastroenterol Clin Biol* 2010;34:17–23.

30 Barbara G, Stanghellini V, Bandi G *et al*. Interaction between commensalbacteria and gut sensorimotor function in health and disease. *Am J Gastroenterol* 2005;100: 2560–2568.

31 Bourdu S, Dapoigny M, Chapuis E *et al*. Rectal instillation of butyrate provides a novel clinically relevant model of non inflammatory hypersensitivity in rats. *Gastroenterology* 2005;128:1996–2008.

32  FAO/WHO. Report of a joint FAO/WHO expert consultation on health and nutritional properties of probiotics in foods including powder milk with live lactic acid bacteria. Cordoba, Argentina, October 2001. ftp://ftp.fao.org/docrep/fao/009/a0512e/a0512e00.pdf (accessed 11 October 2012).

33  Ducrotté P. Microbiota and irritable bowel syndrome. *Gastroenterol Clin Biol* 2010;34:56–60.

34  Romano A, Di Fonso M, Guiffreda F *et al*. Food-dependant exercise-induced anaphylaxis : clinical and laboratories findings in 54 subjects. *Int Arch Allergy Immunol* 2001;125:264–272.

35  Bischoff SC, Herrmann A and Manns MP. Prevalence of adverse reactions to food in patients with gastrointestinal disease. *Allergy* 1996;51:811–818.

36  Nowak-Wegrzyn a, Assa'ad AH, Bahna SL *et al*. Work group report: oral food challenge testing. *J Allergy Clin Immunol* 2009;129:S365–S383.

37  Bock SA, Sampson HA, AtkinsFM *et al*. Double-blind, placebo-controlled food challenge (DBPCFC) as an office procedure: a manual. *J Allergy Clin Immunol* 1988;82: 986–997.

38  Zopf Y, Baenkler HW, Silbermann A *et al*. The differential diagnosis of food intolerance. *Dtsch Arztebl Int* 2009;106:359–370.

39  Eswaran S, Tack J and Chey WD. Food: the forgotten factor in irritable bowel syndrome. *Gastroenterol Clin N Am* 2011;40:141–162.

40  Heizer WD, Southern S and McGovern S. The role of diet in imitable bowel syndrome in adults: a narrative review. *J Am Diet Assoc* 2009;109:1204–1214.

41  Wahnschaffe U, Ullrich R, Riecken EO *et al*. Coeliac disease-like abnormalities in a subgroup of patients with irritable bowel syndrome. *Gastroenterology* 2001;121: 1329–1338.

42  Mein SM and Ladabaum U. Serological testing for coeliac disease in patients with symptoms of irritable bowel syndrome: a cost effectiveness analysis. *Aliment Pharmacol Ther* 2004;19:1199–1210.

43  Adler SN, Jacob h, Lijovetzky G *et al*. Positive coeliac serology in irritable bowel syndrome patients with normal duodenal biopsies: video capsule endoscopy findings and HLA-DQ typing may affect clinical management. *J Gastrointest Liver Dis* 2006;15:221–225.

44  Wahnschaffe U, Schulzke JD, Zeitz M *et al*. Predictors of clinical response to gluten-free diet in patients diagnosed withdiarrhea predominant irritable bowel syndrome. *Clin Gastroenterol Hepatol* 2007;5;844–850.

45  Biesiekierski JR, Newnhham ED, Irving PM *et al*. Gluten causes gastrointestinal symptoms in subjects without coeliac disease : a double blind randomized placebo controlled trial. *Am J Gastroenterol* 2011;106:508–514.

46  Whelan K, Abrahmsohn O, David GJ *et al*. Fructan content of commonly consumed wheat, rye, and gluten-free breads. *Int J Food Sci Nutr* 2011;62:498–503.

47  Fernandez-Benatez F, Esteve-Pardo M, de Leon R *et al*. Sugar malabsorption in functional bowel disease: Clinical implications. *Am J Gastroenterol* l993;88:2044–2050.

48  Vernia P, Ricciardi MR, Frandina C *et al*. Lactose malabsorption and irritable bowel syndrome. Effect of a long-term lactose-free diet. *Ital J Gastroenterol* 1995;27:117–121.

49  Oberacher M, Pohl D, Vavricka SR *et al*. Diagnosing lactase deficiency in three breaths. *Eur J Clin Nutr* 2011;65:614–618.

50  Lomer MC, Parkes GC, Sanderson JD *et al*. Review article: lactose intolerance in clinical practice-myths and realities. *Aliment Pharmacol Ther* 2008;27:93–103.

51  CasellasF, Aparici A, Casaus M *et al*. Subjective perception of lactose intolerancedoes not always indicate lactose malabsorption. *Clin Gastroenterol Hepatol* 2010;8:581–586.

52 Brandt LJ, Chey WD, Foxx-Orenstein AE *et al*. An evidence-based position statementon the management of irritable bowel syndrome. *Am J Gastroenterol* 2009;104;S1–35.

53 Shaukat A, Levitt MD, Taylor BC *et al*. Systematic review: effective management strategies for lactose intolerance. *Ann Intern Med* 2010;152:797–803.

54 Rao SS, Attaluri A, Anderson L *et al*. Ability to the normal human small intestine to absorb fructose: evaluation by breath testing. *Clin Gastroenterol Hepatol* 2007;5:959–963.

55 Gibson PR, Newnham E, Barrettt JS *et al*. Review article: fructose malabsorption and the bigger picture. *Aliment Phamacol Ther* 2007;25:349–363.

56 Fernandez-Banares F, Rosinach M, Esteve M *et al*. Sugar malabsorption in functional abdominal bloating: a pilot study on the long term effect of dietary treatment. *Clin Nutr* 2006;25:824–831.

57 Gibson PR and Dhepherd SJ. Personal view: food for thought – western lifestyle and susceptibility to Crohn's disease. The FODMAP hypothesis. *Aliment Pharmacol Ther* 2005;21:1399–1409.

58 Roberfroid MB and Delzenne NM. Dietary fructans. *Ann Rev Nutr* 1998;18:117–143.

59 Cummings JH and Roberfroid MB. A new look at dietary carbohydrate: chemistry, physiology and health. *Eur J Clin Nutr* 1997;51:417–423.

60 Roberfroid MB. Concepts in functional food: the case of inulin and oligofructose. *J Nutr* 1999;129:S1398–S1401.

61 Moshfegh AJ, Friday JE, Glodmann JP *et al*. Presence of inulin and oligofructose in the diets of Americans. *J Nutr*1999;129:S1407–S1411.

62 European Food Safety Authority (EFSA). Scientific Opinion on the substantiation of health claims related to the sugar replacers xylitol, sorbitol, mannitol, maltitol, lacti-tol, isomalt, erythritol, D-tagatose, isomaltulose, sucralose and polydextrose and maintenance of tooth mineralisation by decreasing tooth demineralisation (ID 463, 464, 563, 618, 647, 1182, 1591, 2907, 2921, 4300), and reduction of post-prandial glycaemic responses (ID 617, 619, 669, 1590, 1762, 2903, 2908, 2920) pursuant to Article 13(1) of Regulation (EC) No 1924/20061. http://www.efsa.europa.eu/en/efsajournal/doc/2076.pdf (accessed 11 October 2012).

63 Biesiekierski JR, Rosella O, Rose R *et al*. Quantification of fructans, galacto-oligosacharides and other short-chain carbohydrates in processed grains and cereals. *Hum J Nutr Diet* 2011;24:154–176.

64 Snook J and Shepherd HA: Bran supplementation in the treatment of irritable bowel syndrome. *Aliment Pharmacol Ther* 1994;8:51l–514.

65 Francis CY and Whorwell PJ: Bran and irritable bowel syndrome: Time for reap-praisal. *Lancet* 1994;344:39–40.

66 Bijkerk CJ, Muris JW, KnottnerusJA *et al*. Systematic review: the role of different types of fibre in the treatment of irritable bowel syndrome. *Aliment Pharmacol Ther* 2004;19:245–251.

67 Bijkerk CJ, deWit NJ, Muris JW *et al*. Soluble or insoluble fibre in irritable bowel syndrome in primary care? Randomised placebo controlled trial. BMJ 2009;339:b3154.

68 Kerckhoffs APM, Samsom M, Van der Rest M *et al*. Lower Bifidobacteria counts in both duodenal mucosa-associated and fecal microbiota in irritable bowel syndrome patients. *World J Gastroenterol* 2009;15(23):2887–2892.

69 Codling C, O'Mahony L, Shanahan F *et al*. A molecular analysis of fecal and mucosal bacterial communities in irritable bowel syndrome. *Dig Dis Sci* 2010;55:392–397.

70 Ohland CL and MacNaughton WK. Probiotic bacteria and intestinal epithelial barrier function. *Am J Physiol Gastrointest Liver Physiol* 2010;298:G807–G819.

71 Moayyedi P, Ford AC, Talley NJ *et al*. The efficacy of probiotics in the treatment of irritable bowel syndrome: a systematic review. *Gut* 2010;59:325–332.

72 Chapman CMC and Gibson GR. Health benefits of probiotics: are mixtures more effective than single strains? *Eur J Nutr* 2011;50:1–17.

73 Choi SC, Kim BJ, Rhee PL *et al*. Probiotic fermented milk containing dietary fiber has additive effects in IBS with constipation compared to plain probiotics fermented milk. *Gut Liver* 2011;5:22–28.

74 Søndergaard B, Olsson J, Ohlson K *et al*. Effects of probiotics fermented milk on symptoms and intestinal flora in patients with irritable bowel syndrome: a randomized, placebo-controlled trial. *Scand J Gastroenterol* 2011;46:663–672.

75 Guglielmetti S, Mora D, Gschwender M *et al*. Randomised clinical trial: Bifidobacterium bifidum MIMBb 75 significantly alleviates irritable bowel syndrome and improves quality of life –a double blind, placebo-controlled study. *Aliment Pharmacol Ther* 2011;33:1123–1132.

76 Gibson GR, Probert HM, Van Loo JAE *et al*. Dietary modulation of the human colonic microbiota: updating the concept of probiotics. *Nutr Res Rev* 2004;17:257–259.

77 Paineau D, Payen F, Panserieu S *et al*. The effects of regular consumption of short chain fructo-oligosaccharides on digestive comfort of subjects with minor functional bowel disorders. *Br J Nutr* 2008;99:311–318.

78 Silk DBA, Davis A, Vulevic J *et al*. Clinical trial: the effects of a trans-galactooligosaccharide prebiotic on faecal microbiota and symptoms in irritable bowel syndrome. *Aliment Pharmacol Ther* 2009;29:508–518.

79 Roberfroid M. Prebiotics: the concept revisited. *J Nutr* 2007;137:830S–837S.

# Multiple Choice Questions

**1** In IBS patients the colonic response to the meal is supposed to trigger abdominal pain or discomfort because:

**A** It is exaggerated as compared to normal subject.

**B** It is decreased as compared to normal subject.

**C** It is absent.

**D** It induces hormonal release that trigger symptoms.

**E** Another answer.

Answer: E

Colonic response to the meal is a physiologic motor function of the colon. But colonic motor disorders have not been accepted anymore as the most important physiopathologic phenomena in IBS.

**2** Among the different diets the IBS patients can be proposed the only efficient one is:

**A** Enriched fibre diet.

**B** Low fibre diet.

**C** No specific diet.

**D** Gluten-free diet.

**E** Lactose-free diet.

Answer: C

Modification of fibre in diet should not be recommended anymore. Coeliac disease and lactose intolerance should be discussed on an individual basis. The most efficient diet advice remains: eat everything!

**3** FODMAPs are:

**A** Found in most meat.

**B** Responsible for true food allergy.

**C** Found in some plants used by the food industry (such as chicory, agave, Jerusalem artichoke).

**D** A triggering of constipation-predominant IBS.

**E** Represented only by fructose, galactose and fructans.

Answer: C

It seems that the food industry is using more and more FODMAPs that are supposed to interact with microbiota to induce IBS like symptoms.

**4** Probiotics are:

**A** A validated treatment of IBS.

**B** Live or dead microorganisms which confer a health benefit for the host.

**C** Nutritional ingredients which improve composition and/or activity of gastrointestinal microflora.

**D** Likely to enhance intestinal barrier function, and to improve immune gut function and competitive adherence to mucus and epithelium.

**E** Mainly represented by lactobacillus and bifidobacter strains.

Answer: D

That is why probiotics are interesting to study from a scientific point of view in IBS patients (and may be in other diseases).

## CHAPTER 9

# Gut Inflammation in Irritable Bowel Syndrome

*Kok-Ann Gwee*

Yong Loo Lin School of Medicine, National University of Singapore and Gleneagles Hospital, Singapore

---

**Key points**

- IBS symptoms do not discriminate IBS from enterocolitides.
- Markers of inflammation and immune activation have been reported in post-infectious IBS and diarrhoea-predominant IBS.
- A sizeable proportion of patients with IBD, coeliac disease and colonic diverticulosis has IBS criteria.
- Potential biomarkers of gut inflammation in IBS are highly sensitive serum C-reactive protein, faecal calprotectin, deamidated antigliadin peptide and duodenal lymphocytosis and mastocytosis.
- Preliminary studies suggest that 5-aminosalicylates, mast cell stabilizers and probiotics may improve IBS symptoms via anti-inflammatory effects.

---

## Introduction

### Historical perspectives

The concept of gut inflammation in IBS raises issues in relation, firstly, to the definition of a functional disorder in that the finding of inflammation would challenge such a diagnosis, and, secondly, to how one defines pathological inflammation given that the normal healthy gut mucosa is populated by lymphocytes, plasma cells, mast cells, eosinophils and macrophages [1]. These latter observations, coupled with the recognition that the gut epithelium is presented, on a daily basis, with antigenic challenge from food and microbial proteins, have suggested that the normal healthy gut is in a state of chronic 'physiological' inflammation.

Faced with this semantic challenge, not surprisingly the role of inflammation in IBS was largely ignored despite hints here and there in the literature. In the 1950s, studies of patients presenting with persistent

---

*Irritable Bowel Syndrome: Diagnosis and Clinical Management,* First Edition.
Edited by Anton Emmanuel and Eamonn M.M. Quigley.
© 2013 John Wiley & Sons, Ltd. Published 2013 by John Wiley & Sons, Ltd.

bowel symptoms after dysentery reported subtle changes in the rectal mucosa, described as granularity and patchy hyperemia [2, 3]. The phenotypic profile of these patients was described as 'irritable colon'. In 1962, Hiatt and Katz examined colonic biopsies taken from four patients with what was referred to as spastic colitis and reported increased numbers of mast cells in the muscularis propria compared with biopsies from normal colons [4]. In the 1962 landmark study of IBS by Chaudhary and Truelove, 34 of 130 patients dated the onset of their IBS to an attack of dysentery [5]. In this series, hyperaemia and excessive mucus secretion were frequently observed on sigmoidoscopy in some of these patients.

## Gut inflammation in IBS

### The post-infectious IBS (PI-IBS) model

In the 1990s, a series of studies of post-infectious IBS (PI-IBS) led to a resurgence of interest in the role of gut inflammation in IBS [6–9]. When patients with acute gastroenteritis were followed up prospectively, those patients who developed IBS post-infection were observed to have had more severe and prolonged symptoms during the acute infection episode [6, 8, 9]. Rectal biopsies taken at the time of the acute illness also supported the presence of more severe inflammation during the infection in those patients who went on to develop IBS, as evidenced by higher inflammatory cell counts and enhanced mucosal expression of the pro-inflammatory cytokine interleukin (IL)-1β m RNA in those who went on to develop IBS, than in those who recovered without IBS. At three months post-infection, the rectal IL-1β m RNA expression remained elevated. The following physiological disturbances have also been reported in patients with PI-IBS: accelerated whole gut transit time, lowered threshold for pain and increased rectal contractility in response to a distension stimulus, reduced rectal compliance and increased intestinal permeability [7, 8, 10]. The accelerated intestinal transit provides a pathophysiological basis for diarrhoea, while the increased rectal sensitivity may relate to abdominal pain and rectal urgency, and the increased intestinal permeability allows for access of bacterial products to the lamina propria, a potential mechanism for perpetuating chronic inflammation. In patients recovering from Campylobacter jejuni gastroenteritis, serial rectal mucosal biopsies demonstrated increased counts of enteroendocrine cells in the immediate post-infection period, that gradually normalized in those who recovered but appeared to persist in patients with PI-IBS [8].

Increased enterochromaffin cell numbers could provide a pathophysiological basis for visceral hypersensitivity via enhanced production of 5-hydroxytryptamine, or serotonin [11, 12]. It was extrapolated that these functional disturbances were due to the infection and associated inflammation, as patients who recovered without IBS sequelae post-infection also demonstrated these disturbances, but to a milder degree [7]. Further support that infection alters the functions of the neuromuscular elements of the gut comes from a series of studies employing a mouse model of post-infective gut dysfunction [13–17]. In these studies, experimental mice were infected with the nematode *Trichinella spiralis* by gavage; longitudinal muscle strips were obtained from the jejunum during and after recovery from the acute infection. Cholinergic and electrical field stimulation of the intramural nerves produced greater contractility in these muscle strips in comparison to noninfested controls. Furthermore, the excitability of these neuromuscular elements correlated with laboratory markers of inflammation.

The PI-IBS studies also provide data to support a role for psychosocial stressors. In a prospective study of patients with acute infectious diarrhoea, it was observed that psychologically traumatic life events preceding the infection and a neurotic personality trait were the best predictors of who might develop IBS post-infection [6]. Putting all these data together we proposed a biopsychosocial model for post-infectious IBS. An episode of infectious diarrhoea may produce changes in gastrointestinal physiology that predispose to symptoms like diarrhoea and pain. The psychosocial factors such as stress and personality would influence the immune response and severity of inflammatory-mediated changes in the functions of the neural and muscular elements of the intestine. At a psychosomatic level, it is also suggested that the occurrence of infection at a stressful time creates an association between stressful situations and bowel symptoms, such that future stressful events may recall in the gut physiological disturbances associated with the index infectious event. However, in this paradigm, the manifestations of IBS will develop when psychological factors exist in association with more severe inflammatory and physiological disturbances. This would explain why only a fraction of patients with infection develop IBS and also why the majority of patients with psychiatric disturbances do not complain of IBS symptoms.

Another role of psychological factors appears to be in influencing the prognosis. During the three months after the infection, PI-IBS patients continued to report more life events, and higher anxiety scores [7, 18]. PI-IBS patients were also observed to have greater anxiety and somatization, and more negative illness beliefs [19]. Looking back at the early study by Chaudhary and Truelove, it is notable that while it was reported that PI-IBS patients were more likely to recover from IBS than non-PI-IBS subjects, they also observed that the presence of anxiety and depression was associated with a poorer outcome, a similar effect to that observed in the non-PI-IBS [5]. However, the prevalence of anxiety and depression in patients with IBS post-*Campylobacter jejuni* infection was less than that found in patients with chronic fatigue syndrome post-Epstein–Barr virus infection [19]. The evidence from PI-IBS supports a psycho-neuro-immunological axis for mediating the phenotypic expression of IBS. In this respect, IBS can be viewed as a psychosomatic condition from a different light [7, 20, 21].

## Gut inflammation in other IBS

There is also evidence supporting an inflammatory diathesis in other groups of IBS patients, most notably in those with diarrhoea [22–32]. Chadwick *et al.* obtained mucosal biopsies from different sections of the colon and consistently found increased intra-epithelial lymphocytes and mucosal CD3+ and CD25+ lymphocytes in a largely diarrhoea-predominant group of IBS patients compared with controls [22]. A study from Sweden demonstrated an augmented cell-mediated intestinal immune response in IBS [23]. Ohman *et al.* simultaneously examined peripheral blood T lymphocytes for expression of integrin β7 and colonic biopsies for endothelial expression of mucosal addressin cell adhesion molecule-1 (MAdCAM-1), and found in IBS patients an increased expression of integrin β7 and MAdCAM-1, resembling that seen in patients with ulcerative colitis [23]. In another study, Liebregts *et al.*, examined peripheral blood mononuclear cells (PBMC) and observed that IBS patients with diarrhoea demonstrated increased basal and E. coli lipopolysaccharide-induced production of TNF-α, with a positive correlation existing between TNF-α production and anxiety scores [24].

Associations between various candidate genes and IBS have been studied. Polymorphisms of the interleukin (IL)-10 and tumour necrosis factor α(TNFα) genes have been associated with some forms of IBS. Two studies have reported lower frequency in IBS patients of genotypes promoting production of IL-10, an anti-inflammatory cytokine [25, 26]. In one study, increased frequency of genotypes that promoted the production of TNF-α, a pro-inflammatory cytokine, was reported in IBS patients [25]. In this study, PI-IBS patients comprised 21% of the study group; comparing PI-IBS with non-PI-IBS patients the frequency of genotypes for IL-10 and TNF-α appeared similar between the two groups. Thus, genetic susceptibility to inflammation could also provide the basis for the role of genetics in the development of IBS.

While the failure of some studies to demonstrate differences in immune and inflammatory markers between IBS and controls appears to be inconsistent with this model, it should be noted that the discordant studies had recruited unspecified IBS subjects with no clear identification of those with diarrhoea and post-infectious features [29, 32].

## Mast cell studies in IBS

Gastrointestinal mast cells have been described as sentinels of the mucosal immune system strategically placed to respond to a variety of stimuli, including allergenic dietary proteins and various intestinal microbes and their associated toxins [33]. Furthermore, inflammation-associated cytokines such as interleukin (IL)-1 and IL-10 have also been implicated in mast cell priming, as well as being mast cell response mediators. In a number of IBS studies, the intestinal mucosa of the duodenum, jejunum, terminal ileum and colon have been reported to contain an increased number of mast cells, and to release higher amounts of the mast cell mediators tryptase and histamine [34–39].

In mucosal biopsies of the proximal descending colon obtained from forty-four IBS patients (half diarrhoea type, half constipation type) Barbara *et al.* found a 150% increase in the number of degranulating mast cells compared with healthy controls [36]. Furthermore, the majority (77%) of IBS patients showed an increased area of mucosa occupied by mast cells, an increased mucosal content of tryptase and enhanced release of mast cell tryptase and histamine. Barbara *et al.* also found that the number of mast cells in close proximity to nerve fibres was 223% greater in IBS patients compared with healthy controls. Furthermore, they found that the concentration of these nerve fibre apposed-mast cells correlated with both the severity and the frequency of abdominal pain. They followed up this study in another group of IBS subjects, replicated their earlier findings on the distribution of mast cells in IBS and went on to provide evidence that the enhanced release of histamine and tryptase in IBS subjects significantly correlated with the number of infiltrating mast cells. They went further to test the relationship of mast cells to the IBS associated phenomenon of visceral hypersensitivity [40]. Using an *ex vivo* model, mucosal supernatants from controls and IBS patients were injected into the mesenteric artery supplying an isolated segment of rat jejunum; supernatants from IBS patients were found to excite rat mesenteric sensory neurons and the dorsal root ganglion nociceptive neurons significantly more than supernatants from controls. This excitation was significantly decreased by the histamine H1 antagonist pyrilamine, but not by granisetron, a 5-HT3 receptor antagonist.

However, some of these mast cell changes have not been replicated in other studies. A number of studies have examined rectal mucosal biopsies and have not found an increase in mast cell counts in IBS patients, including those with PI-IBS [8, 28, 41, 42]. Cenac *et al.* and Klooker *et al.* reported that the number of mast cells was not increased in the ascending colon, descending colon or the rectum, and the latter also reported reduced tryptase release in the rectum of IBS patients [41, 42]. Notwithstanding the apparently discordant results, the study by Cenac *et al.* did demonstrate that supernatants derived from biopsies taken from IBS patients could produce visceral hypersensitivity via a mast cell mediator, protease, when instilled into a mouse model [41]. Two other studies have similarly shown that colonic biopsy specimens taken from IBS patients could activate nociceptive visceral neurons in both rats and human subjects via mucosal mast cell mediators such as histamine and tryptase [40, 43]. These inconsistent data may be due, in part, to the difficulty associated with immunohistochemical staining for mast cells and the uneven distribution of mast cells along the GI tract, as well as patient-related factors. In PI-IBS, Spiller *et al.* and Wang *et al.* both failed to find an increase in rectal mast cell counts, but the latter showed an increased mast cell count in the terminal ileum [8, 34]. Although the sentinel study by Hiatt and Katz had reported increased numbers of mast cells in the muscularis propria layer of colonic biopsies taken from patients with spastic colitis, in the more recent study by Tornblom *et al.*, where full thickness jejunal biopsies were obtained laparoscopically, no mast cells were seen in the myenteric plexus [4, 44]. As an age-related decline in rectal mucosal mast cells has been reported, this also has to be taken into account [45].

## IBS in the inflamed gut

The association of IBS with inflammatory enterocolitides, namely ulcerative colitis, Crohn's disease, diverticulitis and coeliac disease, is presented for a number of reasons. Firstly, these conditions have been associated with IBS-type symptoms and many patients fulfil current diagnostic criteria for IBS. Secondly, studies involving patients with these diagnoses who are thought either to be in the quiescent phase of the disease, or who do not have overt inflammatory activity, provide evidence that gut inflammation can form the basis for the development of IBS-type symptoms. Thirdly, therapeutic studies targeting the underlying inflammatory activity in these diagnoses provide suggestions for treatment of IBS patients with an inflammatory underpinning. Fourthly, observations from these studies provide clues to potential biomarkers for identifying post-inflammatory IBS.

### Inflammatory bowel disease

It has been proposed that patients with inflammatory bowel disease (IBD) can present with IBS-like symptoms when they are in remission. Isgar *et al.* examined 98 patients with ulcerative colitis using sigmoidoscopy to assess activity; 33% of these patients who were in clinical remission fulfilled Manning criteria for IBS compared with 7% of healthy controls [46]. Numerous other studies have reported numerically higher prevalence of

IBS, as defined by various criteria, in ulcerative colitis (33%), Crohn's disease (42–57%) and microscopic colitis (50%) [47–51]. In a study by Barratt *et al.* the symptomatology of IBS and IBD patients was assessed by questionnaires and diary recordings. No differences were found between IBS patients and Crohn's disease patients in the proportion who fulfilled Manning criteria and in their IBS diary scores. Conversely, no differences were found between the two groups on three different inflammatory bowel disease symptom-based indices [52]. Similarly, no differences were apparent between IBS patients and ulcerative colitis patients. This would not be surprising if we recall the study by Thompson which showed that the three symptoms on which the Rome criteria are based had not differentiated IBS from IBD patients; only abdominal distension was observed to occur more frequently in IBS than in IBD [53]. In a study by Keohane *et al.* of 106 IBD (62 Crohn's disease, 44 ulcerative colitis) patients thought to be in clinical remission, 54 patients were found to have IBS criteria; these symptomatic patients were found to have significantly higher faecal calprotectin levels than those who were asymptomatic [54]. The implication is that occult inflammation may underpin IBS symptoms in IBD patients despite apparent clinical remission.

## Coeliac disease

An analogous situation has been observed in coeliac disease, where recent studies suggest that, in certain populations, a substantial number of patients with IBS criteria could have subtle changes associated with gluten sensitivity. In a study from England, Sanders *et al.* found that of 300 patients with IBS criteria, 66 (22%) patients had positive antibody tests for coeliac disease, whereas only 44 of 300 (14.6%) age- and sex-matched asymptomatic controls had a positive test [55]. These patients appear to be extremely sensitive to gluten exposure, as only very mild histological changes were found in 14 patients, of whom only three had any of the complications commonly associated with coeliac disease. In a study from Germany of 102 patients with IBS criteria who were seronegative for antigliadin and tissue transglutaminase (tTg), 30% were found to have increased coeliac disease associated antibodies in the duodenal aspirate, 35% were positive for the coeliac disease associated genotype HLA-DQ2 and 23% had intra-epithelial lymphocytosis on duodenal biopsies [56]. Furthermore, on a gluten-free diet, IBS patients with coeliac disease markers showed significantly greater improvement in stool frequency than IBS patients without these markers [56, 57]. In a study from Ireland of 150 patients with confirmed coeliac disease, 30 (20%) fulfilled the Rome I criteria, compared with 5% in the control group [58]. A particularly intriguing observation was that the duration of coeliac disease had a negative association with IBS-type symptoms; the prevalence of IBS was about 10%

in those who had been diagnosed with coeliac disease for 10 years or shorter, whereas in those who had had coeliac disease longer than 10 years the prevalence of IBS symptoms was less than 5% [58]. The converse was that in those with IBS symptoms the mean duration of coeliac disease was 8.93 years, which was significantly shorter than those without IBS, where the mean duration was 13.6 years. As this was a retrospective study, it is not possible to test the association; however, one could hypothesize that patients with IBS could have a transient form of coeliac disease, with their IBS symptoms persisting even after they lose their gluten sensitivity.

A related hypothesis is that coeliac disease associated gut inflammation could serve to sensitize the gut to develop IBS-type symptoms, which could then persist as IBS even after gluten withdrawal has led to resolution of gluten-induced inflammation, much like in PI-IBS. In a study from Italy, small intestinal bacterial overgrowth was diagnosed in two thirds of a group of 15 patients with confirmed coeliac disease, who had persistent GI symptoms despite compliance with a gluten-free diet [59]. Subsequent treatment with rifaximin resolved the symptoms in all patients, as well as normalised the breath test. Providing further evidence of a possible link between gut microbes and coeliac disease, Verdu *et al.* from Canada reported a patient who developed full blown coeliac disease after she was initially diagnosed with PI-IBS after an episode of acute gastroenteritis [60].

## Diverticular disease

In an early study, Thompson *et al.* had interviewed 97 patients referred to hospital for barium enema and found no differences in the prevalence of IBS symptoms between patients with uncomplicated colonic divertic-ular disease and patients with a normal barium X-ray [61]. Based on this and other uncontrolled studies reporting that the majority of patients were asymptomatic, it was suggested that the occurrence of bowel symp-toms in patients with colonic diverticulosis was due to the co-existence of IBS, rather than due to the diverticular disease. In a more recent com-munity-based study involving 1712 subjects who had undergone a colonic imaging investigation, the presence of IBS, as defined by Rome II criteria, was found to be an independent predictor for diverticulosis but not diverticulitis [62]. This association was found to be particularly strong in those 65 years of age or older, where the presence of IBS was associated with a ninefold increase in odds for diverticulosis. The symp-tom profile of diverticula-associated IBS fulfilled diarrhoea-predominant IBS criteria, similar to post-infectious IBS. An interesting observation from this study was that diverticular disease was associated with a high somatization score.

Analogous to the PI-IBS model, it is possible that an episode of acute diverticulitis could predispose to the development of IBS. In a retrospective study of patients found to have diverticular disease on barium enema, it appeared that those who had had more severe attacks of diverticulitis requiring antibiotic treatment, were more likely to subsequently suffer frequent bouts of short-lived pain as well as abnormal stool form [63]. While it remains possible that these patients could have undetected persistent inflammation, another plausible explanation is that the severe diverticulitis could have produced plastic changes in the neuromuscular elements of the colon resulting in persistent disturbance to the bowel functions. Physiological studies in patients with diverticulosis have also demonstrated motility disturbances and enhanced visceral sensitivity, similar to those reported in IBS, involving even the rectum [64–66].

## Identifying and managing gut inflammation in IBS

The three key symptom descriptors of IBS (abdominal pain or discomfort that is relieved with defecation, or is associated with a change in stool consistency or frequency) originated from the studies by Manning *et al.* and Thompson. These early studies had demonstrated that the three symptoms differentiated IBS subjects from patients with peptic ulcer disease, but not from patients with IBD [53, 67]. Based on this historical perspective and the recent body of evidence that inflammation is a fundamental basis for the development of IBS symptoms, the logical next step in the diagnostic process would be to exclude inflammatory enterocolitides. An endoscopic examination with mucosal biopsies of the small and large intestines would be the obvious choice. However, many patients, and their physicians, are reluctant to undertake this. Therefore, there is a need for a well validated, sensitive and noninvasive test to identify patients at higher risk of inflammation. While the main objective of this test would be to allow for the diagnosis of clear-cut cases of coeliac disease, diverticulitis, Crohn's disease and ulcerative colitis, further investigations could lead to the identification of patients with low grade inflammation who have symptoms and psychological profiles associated with IBS.

The question then arises as to whether treatments targeted at these inflammatory enterocolitides have the potential to improve the patient's well-being. In a proof-of-concept study, prednisolone was employed to treat PI-IBS patients on the premise that increased T lymphocyte counts had been reported in rectal biopsies [68]. Twenty-nine patients with PI-IBS received three weeks of oral prednisolone, 30 mg/day, in a randomized, double-blind, placebo-controlled trial. While mucosal T lymphocyte counts decreased significantly in the prednisolone assigned group compared with the placebo group, their IBS symptoms did not improve. On the other hand, a number of recent studies have reported more promising early experience with the anti-inflammatory effects of aminosalicylates, mast cell stabilizing agents and probiotics in IBS patients. The results from these are still preliminary in nature, as none of these studies has so far been replicated with consistent results, and none of the drugs has so far been subjected to large randomized controlled study. Nonetheless, treatments with anti-inflammatory agents hold strong appeal as they offer the prospect of targeting a potentially fundamental pathophysiological basis for IBS. Furthermore, many of these agents are widely available and, in general, appear to be safe.

## Potential biomarkers for IBS with inflammation

A number of serological, cellular and molecular markers have been employed to study inflammation in IBS. These provide potential biomarkers for identifying IBS patients with gut inflammation. For the purpose of this section, only tests which are usually available in a hospital service laboratory are discussed. The measurement of serum C-reactive protein (CRP) and of faecal calprotectin has been applied to cohorts of IBS, IBD in remission and active IBD patients to assess their performance as inflammatory markers [69–75]. Interestingly, some of these have reported higher than expected values in patients with IBS criteria. In a study by Poullis *et al.* using a highly sensitive CRP, newly presenting cases of Crohn's disease and ulcerative colitis were found to have levels of CRP that were four- to sixfold higher than the upper limit of normal (set at 2.3 mg/l). Interestingly, though, patients with functional diarrhoea had levels of CRP that were significantly higher than those with functional constipation, but were similar to those of quiescent IBD patients [72]. The CRP is an acute phase protein that is produced in response to the release of IL-6, IL-1β and TNF-α at the site of inflammation, and increased expression of these pro-inflammatory cytokines has been reported in IBS [24, 75]. In a study of patients with Crohn's disease and ulcerative colitis who had criteria for clinical remission, those IBD patients who had IBS criteria were found to have higher levels of faecal calprotectin than those who were asymptomatic [54]. Furthermore, in the former group, their levels were comparable to that reported in IBD patients who were about to relapse [76].

Early studies of PI-IBS had explored the potential range of inflammatory cells and mediators associated with the development of IBS largely through the examination of rectal biopsies. Based on their ability to demonstrate increased enteroendocrine cell (EC) and intra-epithelial lymphocyte (IEL) counts in rectal mucosal biopsies taken from PI-IBS patients, Spiller *et al.* suggested rectal biopsy as a possible method to assess inflammation in IBS [8]. While these cells may be relatively easy to assess by routine conventional histopathology, it will be a challenge to draw a line between the subtle changes seen in IBS and low-grade proctitis. The early PI-IBS studies should be viewed as proof-of-concept studies; in this historical context, the rectal biopsy was a reasonable approach. Since then, with the concept of gut inflammation in IBS becoming more widely accepted, other researchers have progressed further afield to examine tissue biopsies from the colon as well as the small intestine. As discussed, increased mast cell numbers have been reported in the jejunum and terminal ileum, but less consistently in the rectum [34–38]. Obviously, the jejunum and terminal ileum are more difficult to access.

Therefore, duodenal biopsies are particularly appealing. Walker *et al.* reported increased mast cell numbers in the duodenum, particularly the second part, in both diarrhoea-predominant and constipation-predominant IBS patients compared to controls [39]. Furthermore, Walker *et al.* also reported a modest increase in duodenal IEL counts in patients with constipation predominant IBS. Recently, duodenal lymphocyte counts of greater than 25 IEL per 100 enterocytes have been defined as the diagnostic criterion for lymphocytic duodenosis [77–79]. Applying this definition, one hundred patients with lymphocytic duodenosis were investigated rigorously for coeliac disease and other known associations; coeliac disease was present in 16%, while 18% had criteria for IBS [80]. In another study, it has been reported that of 102 patients with diarrhoea-predominant IBS, 23% had duodenal lymphocytosis of greater than 40 IEL per 100 enterocytes [56]. Another advantage of duodenal biopsies is that they allow for the detection of the histological changes associated with coeliac disease. This could then be followed up with serology for coeliac disease.

The serological test used to screen for gluten sensitization in IBS needs careful consideration in terms of sensitivity over specificity. Some societies have suggested the use only of endomysial antibody (EMA) testing for IBS patients [81]. As the prevalence of a positive EMA strongly correlates with the severity of mucosal damage, it may not be a sensitive test to detect the milder changes associated with the IBS phenotype[82]. Recent studies suggest that antibodies against deamidated gliadin peptides might appear before the other antibodies and would thus be useful in the diagnosis and follow-up of patients with either gluten sensitization or early-stage coeliac disease [83]. Consistent with the observations that the sensitivity of EMA and tissue trans-glutaminase antibody (tTgA) testing was better for patients with more severe mucosal damage, a meta-analysis by Ford *et al.* found that in studies using IgA antigliadin antibody test, the pooled prevalence among IBS subjects was 4%, whereas in studies using EMA or tTgA testing the pooled prevalence was only 1.6% [84].

## CASE STUDY 9.1

KAS, a 36-year-old Caucasian lady from the United States who had been diagnosed with irritable bowel syndrome since the age of 26, had relocated to the Far East to accompany her husband. Her doctor in the United States had proposed treatment with alosetron, a 5-HT$_3$ antagonist. Her key problem had been chronic diarrhoea for which she had to go as many as 30 times a day and on a good day, at least 10 times. This was associated with urgency and occasionally incontinence. She had not experienced much pain until three months before her move to Singapore; she developed severe right upper quadrant pain, for which she had undergone cholecystectomy because she was found to have gallstones and as her HIDA scan indicated a nonfunctioning gall bladder. Prior to this, she had had extensive investigations in the United States which included repeated CT scans and colonoscopy. At her first colonoscopy four years before, patchy inflammation in the rectum to distal sigmoid colon was noted; visualization had been limited to the caecum. During an episode of right iliac fossa pain the following year, a CT scan of the abdomen reported a thickened appendix with minimal inflammatory changes as well as thickened wall of the sigmoid and distal descending colon with mild inflammatory changes in the adjacent fat. She and her brother have been intolerant of lactose since the age of 20. Her brother also had a history of small intestinal resection. Her father had a history of colon polyps, diverticulitis and oesophageal cancer. There was no known family history of coeliac disease. Her mother had a bipolar mood disorder.

   At the time of her presentation in Singapore she was on a cocktail of an antidiarrhoeal agent, a tranquilizer and an antidepressant. Physical examination revealed a well-nourished individual with red hair and no pallor. A clinical suspicion of coeliac disease was subsequently confirmed by positive tests for antigliadin IgA and anti-endomysium IgA, and the presence of mild villous atrophy and intra-epithelial lymphocytosis on duodenal biopsies. Serum levels of vitamin B12 (350 pmol/l, normal 150–700), folate (49.4 nmol/l, normal 2.5–45.4) and ferritin (28 ug/l, normal 10–291) were within normal reference ranges. When the diagnosis of coeliac disease was presented to her, she was initially incredulous; she had previously always felt comforted by eating bread during her attacks. However, after her first week on a gluten-free diet, her diarrhoea had reduced to three times a day and since then she has even experienced constipation on some days. She was able to discontinue her psychotropic drugs.

   During the year that she was in Singapore she experienced a number of short-lived acute but mild diarrhoeal episodes, usually triggered by antibiotics for upper respiratory tract infections. These antibiotic associated episodes have diminished in frequency and severity since she was maintained on a Lactobacillus-containing preparation. About six months after the diagnosis of coeliac disease, she began experiencing lower abdominal pains alternating between the right and left iliac fossa usually in association with mild diarrhoea. Three months after the onset of these episodes a check gastroscopy as well as colonoscopy was performed. Biopsies from the distal duodenum this time did not reveal villous atrophy and previous inflammatory changes had resolved. The colonoscopy revealed erythematous proctitis, multiple ring-like red spots in the caecum and multiple small erosions in the terminal ileum. Respective biopsies showed reactive lymphoid hyperplasia in general with small number of polymorphs around and between crypts in the caecum, and some ulceration over the lymphoid aggregates was present in the terminal ileum. In the course of the next four months she received three courses of tinidazole 500 mg b.d. for diarrhoea; each time her diarrhoea resolved rapidly on the nitroimidazole antibiotic. After her last course of antibiotic, she was placed on a 5-aminosalicylate 3 g daily as for possible Crohn's disease. She seemed to derive benefit from this treatment. She reported that she had felt better in the year following the diagnosis of coeliac disease than in the 10 years before.

## Potential anti-inflammatory agents for IBS
### Aminosalicylates

5-Aminosalicylic acid (mesalazine) is an anti-inflammatory agent widely used in the treatment of ulcerative colitis and Crohn's disease. Three preliminary uncontrolled trials had suggested that mesalazine could reduce pain and stool frequency, and improve stool consistency in patients with post-infectious and nonspecific IBS [85, 86]. In a small randomized, double-blind, placebo-controlled trial, Corinaldesi *et al.* tested the efficacy of mesalazine (800 mg three times daily for eight weeks) on intestinal immune cells and symptom perception in a mixed group of twenty IBS patients [87]. A significant improvement in general well-being was observed, with a trend for improvement in abdominal pain and frequency of bowel movement. No serious adverse drug reactions were observed. Given the small sample size and the pilot nature of the study, further studies are required to confirm the efficacy of mesalazine on IBS symptoms. Nonetheless, this study is particularly encouraging because mesalazine treatment was associated with markedly reduced mucosal immune cells and, in particular, mast cells, suggesting that mesalazine acted through an immune-mediated anti-inflammatory effect in this group of IBS patients. Barbara *et al.* have also proposed other actions of mesalazine that could operate in IBS patients with an inflammatory underpinning: alterations in the gut flora, modulation of protease release and enhancement of epithelial barrier function [41, 85, 88, 89].

### Mast cell stabilisers

Barbara *et al.* had shown in 2004 [36] that activated mast cells were present in close proximity to colonic neurons and that the density correlated with the severity of abdominal pain reported by the IBS patients. The therapeutic potential of agents with activity on mast cells has been reviewed [89]. Chromones (e.g. cromolyn sodium, nedocromil sodium) are compounds that act primarily by stabilizing the plasma membrane of mast cells, controlling the release of mast cell mediators such as histamine. In the 1980s, disodium cromoglycate was tested in twenty IBS patients with diarrhoea and observed to have a 40% therapeutic advantage over placebo in improving symptom scores [90]. The benefit appeared to be independent of the presence of atopy, food intolerance or lactase deficiency. On the other hand, in another small double-blind, placebo-controlled study, sodium cromoglycate significantly improved abdominal pain and diarrhoea in patients with IBS-D who also reported food intolerance [91]. Similarly, two uncontrolled, unblinded studies comparing oral cromoglycate against elimination diet therapy in patients with IBS-D reported high response rates of over 60% with both treatments; in both treatment arms it was suggested that patients with positive skin tests for dietary antigens were more likely to respond favourably [92, 93]. Two other unblinded studies which purported that cromoglycate improved symptoms in IBS-D patients provided some mechanistic insights by suggesting effects via enhancement of mucosal barrier function and reduction in mucosal tryptase release [94, 95]. One potential limitation to the role of cromoglycate is that in many countries it is available only as an inhaler for the treatment of asthma; the reason is that cromoglycate is not amenable to absorption when ingested orally, although this actually makes it an excellent compound for targeting mast cells in the gastrointestinal mucosa, without incurring systemic side effects.

Another mast cell stabilizing agent that has oral bioavailability is ketotifen. In a recent well-designed study, 60 patients with IBS underwent a barostat study to assess rectal sensitivity before and after eight weeks of treatment with ketotifen [42]. All patients were randomized to receive ketotifen starting with 2 mg twice daily for two weeks, after which the dose was increased to 4 mg twice daily for another two weeks to reach a final dose of 6 mg twice daily during the last four weeks of the study. Of the patients with IBS, 22% indicated that symptoms started following an episode of acute gastroenteritis. After eight weeks of treatment 20% of patients on ketotifen reported at least considerable relief of symptoms compared with only 10% on placebo. Univariate analysis suggested that there were improvements in abdominal pain, bloating, flatulence, diarrhoea and incomplete evacuation. Intriguingly, in this study, the number of mast cells was even lower in patients with IBS than in age-matched controls. Furthermore, no effect on the release of tryptase and histamine from rectal biopsies could be demonstrated, suggesting that mechanisms other than mast cell stabilization could have been operating.

Ketotifen is also recognised to be a relatively selective noncompetitive histamine H1 receptor antagonist. In the gastrointestinal tract, H1 receptors are expressed in the muscularis, mucosa and submucosa and, interestingly, are more expressed in the colonic mucosa of patients with IBS [96]. H1 receptors are also widely expressed in the brain, mediating nociception, arousal, locomotor activity and appetite control, which could potentially contribute improvement in terms of sleep, appetite and energy [97]. In a novel *ex vivo* model to test the role of mast cells in the development of visceral hypersensitivity, Barbara *et al.* demonstrated that the excitation of rat sensory neurons by colonic supernatant derived from patients with IBS was inhibited by H1 receptor blockade [40]. Barbara *et al.* had shown in 2004 [36] that activated mast cells were present in close proximity to colonic neurons and that the density correlated with the severity of abdominal pain reported by the IBS patients. In a recent uncontrolled study, 33 patients with intractable diarrhoea who had increased mucosal mast cell counts (defined as greater than 20 mast cells per high power field) in either duodenal or colonic biopsies, were treated with a combination of cetirizine (H1 receptor antagonist) 10 mg daily and ranitidine (H2 receptor antagonist) 300 mg twice daily with or without cromolyn sodium 200 mg four times daily for four weeks, 22 (67%) had either cessation or significant reduction in diarrhoea [98].

### Probiotics

There is growing evidence for the role of the gut microflora in IBS and for the use of probiotics in treating IBS [99]. A number of studies suggest that the therapeutic effect of probiotics in IBS could be mediated by an immunomodulatory effect. In a study from Cork, Ireland, a mixed group of 67 IBS patients completed a randomized controlled trial of one of three treatments – *Bifibacterium infantis 35624*, *Lactobacillus salivarius UCC4331* or placebo [100]. Patients treated with *B infantis* achieved the most favourable response with respect to composite symptom score, abdominal pain and bloating. In this study, blood samples were obtained for measurement of peripheral blood mononuclear cell (PBMC) release of cytokines interleukin (IL)-10 and IL-12 at baseline and end of treatment. At baseline, IBS patients were found to have a significantly lower IL-10:IL-12 ratio (indicative of a skew towards a Th1 pro-inflammatory profile) than healthy controls. This low IL-10:IL-12 ratio normalized after treatment with *B infantis* but not with *L salivarius* or placebo, supporting an anti-inflammatory effect for the former. In a study using a mouse model of post-*Trichinella spiralis* infection, *Lactobacillus paracasei* treatment was shown to attenuate the development of intestinal smooth muscle hypercontractility. It was also demonstrated that this effect was associated with reductions in the associated *T spiralis* Th2 response, transforming growth factor (TGF)-$\beta$1 and other inflammatory markers in the smooth muscle [101].

## Conclusions

How has the appreciation of the presence of gut inflammation in IBS affected clinical practice? What are the implications, if any, for biochemical and histopathological markers of inflammation? How do we apply this awareness of gut inflammation in our management of IBS?

Firstly, this appreciation of gut inflammation has changed our perception of the psychosomatic label we affix to IBS. We can now better visualize how immunological events may lead to the development of IBS and how environmental, genetic and psychological factors may modulate the outcome. We are also seeing a blurring of the boundaries between functional and organic.

Secondly, with this new understanding, we can also appreciate how patients with diagnoses that are traditionally labelled as inflammatory conditions of the gut could also 'develop' IBS. In this respect, we can consider IBS in patients with infectious gastroenteritis, inflammatory bowel disease, microscopic colitis, coeliac disease and colonic diverticular disease. With this compelling data that gut inflammation underpins the manifestation of these 'IBS' type symptoms, we should also be mindful that it is difficult to differentiate the inflamed gut from the irritable gut based on symptoms alone. Thus, we need to be more careful to exclude occult inflammatory activity before making a diagnosis of IBS.

Thirdly, we should reconsider the need to carry out tests of inflammatory activity in all patients with IBS criteria to exclude an inflamed gut. In this respect, we should emphasize high test sensitivity over specificity. Thus, tests that we can consider are a highly sensitive assay for C-reactive protein, faecal calprotectin, second-generation antigliadin IgA to deamidated gliadin peptides, and duodenal and rectal biopsies for intra-epithelial lymphocyte counts.

Fourthly, the hope is that with this new perspective and greater attention to the detection of inflammation, we can begin to move treatments to a more pathophysiolocally-based level. In this respect, we could consider the use of certain pharmacological agents with anti-inflammatory properties. The potential drugs to consider are mast cell stabilizing compounds, amino-salicylic acid containing compounds and probiotic preparations. While, admittedly, the evidence is preliminary, the results are encouraging, and provide for an optimistic outlook.

'There remains a tendency for investigators exploring the nature of IBS to divide themselves, in Cartesian fashion, into those who seek a cause for the problem in the mind and those who seek a cause in the gastrointestinal tract. Such a division is undoubtedly artificial and often seems dependent on the philosophical viewpoint of the clinician and of the patient [102].'

# References

1 Kirsch R, Kirsch RH, Riddell RH and Riddell R. Histopathological alterations in irritable bowel syndrome. *Mod Pathol* 2006;19(12):1638–1645.
2 Bockus HL, Kalser MH and Zion DE. Functional diarrhea: an analysis of the clinical and roentgen manifestations. *Gastroenterology* 1956;31(6):629–646; discussion, 646.
3 Stewart G. Post-dysenteric colitis. *Br Med J.* 1950;1(4650):405.

4 Hiatt RB and Katz L. Mast cells in inflammatory conditions of the gastrointestinal tract. *Am J Gastroenterol* 1962;37:541–545.

5 Chaudhary NA and Truelove SC. The irritable colon syndrome. A study of the clinical features, predisposing causes, and prognosis in 130 cases. *Q J Med* 1962;31: 307–322.

6 Gwee KA, Graham JC, McKendrick MW *et al*. Psychometric scores and persistence of irritable bowel after infectious diarrhoea. *Lancet* 1996;347(8995):150–153.

7 Gwee KA, Leong YL, Graham C *et al*. The role of psychological and biological factors in postinfective gut dysfunction. *Gut* 1999;44(3):400–406.

8 Spiller RC, Jenkins D, Thornley JP *et al*. Increased rectal mucosal enteroendocrine cells, T lymphocytes, and increased gut permeability following acute Campylobacter enteritis and in post-dysenteric irritable bowel syndrome. *Gut* 2000;47(6):804–811.

9 Gwee KA, Collins SM, Read NW *et al*. Increased rectal mucosal expression of interleukin 1beta in recently acquired post-infectious irritable bowel syndrome. *Gut* 2003;52(4):523–526.

10 Marshall JK, Thabane M, Garg AX *et al*. Intestinal permeability in patients with irritable bowel syndrome after a waterborne outbreak of acute gastroenteritis in Walkerton, Ontario. *Aliment Pharmacol Ther* 2004;20(11–12):1317–1322.

11 Dunlop SP, Coleman NS, Blackshaw E *et al*. Abnormalities of 5-hydroxytryptamine metabolism in irritable bowel syndrome. *Clin Gastroenterol Hepatol* 2005;3(4): 349–357.

12 Atkinson W, Lockhart S, Whorwell PJ *et al*. Altered 5-hydroxytryptamine signaling in patients with constipation- and diarrhea-predominant irritable bowel syndrome. *Gastroenterology* 2006;130(1):34–43.

13 Barbara G, Vallance BA and Collins SM. Persistent intestinal neuromuscular dysfunction after acute nematode infection in mice. *Gastroenterology* 1997;113(4): 1224–1232.

14 Collins SM, McHugh K, Jacobson K *et al*. Previous inflammation alters the response of the rat colon to stress. *Gastroenterology* 1996;111(6):1509–1515.

15 Barbara G, De Giorgio R, Deng Y *et al*. Role of immunologic factors and cyclooxygenase 2 in persistent postinfective enteric muscle dysfunction in mice. *Gastroenterology* 2001;120(7):1729–1736.

16 Bercík P, Wang L, Verdú EF *et al*. Visceral hyperalgesia and intestinal dysmotility in a mouse model of postinfective gut dysfunction. *Gastroenterology* 2004;127(1):179–187.

17 MacQueen G, Marshall J, Perdue M *et al*. Pavlovian conditioning of rat mucosal mast cells to secrete rat mast cell protease II. *Science* 1989;243(4887):83–85.

18 Dunlop SP, Jenkins D and Spiller RC. Distinctive clinical, psychological, and histological features of postinfective irritable bowel syndrome. *Am J Gastroenterol* 2003;98(7):1578–1583.

19 Spence MJ and Moss-Morris R. The cognitive behavioural model of irritable bowel syndrome: a prospective investigation of patients with gastroenteritis. *Gut* 2007;56(8):1066–1071.

20 Mayer EA. Breaking down the functional and organic paradigm. *Curr Opin Gastroenterol* 1996;12(1): 3–7.

21 Gwee KA. Irritable bowel syndrome: psychology, biology, and warfare between false dichotomies. *Lancet* 1996;347(9010):1267.

22 Chadwick VS, Chen W, Shu D *et al*. Activation of the mucosal immune system in irritable bowel syndrome. *Gastroenterology* 2002;122(7):1778–1783.

23 Ohman L, Isaksson S, Lundgren A *et al*. A controlled study of colonic immune activity and beta7+ blood T lymphocytes in patients with irritable bowel syndrome. *Clin Gastroenterol Hepatol* 2005;3(10):980–986.

24 Liebregts T, Adam B, Bredack C *et al.* Immune activation in patients with irritable bowel syndrome. *Gastroenterology* 2007;132(3):913–920.

25 van der Veek PPJ, van den Berg M, de Kroon YE *et al.* Role of tumor necrosis factor-alpha and interleukin-10 gene polymorphisms in irritable bowel syndrome. *Am J Gastroenterol* 2005;100(11):2510–2516.

26 Gonsalkorale W, Perrey C, Pravica V *et al.* Interleukin 10 genotypes in irritable bowel syndrome: evidence for an inflammatory component? *Gut* 2003;52(1):91–93.

27 O'Mahony L, McCarthy J, Kelly P *et al.* Lactobacillus and bifidobacterium in irritable bowel syndrome: symptom responses and relationship to cytokine profiles. *Gastroenterology* 2005;128(3):541–551.

28 Dinan TG, Quigley EM, Ahmed SM *et al.* Hypothalamic-pituitary-gut axis dysregulation in irritable bowel syndrome: plasma cytokines as a potential biomarker? *Gastroenterology* 2006;130(2):304–311.

29 Macsharry J, O'Mahony L, Fanning A *et al.* Mucosal cytokine imbalance in irritable bowel syndrome. *Scand J Gastroenterol* 2008;43(12):1467–1476.

30 Aerssens J, Camilleri M, Talloen W *et al.* Alterations in mucosal immunity identified in the colon of patients with irritable bowel syndrome. *Clin Gastroenterol Hepatol* 2008;6(2):194–205.

31 Scully P, McKernan DP, Keohane J *et al.* Plasma cytokine profiles in females with irritable bowel syndrome and extra-intestinal co-morbidity. *Am J Gastroenterol* 2010;105(10):2235–2243.

32 Chang L, Adeyemo M, Karagiannidis I *et al.* Serum and colonic mucosal immune markers in irritable bowel syndrome. *Am J Gastroenterol* 2012;107(2):262–272.

33 Barbara G, Stanghellini V, De Giorgio R and Corinaldesi R. Functional gastrointestinal disorders and mast cells: implications for therapy. *Neurogastroenterol Motil* 2006;18(1):6–17.

34 Wang LH, Fang XC and Pan GZ. Bacillary dysentery as a causative factor of irritable bowel syndrome and its pathogenesis. *Gut* 2004;53(8):1096–1101.

35 Guilarte M, Santos J, de Torres I *et al.* Diarrhoea-predominant IBS patients show mast cell activation and hyperplasia in the jejunum. *Gut* 2007;56(2):203–209.

36 Barbara G, Stanghellini V, De Giorgio R *et al.* Activated mast cells in proximity to colonic nerves correlate with abdominal pain in irritable bowel syndrome. *Gastroenterology* 2004;126(3):693–702.

37 Weston AP, Biddle WL, Bhatia PS and Miner PB. Terminal ileal mucosal mast cells in irritable bowel syndrome. *Dig Dis Sci* 1993;38(9):1590–1595.

38 O'Sullivan M, Clayton N, Breslin NP *et al.* Increased mast cells in the irritable bowel syndrome. *Neurogastroenterol Motil* 2000;12(5):449–457.

39 Walker MM, Talley NJ, Prabhakar M *et al.* Duodenal mastocytosis, eosinophilia and intraepithelial lymphocytosis as possible disease markers in the irritable bowel syndrome and functional dyspepsia. *Aliment Pharmacol Ther* 2009;29(7):765–773.

40 Barbara G, Wang B, Stanghellini V *et al.* Mast cell-dependent excitation of visceral-nociceptive sensory neurons in irritable bowel syndrome. *Gastroenterology* 2007;132(1):26–37.

41 Cenac N, Andrews CN, Holzhausen M *et al.* Role for protease activity in visceral pain in irritable bowel syndrome. *J Clin Invest* 2007;117(3):636–647.

42 Klooker TK, Braak B, Koopman KE *et al.* The mast cell stabiliser ketotifen decreases visceral hypersensitivity and improves intestinal symptoms in patients with irritable bowel syndrome. *Gut* 2010;59(9):1213–1221.

43 Buhner S, Li Q, Vignali S *et al.* Activation of human enteric neurons by supernatants of colonic biopsy specimens from patients with irritable bowel syndrome. *Gastroenterology* 2009;137(4):1425–1434.

44  Törnblom H, Lindberg G, Nyberg B and Veress B. Full-thickness biopsy of the jejunum reveals inflammation and enteric neuropathy in irritable bowel syndrome. *Gastroenterology* 2002;123(6):1972–9.

45  Dunlop SP, Jenkins D and Spiller RC. Age-related decline in rectal mucosal lymphocytes and mast cells. *Eur J Gastroenterol Hepatol.* 2004;16(10):1011–1015.

46  Isgar B, Harman M, Kaye MD and Whorwell PJ. Symptoms of irritable bowel syndrome in ulcerative colitis in remission. *Gut* 1983;24(3):190–192.

47  Minderhoud IM, Oldenburg B, Wismeijer JA *et al*. IBS-like symptoms in patients with inflammatory bowel disease in remission; relationships with quality of life and coping behavior. *Dig Dis Sci* 2004;49(3):469–474.

48  Rogala L, Miller N, Graff LA *et al*. Population-based controlled study of social support, self-perceived stress, activity and work issues, and access to health care in inflammatory bowel disease. *Inflamm Bowel Dis* 2008;14(4):526–535.

49  Hungin APS, Chang L, Locke GR *et al*. Irritable bowel syndrome in the United States: prevalence, symptom patterns and impact. *Aliment Pharmacol Ther* 2005;21(11):1365–1375.

50  Longobardi T, Jacobs P and Bernstein CN. Work losses related to inflammatory bowel disease in the United States: results from the National Health Interview Survey. *Am J Gastroenterol* 2003;98(5):1064–1072.

51  Simren M, Axelsson J, Gillberg R *et al*. Quality of life in inflammatory bowel disease in remission: the impact of IBS-like symptoms and associated psychological factors. *Am J Gastroenterol* 2002;97(2):389–396.

52  Barratt HS, Kalantzis C, Polymeros D and Forbes A. Functional symptoms in inflammatory bowel disease and their potential influence in misclassification of clinical status. *Aliment Pharmacol Ther* 2005;21(2):141–147.

53  Thompson WG. Gastrointestinal symptoms in the irritable bowel compared with peptic ulcer and inflammatory bowel disease. *Gut* 1984;25(10):1089–1092.

54  Keohane J, O'Mahony C, O'Mahony L *et al*. Irritable bowel syndrome-type symptoms in patients with inflammatory bowel disease: a real association or reflection of occult inflammation? *Am J Gastroenterol* 2010;105(8):1788–1794; quiz 1795.

55  Sanders DS, Carter MJ, Hurlstone DP *et al*. Association of adult coeliac disease with irritable bowel syndrome: a case-control study in patients fulfilling ROME II criteria referred to secondary care. *Lancet* 2001;358(9292):1504–1508.

56  Wahnschaffe U, Ullrich R, Riecken EO and Schulzke JD. Coeliac disease-like abnormalities in a subgroup of patients with irritable bowel syndrome. *Gastroenterology* 2001;121(6):1329–1338.

57  Wahnschaffe U, Schulzke JD, Zeitz M and Ullrich R. Predictors of clinical response to gluten-free diet in patients diagnosed with diarrhea-predominant irritable bowel syndrome. *Clin Gastroenterol Hepatol* 2007;5(7):844–850; quiz 769.

58  O'Leary C, Wieneke P, Buckley S *et al*. Coeliac disease and irritable bowel-type symptoms. *Am J Gastroenterol* 2002;97(6):1463–1467.

59  Tursi A, Brandimarte G and Giorgetti G. High prevalence of small intestinal bacterial overgrowth in coeliac patients with persistence of gastrointestinal symptoms after gluten withdrawal. *Am J Gastroenterol* 2003;98(4):839–843.

60  Verdu EF, Mauro M, Bourgeois J and Armstrong D. Clinical onset of coeliac disease after an episode of Campylobacter jejuni enteritis. *Can J Gastroenterol* 2007;21(7):453–455.

61  Thompson WG, Patel DG, Tao H and Nair RC. Does uncomplicated diverticular disease produce symptoms? *Dig Dis Sci* 1982;27(7):605–608.

62  Jung H, Choung R, Locke III G *et al*. Diarrhea-predominant irritable bowel syndrome is associated with diverticular disease: a population-based study. *Am J Gastroenterol* 2010;105(3):652.

63  Simpson J, Neal K, Scholefield J and Spiller R. Patterns of pain in diverticular disease and the influence of acute diverticulitis. *Eur J Gastroenterol Hepatol* 2003;15(9):1005.

64  Bassotti G, Battaglia E, Spinozzi F *et al*. Twenty-four hour recordings of colonic motility in patients with diverticular disease: evidence for abnormal motility and propulsive activity. *Dis Colon Rectum* 2001;44(12):1814–1820.

65  Clemens CHM, Samsom M, Roelofs J *et al*. Colorectal visceral perception in diverticular disease. *Gut* 2004;53(5):717–722.

66  Trotman IF and Misiewicz JJ. Sigmoid motility in diverticular disease and the irritable bowel syndrome. *Gut* 1988;29(2):218–222.

67  Manning AP, Thompson WG, Heaton KW and Morris AF. Towards positive diagnosis of the irritable bowel. *BMJ* 1978;2(6138):653–654.

68  Dunlop SP, Jenkins D, Neal KR *et al*. Randomized, double-blind, placebo-controlled trial of prednisolone in post-infectious irritable bowel syndrome. *Aliment Pharmacol Ther* 2003;18(1):77–84.

69  Sidhu R, Wilson P, Wright A *et al*. Faecal lactoferrin--a novel test to differentiate between the irritable and inflamed bowel? *Aliment Pharmacol Ther* 2010;31(12): 1365–1370.

70  Schoepfer AM, Trummler M, Seeholzer P *et al*. Discriminating IBD from IBS: comparison of the test performance of fecal markers, blood leukocytes, CRP, and IBD antibodies. *Inflamm Bowel Dis* 2008;14(1):32–39.

71  Langhorst J, Junge A, Rueffer A *et al*. Elevated human beta-defensin-2 levels indicate an activation of the innate immune system in patients with irritable bowel syndrome. *Am J Gastroenterol* 2009;104(2):404–410.

72  Poullis AP, Zar S, Sundaram KK *et al*. A new, highly sensitive assay for C-reactive protein can aid the differentiation of inflammatory bowel disorders from constipation- and diarrhoea-predominant functional bowel disorders. *Eur J Gastroenterol Hepatol* 2002;14(4):409–412.

73  Otten CMT, Kok L, Witteman BJM *et al*. Diagnostic performance of rapid tests for detection of fecal calprotectin and lactoferrin and their ability to discriminate inflammatory from irritable bowel syndrome. *Clin Chem Lab Med* 2008;46(9): 1275–1280.

74  Tibble JA, Sigthorsson G, Foster R *et al*. Use of surrogate markers of inflammation and Rome criteria to distinguish organic from nonorganic intestinal disease. *Gastroenterology* 2002;123(2):450–460.

75  Solem CA, Loftus EV, Tremaine WJ *et al*. Correlation of C-reactive protein with clinical, endoscopic, histologic, and radiographic activity in inflammatory bowel disease. *Inflamm Bowel Dis* 2005;11(8):707–712.

76  Tibble JA, Sigthorsson G, Bridger S *et al*. Surrogate markers of intestinal inflammation are predictive of relapse in patients with inflammatory bowel disease. *Gastroenterology* 2000;119(1):15–22.

77  Walker MM, Murray JA, Ronkainen J *et al*. Detection of coeliac disease and lymphocytic enteropathy by parallel serology and histopathology in a population-based study. *Gastroenterology* 2010;139(1):112–119.

78  Veress B, Franzén L, Bodin L and Borch K. Duodenal intraepithelial lymphocyte-count revisited. *Scand J Gastroenterol* 2004;39(2):138–144.

79  Hayat M, Cairns A, Dixon MF and O'Mahony S. Quantitation of intraepithelial lymphocytes in human duodenum: what is normal? *J Clin Pathol* 2002;55(5): 393–394.

80  Aziz I, Evans KE, Hopper AD *et al*. A prospective study into the aetiology of lymphocytic duodenosis. *Aliment Pharmacol Ther* 2010;32(11–12):1392–1397.

81 Spiller R, Aziz Q, Creed F *et al.* Guidelines on the irritable bowel syndrome: mechanisms and practical management. *Gut* 2007;56(12):1770–1798.

82 Tursi A, Brandimarte G, Giorgetti G *et al.* Low prevalence of antigliadin and anti-endomysium antibodies in subclinical/silent coeliac disease. *Am J Gastroenterol* 2001;96(5):1507–1510.

83 Kurppa K, Lindfors K, Collin P *et al.* Antibodies against deamidated gliadin peptides in early-stage coeliac disease. *J Clin Gastroenterol* 2011;45(8):673–678.

84 Ford AC, Chey WD, Talley NJ *et al.* Yield of diagnostic tests for coeliac disease in individuals with symptoms suggestive of irritable bowel syndrome: systematic review and meta-analysis. *Arch Intern Med* 2009;169(7):651–658.

85 Andrews C, Petcu R, Griffiths T *et al.* Mesalamine alters colonic mucosal proteolytic activity and fecal bacterial profiles in diarrhea-predominant irritable bowel syndrome. *Gastroenterology* 2008;4(suppl 1):A548.

86 Bafutto M, Almeida J, Leite NV and Filho JR. Treatment of diarrhea-predominant irritable bowel syndrome with mesalazine and/or Saccharomyces boulardii. *Gastroenterology* 2008;4(suppl 1):A527.

87 Corinaldesi R, Stanghellini V, Cremon C *et al.* Effect of mesalazine on mucosal immune biomarkers in irritable bowel syndrome: a randomized controlled proof-of-concept study. *Aliment Pharmacol Ther* 2009;30(3):245–252.

88 Di Paolo MC, Merrett MN and Crotty B, Jewell DP. 5-Aminosalicylic acid inhibits the impaired epithelial barrier function induced by gamma interferon. *Gut* 1996;38(1):115–119.

89 Barbara G, Stanghellini V, Cremon C *et al.* Aminosalicylates and other anti-inflammatory compounds for irritable bowel syndrome. *Digestive Diseases* 2009;27(1):115–121.

90 Bolin T. Use of oral sodium cromoglycate in persistent diarrhoea. *Gut* 1980;21(10): 848–850.

91 Lunardi C, Bambara LM, Biasi D *et al.* Double-blind cross-over trial of oral sodium cromoglycate in patients with irritable bowel syndrome due to food intolerance. *Clin Exp Allergy* 1991;21(5):569–572.

92 Stefanini GF, Saggioro A, Alvisi V *et al.* Oral cromolyn sodium in comparison with elimination diet in the irritable bowel syndrome, diarrheic type. Multicenter study of 428 patients. *Scand J Gastroenterol* 1995;30(6):535–541.

93 Stefanini GF, Prati E, Albini MC *et al.* Oral disodium cromoglycate treatment on irritable bowel syndrome: an open study on 101 subjects with diarrheic type. *Am J Gastroenterol* 1992;87(1):55–57.

94 Martinez C, Ramos L, Mosquera J *et al.* Relevant transcriptional changes after long-term mast cell stabilization in the jejunal mucosa of diarrhea-prone irritable bowel syndrome. *Gastroenterology* 2008;4(suppl):A28.

95 Paganelli R, Fagiolo U, Cancian M *et al.* Intestinal permeability in irritable bowel syndrome. *Effect of diet and sodium cromoglycate administration. Ann Allergy* 1990;64(4):377–380.

96 Sander LE, Lorentz A, Sellge G *et al.* Selective expression of histamine receptors H1R, H2R, and H4R, but not H3R, in the human intestinal tract. *Gut* 2006;55(4): 498–504.

97 Watanabe S, Hattori T, Kanazawa M *et al.* Role of histaminergic neurons in hypnotic modulation of brain processing of visceral perception. *Neurogastroenterol Motil* 2007;19(10):831–838.

98 Jakate S, Demeo M, John R *et al.* Mastocytic enterocolitis: increased mucosal mast cells in chronic intractable diarrhea. *Archives of pathology \& laboratory medicine* 2006;130(3):362–367.

99 Quigley EMM and Flourie B. Probiotics and irritable bowel syndrome: a rationale for their use and an assessment of the evidence to date. *Neurogastroenterol Motil* 2007;19(3):166–172.

100 O'Mahony L, McCarthy J, Kelly P *et al.* Lactobacillus and bifidobacterium in irritable bowel syndrome: symptom responses and relationship to cytokine profiles. *Gastroenterology* 2005;128(3):541–551.

101 Verdú EF, Bercík P, Bergonzelli GE *et al.* Lactobacillus paracasei normalizes muscle hypercontractility in a murine model of postinfective gut dysfunction. *Gastroenterology* 2004;127(3):826–837.

102 Thompson DG. IBS – the irritation of inflammation. *Gastroenterology* 2005;129(1): 378–380.

# Multiple Choice Questions

1 Which of the following cells have **not** been reported to be increased in mucosal biopsies taken from IBS patients?
   A Lymphocytes
   B Enteroendocine cells
   C Polymorphonuclear neutrophils

Answer: C

Intra-epithelial lymphocytosis has been observed in mucosal biopsies taken from the duodenum, rectum and colon in IBS subjects. Increased enteroendocrine cell counts have been observed in rectal biopsies from post-Campylobacter infection IBS subjects. Polypmorphonuclear neutrophils are acute inflammatory cells usually associated with active colitis.

2 A 50-year-old patient presents with recurrent episodes of abdominal pain associated with mild diarrhoea since he had his first episode of acute diverticulitis six months ago.
   A Inflammatory markers should be done to exclude recurrent diverticulitis.
   B Patient should be treated empirically with antibiotics.
   C A colonoscopy should be performed.

Answer: A

The pain in this situation could be IBS in co-existing colonic diverticulosis, or the manifestation of a post-inflammatory form of IBS. Therefore, evidence of inflammation should be sought before prescribing antimicrobial or anti-inflammatory therapy. Colonoscopy should be deferred if severe acute diverticulitis is present.

## CHAPTER 10

# Psychological Factors and Treatments in Irritable Bowel Syndrome

*Stephan R. Weinland[1] and Douglas A. Drossman[2]*

[1]UNC Center for Functional GI and Motility Disorders, University of North Carolina at Chapel Hill, Chapel Hill, NC, USA

[2]Drossman Center for Education and Practice of Biopsychosocial Care and Center for Functional GI and Motility Disorders, University of North Carolina at Chapel Hill, Chapel Hill, NC, USA

---

### Key points

- Severity of irritable bowel syndrome (IBS) symptoms is associated with greater frequency of, and interplay between, biopsychosocial factors.
- Familial clustering of IBS symptoms may relate to learned patterns of illness behaviour, clustering of personality types and early-life abuse factors, as much as – or more than – genetics.
- Precipitating factors which help maintain symptoms are increasingly being recognized and used as foci of treatment: in particular, post-infectious symptoms and stress-induced ones.
- Factors that maintain symptom persistence are maladaptive and can include ineffective/incomplete treatment, poor physician–patient relationship and factors related to potential secondary gain.
- Psychological treatment works on prefrontal cortical regions (top-down) while antidepressants mediate their effect through deeper limbic regions (bottom-up). Whilst the latter may be prescribed by physicians acting alone, the former treatments encompass a range of options which need to be chosen based on close working involvement between patient, physician and psychologist.

---

*The greatest mistake in the treatment of diseases is that there are physicians for the body and physicians for the soul, although the two cannot be separated.*

– Plato, 400 BC

Gastroenterologists are keenly aware that psychological factors can affect GI conditions. Patients with functional GI disorders have been identified as having a larger proportion of psychological comorbidities

---

*Irritable Bowel Syndrome: Diagnosis and Clinical Management*, First Edition.
Edited by Anton Emmanuel and Eamonn M.M. Quigley.
© 2013 John Wiley & Sons, Ltd. Published 2013 by John Wiley & Sons, Ltd.

than with other GI conditions [1]. Often, clinicians find the psychosocial contributions and comorbidities in this population to be frustrating, anxiety provoking and difficult to understand and manage  [2]. One possible reason for this response relates to their limited training and level of understanding of how psychological factors affect irritable bowel syndrome (IBS) and how to best manage this condition from a biopsychosocial perspective [3]. This chapter provides a framework to understand psychological factors as they relate to their predisposing, precipitating and perpetuating influences in IBS. We will also discuss the role of psychological interventions that can result in symptom improvement. With greater understanding of the psychosocial aspects of IBS, the clinician becomes increasingly able to personally manage patients with greater satisfaction  [4].

The Rome III criteria for irritable bowel syndrome [5, 6] require symptoms of recurrent abdominal pain or discomfort associated with change in bowel habit. The pain or discomfort must be at least somewhat relieved by bowel movement and its onset associated with a change in the frequency or appearance of stool. This symptom-based definition does not address the rich interplay with psychological factors and the mind/body interaction that contribute to symptom experience and its clinical expression. At its heart, IBS is an increased reactivity of the gut arising from several sources, both central and peripheral. Naliboff has proposed an integrated neurobiological process [7]of peripheral and central vulnerability to precipitating factors. It is this interaction that adds dimensionality to IBS, its severity, degree of disability and the perceptions and behaviours associated with the symptoms. These factors must be properly understood to decide on proper treatment and to affect an optimal treatment response.

## Common problems in psychological treatment of IBS

- Identifying the presence of situational or chronic issues that may be contributing to patient symptoms.
- Addressing psychological concerns in a clinic setting.
- Introducing psychological management of IBS symptoms to patients.
- Locating clinicians who can provide psychological and related services
  - Cognitive Behavioural Therapy
  - Biofeedback
  - Hypnosis
  - Relaxation strategies
  - Interpersonal Psychotherapy

- Assessing patients' progress with psychological therapies and maintaining communication among practitioners.
- Familiarity with psychological treatment strategies and different specializations in psychology.

---

### CASE STUDY 10.1

Ms S, a 32-year-old bank branch employee, developed her first symptoms approximately ten months prior to her visit, though she states she's always had a 'nervous stomach' since childhood. She reports at least two times a week mild to moderate (3–4/10) abdominal pain associated with more frequent looser stools which improve with defecation. She believes Mexican food and other spicy meals caused her symptoms and as a result she has restricted eating out in restaurants. Ms S has been married for eight years and has two children, aged four and seven. In college Ms S had panic attacks and anxiety. She sought treatment from the university counsellor who saw her for one session. She was given no formal psychiatric diagnosis, though her symptoms were severe enough that she dropped out of college after her third year. There was some improvement; however, 10 months ago her abdominal pain and loose stools recurred after getting an acute gastroenteritis that coincided with her stepfather's funeral. Since that time her symptoms have fluctuated in intensity (0–6/10) with some progressive worsening. She was treated with an anticholinergic medication to take when needed and invited to return back in two months for follow up.

---

IBS exists in a range of severities with varying medical and psychological comorbidities and dysfunction. It is understood to be a condition with increased gut reactivity (altered motility and visceral sensation and/or dysregulation of brain–gut function) to stimuli. Therefore, stress and psychosocial issues as well as physiological perturbations, include eating and hormonal changes such as menses or physical activity, can affect symptom experience, although the triggering factors are not always apparent.

The severity of the symptoms influences patient experience and associated cognitions and behaviours including medication taking, the degree of physical activity or social functioning and health care use. In its mildest form, there may be no evident psychological correlates of dysfunction and patients experience only mild gut symptoms on occasion. As severity of symptoms increase, the interplay between biopsychosocial components of the disorder becomes more pronounced.

Those with more severe symptoms differ from those with milder symptoms by having greater psychosocial comorbidities, greater pain, more varied symptoms and greater health care seeking. Ms S, who might be classified as moderate IBS, has had some distress and reduced functioning from symptoms in the past and recently experienced increasing distress in association with an acute gastroenteritis, considered to be post-infectious IBS [8]. Prevalence rates of IBS paired with at least one additional psychiatric diagnosis range from 40 to 90%. Population-based surveys identifying rates of 18–40% with a lifetime psychiatric diagnosis possibility being 10–20% higher than momentary levels [9–11]. In terms of specific psycho-pathology, Lydiard and Falsetti found rates of mood disorders near 60% and rates of panic disorder, social anxiety disorder, PTSD and somatization disorder near 30% [12] in patients with IBS. However, as noted, the prev-alence of psychiatric comorbidities varies with the severity of the condi-tion, whether the individual has sought health care and the nature of the clinical practice, being more prevalent in referral practices [13].

The biopsychosocial model as developed by Engel and adapted for FGID by Drossman (Figure 10.1) emphasizes the integration of biological and psychological factors into the development and maintenance of IBS symp-toms [5].This model provides a foundation from which to examine the predisposing, precipitating and perpetuating psychosocial factors in IBS and how they relate to symptom experiences.

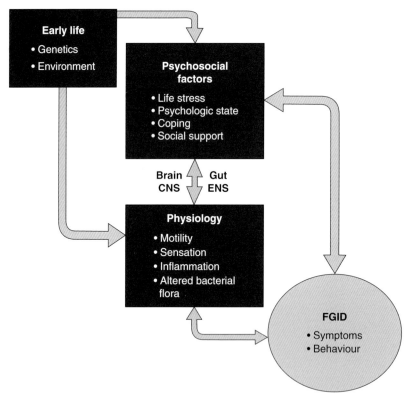

CNS: central nervous system; ENS: enteric nervous system; FGID: functional gastrointestinal disorder.

**Figure 10.1** A biopsychosocial conceptualization of the pathogenesis and clinical expression of irritable bowel syndrome (IBS). It shows the relationships between psychosocial and physiological factors and IBS symptoms.
(Adapted from Drossman[14] with permission from Lippincott Williams & Wilkins.)

# Predisposing psychological factors in IBS

---

### CASE EXAMPLE 10.1 (CONTINUED)

At her second visit, Ms S reports no improvement. She reports sporadically taking the medication prescribed and now communicates frustration with her continued symptoms. Ms S feels hopelessness believing it's just her time to 'have to live with symptoms like her mother and grandmother did'. When inquiring about how she experiences her symptoms, Ms S notes an association that as a child her mother was not employed outside of the home because she was frequently ill with GI symptoms as well. As the visit is drawing to a close she hesitatingly relates a troubled childhood alluding to abuse; you choose not to engage her on these issues at this time because of time constraints and a need to decide on proper follow-up care. However, you express your understanding of the difficulty she experienced and a willingness to discuss it further in the future.

   Because Ms S's issues may be important in treating her condition, you later phone her offering to find someone to explore her thoughts and concerns further. When you make this recommendation, Ms S is reluctant to re-engage with therapy but as an alternative agrees to meet with a psychologist who specializes in behavioural medicine to help her learn strategies to reduce symptom intensity. You agree to make the consultation to the psychologist and follow up again with the patient in two months time.

---

## Parental influence on IBS development in children

Early life events or triggering situations may predispose individuals to develop symptoms of IBS. Parental reinforcement of patterns of illness in children may make children more likely to consistently report painful conditions and focus more on abdominal pain [15–17]. In the study by Walker *et al.* parents of children diagnosed with functional abdominal pain were challenged to either pay attention to, or distract their children from, abdominal pain induced by a water load test. Parents who paid attention to their child's pain report noted that they felt like better parents – however, their children reported higher levels of pain and discomfort. Children whose parents distracted them from the pain induced by the water load test reported experiencing lower levels of pain for shorter periods. These children reported experiencing less discomfort than the attention focused group. Additionally, parents who have been diagnosed with a GI condition are more likely to have children who evidenced significantly more absences from school over a three-month observation period [18]. Thus, greater parental attention to the illness behaviours of their children amplifies these behaviours, and distraction reduces this effect. These early influences may affect illness experience and behaviours in patients later in life [19].

   Here, Ms S notes a family history of GI complaints in both her mother and grandmother. This is notable not just for the influence of biological and genetic predisposing factors but also for the behavioural and learned factors that contribute to how Ms S reacts to her abdominal symptoms. When going to the doctor for nonspecific stomach discomfort is modelled by parents, adult children are more likely to follow behaviourally in their parents footsteps.

## Bodily learning and IBS symptom development

Much like Ms S, patients who experience acute gastroenteritis symptoms in the presence of psychological distress are more likely to develop symptoms of post-infectious irritable bowel syndrome [20]. Here the cooccurrence of an acute infectious episode, most often bacterial, linked to psychological distress likely leads to alteration of mucosal immune functioning, via brain–gut (e.g., hypothalamic pituitary adrenal) pathways which prolong the gastrointestinal symptoms even after the infection is gone [21]. This can also occur in the setting of other types of trauma to the bowel, including surgical procedures. Among a cohort of patients with pelvic surgery evaluated prospectively by Sperber *et al.* [22], psychological factors significantly predicted the onset of abdominal pain relative to gynecological patients not having surgery. Furthermore, IBS developed in three post-surgical patients at 12 months compared to none in the control group. The cooccurrence of physical infection or, in the case of Ms S, significant stressors, along with cognitive enabling factors may increase the probability of abdominal pain developing, thereby facilitating the development of IBS.

Once established, pain pathways that are activated between the gut and the brain form neural connections that become ever stronger with repeated activation. In neuroscience, according to Hebb's dual trace hypothesis, neurons that are activated together repeatedly and persistently change the efficiency with which they activate. Learning in pain sensation, just as in voluntary motor learning, takes place at a neuronal level [23]. When Ms S discussed vague ideation relating to childhood abuse and the concurrence of GI distress with an acute emotional experience, one can suspect that brain–gut linkages exist. Over the course of repeated experiences with GI symptoms and cognition around those symptoms, less and less activation is required for a dysfunctional symptom pattern to develop. The threshold for IBS symptom activation therefore becomes ever more decreased, concurrent with the amount of abdominal trauma the patient presents with, as well as with the length of time experiencing IBS symptoms. From a neurophysiological perspective we have found that a history of abuse leads to increased activation of the anterior mid-cingulate cortex after rectal distension; this correlates with increased abdominal pain reporting [24].

## Abuse and IBS symptom development

Our understanding of the relationship of abuse history with medical disorders has evolved from being seen as causing psychiatric difficulties, to having multiple effects on symptoms experience, patient illness behaviours and clinical outcomes [25]. The prevalence of abuse history increases among those who have more severe symptoms and who are seen in referral settings [26]. Within gastroenterology, where a great deal of the investigation has been done, comorbid abuse history has overarching effects on all disorders, leading to more severe pain, hospitalizations and even surgeries regardless of diagnosis. More severe abuse seems to occur in patients with IBS and other functional GI diagnoses than for other GI disorders [14]. The pathophysiological features to explain this association relate to stress mediated brain–gut dysfunction and can range from altered stress induced mucosal immune function to impaired CNS ability to down regulate incoming visceral or somatic afferent signals [27]. The increased pain and GI symptoms then lead to increased pain and other GI symptoms, which in turn lead to greater health care seeking. More recently, brain imaging studies have shown that in response to rectal distension (thereby mimicking GI symptoms in IBS) there is an associated activation of the anterior cingulate cortex. Furthermore, patients who have an abuse history have a greater pain response to rectal distension that correlates with increased activation of the cingulate cortex, thus providing a putative pathophysiological mechanism [24, 28]. Also, there is growing evidence that centrally targeted interventions like antidepressants and psychotherapy may have palliative effects on reducing symptoms, altering brain–gut dysregulation and structures and improving the clinical outcome [29].

## Personality and acute psychopathology

Personality components that predispose patients to IBS are trait characteristics that may contribute to the development and enhanced perception of IBS symptoms. Trait characteristics are understood to be habitual patters of thoughts, behaviours and emotions that individuals maintain and are often resistant to change. Trait characteristics are contrasted with state characteristics which are often situationally determined attributes that are directly influenced by cognitions and bodily reactions. Acute psychosocial distress is believed to represent the more state dependent characteristics of the individual. Certain state and trait features of patients with IBS have been observed in patients. For example, Koloski *et al.* [30] conducted a population-based study looking for predictors of IBS in a sample of 361 subjects who reported new onset abdominal pain for greater than one month. Subjects were contacted every four months for one year. A control population of 120 patients without abdominal pain was also followed. At each contact point subjects were assessed for the presence of GI symptoms, psychological variables and healthcare seeking behaviours. Several psychological factors measured at baseline were predictors of IBS. Specifically, trait neuroticism, somatic fear, anxiety and persistence of GI symptoms were significant predictors of a new diagnosis of irritable bowel syndrome sometime during the twelve month observation period.

Nicholl *et al.* have identified that psychosocial risk factors can increase the percentage of new cases of IBS onset in an increasing number correlating with the number of factors [31]. In a 15-month prospective study of primary care subjects aged 25–65, 3.5% of all subjects (n=86) developed IBS. The presence of two or more of the following factors: HADS anxiety, sleep disturbance, illness behaviour and somatic symptoms, increased the odds ratio of having IBS symptom onset from 2.59 to 6.33. With patients evidencing all four factors being six times more likely to experience IBS symptom onset than patients experiencing zero or one factor. Ms S's past history of GI symptoms, past history of anxiety pathology and trauma all likely contributed to establishing the basis for her symptom development.

This relationship between state and trait psychological factors in IBS requires further study, as correlation with IBS symptoms may not indicate causation. IBS symptom experience can in and of itself lead to the development of acute psychosocial distress and may also resemble psychopathological states and traits in patients.

## Precipitating psychological variables associated with IBS symptom onset

---

**CASE EXAMPLE 10.1 (CONTINUED)**

In meeting with the psychologist the following week, Ms S provides additional information relating to her symptom onset and experience. As previously noted with the gastroenterologist, the patient's symptoms began acting up ten months prior to her clinical visit. At that time Ms S developed acute gastroenteritis while on a multiday car trip to her stepfather's funeral. The gastroenteritis was believed to be food-borne in nature and resulted in fever, vomiting and significant diarrhoea that prevented Ms S from attending the actual funeral ceremony or leaving her hotel room. Later psychotherapy sessions provided the opportunity for Ms S to elaborate further on the abuse history. When she was five years old her mother and father separated and she lived with her mother. Her mother eventually remarried to another man that Ms S never liked. Over the ensuing sessions Ms S tearfully recounted and worked through her feelings relating to a three-year history of sexual abuse at the hands of her stepfather.

---

The precipitating events for this symptom flare for Ms S is most likely the combination of acute gastroenteritis mixed with the extreme stressor of having to travel to a funeral for a relative that Ms S has significantly conflicted feelings about. In fact, the stress of the experience may have increased her susceptibility to getting an enteric infection [32]. This combination of a psychological distressing situation mixed with increased physiologic vulnerability leading to infection is seen in about 25% of patients with IBS at the time of symptom onset. Indeed, for veterans the stresses of deployment to a war zone usually in association with a gastroenteritis can precipitate symptom onset [33, 34]. This observation led to the Institute of Medicine report on the Gulf War and Health in 2010 to conclude a probable association of deployment in a war zone to the development of IBS and other functional GI disorders [35]. Subsequently, the US Veterans Administration issued a directive that allowed veterans who develop IBS during or after deployment to be eligible for disability benefits. It should be noted also that predisposing factors, as discussed, increase vulnerability to developing IBS, which is often related to a precipitating event that is uniquely stressing for the individual, possibly related to the predisposing event, which together lead to the clinical expression of the IBS or its exacerbation. As with Ms S., attending the stepfather's funeral along with the background history of the abuse experience with him precipitated the clinical exacerbation.

Acute research stressors have been shown by Dickhaus *et al.* to play a role in modulation of visceral pain sensation and emotional activation in IBS. Stronger emotional responses were observed in IBS patients during research stressors when compared to controls. IBS patients demonstrated significantly increased unpleasantness ratings as well as significant correlations between anxiety, anger and stress with levels of rectal distension during a stressor. Correlations between rectal distension ratings and emotional responses to stresses were not observed in control subjects. Stresses in these studies appeared to increase visceral pain sensitivity and emotional activation acutely in patients diagnosed with IBS-D [36, 37]. Similar findings were echoed by Murray *et al.* in working with patients with IBS-C who also demonstrated heightened visceral sensation when compared to controls in response to acute physical and psychological stressors [38].

As discussed earlier in this chapter, neuronal pathways once established become learned and 'hard wired' within the body over time and with repeated activation. Acute stresses and their effects can, therefore, often become chronic stressors that change the emotional valence associated with that stressor over time. These chronic stressors then may manifest into chronic changes in visceral sensitivity, contributing to IBS symptom experiences that perpetuate. It becomes important in treatment, therefore, to help patients see how what may now be perceived as 'routine' stressors can effect IBS symptom experiences that may have developed during previous periods of acute stress .

Patients with more severe predisposing factors may require less severe precipitating events or may have more frequent precipitating stressors that contribute to flare up of symptoms [37]. Additionally, patients who have had symptoms for longer periods are more likely to experience symptoms at lower thresholds of precipitating stressors. Therefore, any experiences that up regulate other systems in the body (exercise, relationship distress, workplace distress) can also precipitate the onset of an IBS episode.

## Perpetuating psychological factors

Once the disorder is established, clinical (recovery from an infection) or psychosocial adaptations (coping mechanisms) can lead to recovery. However, there may be other, perpetuating factors that tend to maintain the illness state.

---

### CASE EXAMPLE 10.1 (CONTINUED)

Ms S works with her psychologist to direct the focus of the therapeutic relationship on working to manage daily symptoms. In the process of this collaborative effort Ms S acknowledges depressive symptoms which may be impairing her ability to function. Accordingly, the psychologist discusses with the gastroenterologist the possibility of prescribing an antidepressant, which is done. The psychologist continues to teach Ms S relaxation strategies and asks her to track her symptoms between sessions. This tracking shows a pattern of increased symptoms on the weekend that needs to be further understood. The psychologist also uses motivational interviewing strategies to help the patient better understand how her symptoms are affecting her behaviourally and psychosocially. In doing so, the psychologist is also examining the role of positive aspects of symptom experience such as primary or secondary gain that may contribute to the maintenance of symptoms.

After four sessions, Ms S notes some clinical improvement. The focus of the sessions then shifts from addressing current symptom experience to providing cognitive tools to change the way Ms S views and manages situations that exacerbate her symptoms. In this way, the session process moves from symptom monitoring and nonspecific relaxation methods toward a more active process of cognitive behavioural therapy. By using her symptom log as a way to access cognitions, Ms S becomes aware of inaccurate ways of thinking that may perpetuate her symptom experience, and she then learns of new ways that increase more accurate and adaptive cognitive methods that can improve them. She returns to the gastroenterologist's follow-up appointment noting significant improvement in all of her symptoms. Depressive features are no longer present, she finds that she is better able to manage with her sense of anxiety and she is not experiencing as many episodes of IBS as she was previously.

---

At this point we are seeing the benefit of a combined treatment strategy that synergistically enhances clinical recovery. This is done pharmacologically by treating the depression and raising symptom threshold, and psychologically by reducing stress enhancing bodily effects via relaxation methods and increasing cognitive strategies to regain self-confidence and reinterpretation of the symptoms as less threatening. From a neurophysiological standpoint the psychological treatment works on prefrontal cortical regions (top-down) while the antidepressants work on deeper limbic regions (bottom-up) [27, 39].

Patients who have had symptoms for a prolonged period learn ways of accommodating the symptom experience cognitively and behaviourally into their lives. This can be adaptive or maladaptive. Factors that perpetuate symptom experience in IBS are considered maladaptive and can include ineffective/incomplete treatment, poor physician patient relationship and factors related to potential secondary gain.

Perpetuating psychological factors can sometimes be effortful thought based factors relating to obtaining disability compensation while staying out of work, receiving more help around the home or obtaining narcotic pain medication. Identifying these factors in therapy can be difficult, as patients are aware of these benefits and will guard against removal of them without adequate replacement. It becomes the therapist's task to teach a different skill set for approaching or dealing with this type of benefit removal. Ms S noted to her psychologist that her symptoms were worse on the weekends. When examined in session she noted that her symptom experience was at its worst on Sunday evenings before she started another work week. Understanding the role that job stress was playing in her symptoms allowed Ms S take steps to compensate for it by scheduling distracting or pleasurable activities during that time and look for how she could learn problem solving skills to help her affect change at work to make it a place she felt less anxious about.

Even more difficult and outside of the scope of this chapter is dealing with perpetuating factors that are unconscious or noneffortful motivations. Patients who are motivated by attention and appreciation they may feel during their illness are not necessarily aware of the benefit to their sense of self that they are receiving. In therapy, the task becomes exploring these benefits called 'secondary gain' in a nonconfrontational fashion. With Ms S one issue was addressed later in therapy. She did not consciously deal with the negative thoughts resulting from the abuse experience toward her stepfather. However, with his death these feelings and thoughts became more effortful and were difficult to tolerate. The onset of symptoms occurring at the time of the funeral could adaptively 'mask' these feelings and, at the same time, through suffering from the symptoms, expiate the sense of guilt and mental anguish that occurred [40].

## Perpetuating cognitive factors

Ms S worked with the psychologist to look at cognitions that were contributing to increased autonomic arousal during the CBT portion of her therapy. The cognitive model proposed by Beck hypothesizes that all human emotions and behaviours have cognitive precursors that are either cognitively effortful or noneffortful. As maladaptive cognitions occur repeatedly they move from being effortful to noneffortful, that is 'automatic' cognitions or thoughts. Automatic thoughts relating to the symptoms of IBS manifest themselves in behaviours and emotions and can adversely affect symptom experience.

One form of automatic thought is catastrophization, a maladaptive coping strategy. Patients have the belief that by planning or focusing on the possible negative outcomes they will be more prepared for them and better able to cope with their symptoms. While a certain amount of planning around symptom experience is useful, coping by focusing on negative catastrophization actually can lead to poorer health outcomes [41]. Examples of catastrophizing thoughts are 'It's terrible and I feel it will never get better', 'I worry all the time whether it will end'. Focusing on these areas during the course of daily symptom experience does not allow patients to recognize situations and times when they do have improved control over symptom experience and when they have been able to decrease their symptom experience. Cognitive factors play a pivotal role in the experience of IBS symptoms [42].

## Psychological and behavioural treatments for IBS

To address predisposing, precipitating and perpetuating factors in IBS, a number of psychological and behavioural treatment strategies can be implemented by trained clinicians. This section introduces some of the treatments used in the care of patients with IBS and other functional GI disorders (Table 10.1)

### Cognitive behavioural therapy (CBT)

CBT comprises a form of interpersonal psychotherapy that focuses on the accuracy of cognitions and core beliefs that drive patient behaviour and emotion. Developed by Aaron Beck initially for treatment of anxiety disorders and depression, it has become a staple in psychological treatments because of its effectiveness in helping people feel better. Traditional CBT follows a rigid schedule in each session with time allotted for patients to discuss homework and to practice skills of examining cognitions in session. Typically, however, clinicians do not follow the strict CBT model and are more likely to practice a variant that uses from 8 to 10 sessions to help patients examine cognitions as they relate to both symptom and wellness experiences.

CBT focuses on identifying unhelpful or nonaccurate cognitions. Patients are asked to examine their evidence for thinking a certain way. Cognitive distortions of all or none thinking, catastrophizing and so on are challenged in session. Patients are asked to examine 'What is your evidence?' for thinking a certain way, 'What else could be going on', 'What if the thought you have isn't true' and 'What if the worst thing that could happen does happen'. Through use of appropriate Socratic questioning techniques and engagement in therapy, patients are taught to persist in finding answers to

**Table 10.1** Psychological and behavioural treatments for IBS and other FGIDs.

| Psychological Method | Explanation |
| --- | --- |
| Cognitive behavioural therapy (CBT) | Therapist and patient work together to examine accuracy of cognitions as they relate to symptom experience. Strategies for challenging dysfunctional thinking patterns and styles are taught and practiced in structured fashion. |
| Trauma-focused interpersonal psychotherapy (prolonged exposure & eye movement desensitization and reprocessing – EMDR) | Prolonged exposure (PE) – Patient learns centring strategies and relaxation and is then guided in real or imagined exposure to traumatic memories. EMDR combines aspects of prolonged exposure with physical activity reminders to maintain a present focus (eye movement instructions, tapping etc.) |
| Hypnosis | Patient and therapist engage in hypnotic induction exercise followed by combination of suggestions that alter perception of symptoms and instructions for better management of symptoms. |
| Relaxation therapies (diaphragmatic breathing (DB), progressive muscle relaxation (PMR)) | Increasing parasympathetic activity and relaxation by instructing patients on slowing breathing (DB). PMR highlights the difference between tense and relaxed muscles and teaches patients to identify either state and engage in muscle relaxation. |
| Generalized biofeedback | Helps patients learn relaxation strategies by highlighting tension/relaxation via visual or auditory feedback mechanisms (EMG, GSR, breathing rate or heart rate variability) |
| Mindfulness-based meditation | Therapist-guided focus on cognitions and approaching oneself and one's symptom experience from a nonjudgmental perspective. Reduces anxiety and autonomic activation by focusing on the present moment. |
| Motivational interviewing | Therapy focusing on patient behaviours that may be contributing to unhealthy status. Traditionally applied in substance abuse counselling formats but finding increasing effectiveness in improving adherence to biomedical treatment of chronic conditions. |

all of these questions in an effort to think accurately about each possible situation to its logical conclusion. Once the goal of thinking accurately about situations is achieved, it is hypothesized that the patient's bodily and emotional symptoms will also reflect this accurate way of thinking. Traditional CBT has been shown to be an effective treatment in IBS [43–45].

More recently, Lackner *et al.* [46, 47] have developed a more succinct four-session CBT-based intervention that has been shown to be effective and improve on treatment gains seen in longer forms of CBT. This minimal contact CBT allows patients to monitor and challenge symptom experience on their own and within their home environment. This may help patients rely on their own skill development rather than those of a therapist.

Also engaging in therapy in the home may help people make changes to that environment more easily and view themselves as more effective in managing their symptoms and experiences on their own.

### Trauma-focused interpersonal psychotherapy

Given the high prevalence of experienced trauma and the relationship between trauma and symptoms in IBS, therapy to address this area is an important component of treatment as well [48]. Trauma therapy practice requires appropriate training and is not an area of focus for this chapter. If handled incorrectly a significant risk of re-traumatizing patients is possible. This does not mean that talking about trauma itself is off limits in clinical interactions, rather that it needs to be a conscious choice to discuss past trauma in a safe environment and with patients being fully prepared to process that history.

Exposure-based treatments and eye movement desensitization and reprocessing (EMDR) therapies have been shown to be effective in teaching patients new ways to think about their experiences and to process them with an increased sense of personal control [49]. As with all psychotherapies, a good relationship with the practitioner is critically important in establishing trust enough to activate highly emotional memories and felt experiences.

### Relaxation-based therapies – resetting the body's overall level of activation

The relaxation response characterized by Benson in 1975 [50] has been applied to a variety of fields in medicine with generally positive findings. As IBS is characterized by hyperactivity and reactivity in the enteric nervous system, decreasing activation of the entire autonomic nervous system can therefore have a calming effect on the gut as well. Relaxation techniques have the effect of slowing down bodily processes in general. In a small study, Blanchard *et al.* looked at the effects of relaxation training in patients with IBS with positive findings [51]. Practitioners often instruct patients that we can learn to develop control over many body physiological processes over time but relaxation encouraged through breathing exercises is the most direct way to access relaxation.

### Breathing exercises – diaphragmatic breathing

In this exercise patients are instructed to place one hand on their upper chest and one hand on their abdomen. They are then instructed to breathe slowly and deeply at their own pace while observing which of their hands is moving the most. Patients are instructed that the hand on their abdomen should move more than the hand on their chest indicating a more diaphragmatic breathing pattern rather than a shallower breathing pattern.

Therapists will usually demonstrate the breathing pattern first and may exaggerate the abdominal motions to show patients a relaxed breathing pattern. By slowing the breathing down, patients slow down heart rate and a number of other physiological processes as well. The hypothesis that is communicated to the patient is that this slowing of bodily functioning will affect gut functioning as well [52, 53].

Other breathing exercises include guiding a patient while slowly counting to a pre-designated number on the inbreath and outbreath. Breathing in through the mouth and out through the nose or using fingers to alternate between breathing in and out from different nostrils. All of these exercises have the effect of slowing breathing down but also have the effect of forcing people to be mindful of their breathing and of purposefully slowing down.

## Progressive muscle relaxation

Sometimes patients become insensitive to or unaware of the tension in their bodies. Progressive muscle relaxation (PMR) exercises help patients understand and reset this level of bodily tension. PMR is a guided exercise in which the therapist will walk a patient through each of their general muscle groups from their feet to their head in order [54]. At each major muscle group, patients are instructed to tense as tight as possible, hold the tension for a few seconds, then release the tension all at once and notice the difference between feeling fully tensed and fully relaxed in that muscle group. As with all relaxation exercises, over time and with repeated practice the patient will become better at being aware of tension and its effects on the body and how they can release that tension [51]. Treatments using relaxation techniques have shown sustained positive effects on patients with irritable bowel syndrome though further study is needed [55–58].

## Hypnosis

Gut-focused hypnotherapy is particularly effective for reducing symptoms of IBS. Whorwell *et al.* have shown improvement rates between 40 and 100% of patients using a course of gut-focused hypnotherapy [59]. In his study, patients over 50 years of age, who had IBS symptoms, experienced the lowest level of improvement; however, 100% of patients under age 50 evidenced at least 50% improvement in symptoms. What is most impressive about this study is that symptom benefit was seen as significantly improved even at 18 months post treatment.

Due to difficulty in locating hypnotherapy practitioners as well as difficulties with standardizing research on the topic, Pallson *et al.* have developed a manual gut-focused hypnotherapy treatment consisting of eight gut-focused hypnotherapy sessions [60, 61]. The treatment has been shown to be effective in reducing symptoms and has even been converted to audio recorded format for use in self-hypnosis practice in the home.

At its core, hypnosis is very focused attention paired with a state of intense relaxation that allows the therapist to address cognitive issues and circumvent typical patient defensive reactions. The hypnosis practitioner uses the patient's suggestible state to practice relaxation and examine cognitions that may contribute to symptom experience. Visualization is also often used to provide metaphors that patients can use to change the way they think about their symptom experience. Multiple components of hypnotherapy address multiple possible methods of action in symptom improvement. Indeed, hypnotherapy may be the most efficient form of psychotherapy for evidencing symptom improvement, as it addresses many of the other components of CBT and relaxation therapy strategies.

Finding an appropriate hypnotherapist can be difficult. Obtaining credentials in medical hypnotherapy takes between one and three years and involves supervised hypnotherapy practice. Working with a accrediting body such as the American Society for Clinical Hypnosis to find a practitioner in your area is particularly advisable. Look for hypnotherapy providers that have additional credentials or licenses as psychologists or psychotherapists in addition to a hypnosis credential.

## Generalized biofeedback

Generalized biofeedback is a treatment modality where patients learn to bring autonomic arousal activity under conscious control. It is in contrast to anorectal biofeedback, which is a common treatment for outlet dysfunction. Generalized biofeedback involves the use of a series of sensors (commonly respiration, galvanic skin response, muscle tension, skin temperature and heart rate) which then present information back to the patient on a computer screen about the status of all of these measures of bodily function. Patients then work with a biofeedback practitioner to practice making changes that affect these autonomic variables. Commonly, changes in breathing that affect heart rate and all of the other variables are suggested. Additionally, exercises relating to progressive muscle relaxation can also be implemented to show patients how they can affect change in their bodies [62–64].

Once again, finding a practitioner who uses biofeedback for functional GI concerns may be difficult. However, the Biofeedback Certification Institute of America offers a list of qualified and licensed providers across the country that are able to work with patients with a variety of medical illnesses.

## Mindfulness-based stress reduction

Mindfulness-based stress reduction (MBSR) is a structured therapy programme that teaches patients ways of devoting intentional focus on present-moment experiences and nonjudgmental awareness of body sensations and emotions. This skill is particularly useful in teaching patients ways of decreasing autonomic arousal. First developed by Jon Kabat-Zinn

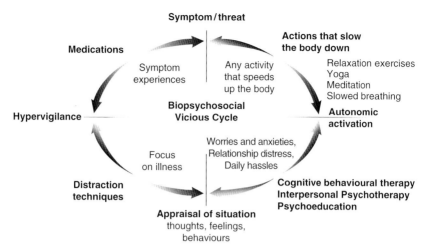

**Figure 10.2** A cycle of patient IBS symptom experience in which symptom experience alters physiologic arousal, moods and cognitions and situation appraisals that can then lead to hypervigilance. Once patients become hypervigilant about their symptom experience, those fears can lead to symptom onset or exacerbation via autonomic activation.

in 1979, it is now used in more than 250 hospitals across the United States and has been shown to have beneficial effects in treatment of cardiac disease, fibromyalgia and depression [65].

When compared against an attention control condition in an eight-week study, Gaylord *et al.* found that a mindfulness-based stress reduction training programme significantly improved IBS symptom severity and quality of life at three-month follow up [66]. Interestingly, results seemed to improve over time, indicating that participants may have learned a new skill set that allowed them to improve their symptoms experience in their home environment, similar to that Lackner *et al.* found in the CBT treatment study.

A good understanding of predisposing, precipitating and perpetuating factors in IBS combined with a basic understanding of psychological treatments can help the clinician communicate with patients about their IBS effectively. The next step involves understanding the integration of those factors into a unifying treatment strategy. The Biopsychosocial Vicious Cycle (Figure 10.2) provides an excellent graphic for communicating a shared understanding between the treating clinician and patient with IBS. It visually identifies how and why symptoms are perpetuated and what patients can do to engage in more effective symptom management strategies. Patients are introduced to the graphic by highlighting the relationships between symptom experiences in each of four quadrants. This is followed by an explanation of the steps that can ameliorate IBS symptom experience on the outside of each quadrant [67]. Each of the four quadrants can be described using the case example of Ms S.

### Symptom/threat to arousal quadrant

Recall that Ms S readily acknowledged that she felt threatened by her GI symptoms and wanted them to go away. She understood that her body interprets symptoms as triggering events that result in feelings of arousal. This activation can occur on an unconscious or noneffortful level of thought. It is outlined to patients that the body reacts to these symptoms with autonomic arousal and activation. Heart rate may speed up, blood pressure may rise, galvanic skin response may increase and respiration rate may increase. As the GI tract is connected to all of these systems, increases in gut activation are likely also occurring. This may happen imperceptibly to Ms S due to what has happened in the past through predisposing or precipitating factors. The frequency with which symptoms occur or recur cause the activated pathways to become 'learned'. This autonomic arousal was discussed with Ms S as being the body's way of being 'keyed up to act' and is understood by the lay person as being part of the fight or flight stress response.

Addressing issues in this quadrant with Ms S occurred by finding and implementing ways of interrupting the body's process of automatic autonomic activation and finding ways of slowing the body's reaction to threat of symptoms. Ms S learned steps she can take to purposefully and thoughtfully slow her body down. Relaxation exercises, breathing exercises, yoga, meditation, calming activities such as taking a hot bath or shower, or practicing an imagery exercise are all effective strategies that can decrease autonomic arousal. Many times a clinician will be the first to suggest such strategies. In doing so, it is critical to discuss the importance of home exercises with these strategies and to provide means of recording home exercise. If patients do not practice decreasing autonomic arousal, many of the later steps required for improvement in symptom experience will also not be effective.

### Autonomic activation to appraisal of situation quadrant

Once the autonomic nervous system was activated it shaped the way Ms S interpreted situations and events. Indeed, it directly affected her mood and cognitions relating to problem solving and catastrophization. Patients are familiar with this state of being when the clinician points out that irritable mood is a common cooccurrence with pain onset and autonomic activation. Ms S noted that she often would not make the best decisions for herself when she was experiencing symptoms. Symptom experience can also provide a lens through which patients look towards future experiences. With Ms S, the fact that symptoms occurred at a distressingly inconvenient time coloured her perception of when her symptoms may occur in the future. This directly affected her sense of self-efficacy and contributed to depressive cognitions activated during the course of her illness experience.

Addressing this quadrant is done through engaging Ms S in cognitive behavioural therapy and interpersonal psychotherapy. The goal of these treatments is not to impute a false positive outlook or to cancel out negative thought processes. Rather, the goal of interventions in this quadrant is to take steps that help patients see situations and symptom experiences accurately. Ms S engaged in this quadrant by keeping symptom diaries and noting precursors and subsequent effects of symptom experiences. Maintaining an accurate view of symptoms and experiences makes it more likely that the bodily reactions to these emotions and situations will also be accurate. For example, with Ms S the therapist was able to identify thought distortions of 'all or nothing' thinking – 'My symptoms are either great or they are horrible', Overgeneralization – 'I'm never able to do anything I enjoy'. These cognitions were challenged in session and Ms S was able to identify a more accurate view of her symptom experience that helped her emotional and bodily reactions become more accurate as well.

## Appraisal of situation – development of hypervigilance quadrant

Once Ms S was fully engaged in her symptom experience she became hypervigilant to situations that resulted in symptom activation. Hypervigilance is a general state of heightened awareness that often accompanies autonomic arousal and activation. Ms S began limiting her exposure to novel situations and environments. She ventured out only to places and things that she was ultimately familiar with and reported always wanting to be close to a familiar bathroom. Hypervigilance often expands to eating behaviours that relate to superstitious beliefs based on unrelated pairings of food experiences to symptom experience. For example Ms S believed that eating at a Mexican restaurant caused her food-borne gastroenteritis; she then developed a belief that she had sensitivity to all Mexican food and would no longer eat at any Mexican restaurants.

To address this quadrant in the diagram, Ms S was instructed on effective ways of engaging in distraction. Did she have any activities that she engaged in during which she experienced what appeared to be a loss of time? An example of driving home on a long car ride or reading a pleasurable book are often listed as times when people may lose track of time. Patient-offered experiences of this mental state are an excellent place to start looking for behaviours that can interrupt symptom experiences. Ms S noted that she enjoyed watching black and white movies and that she regularly engaged in this activity in an effort to manage with her symptoms. Finding distracting activities and determining how to engage in more of them became a goal in her therapy. Event-scheduling strategies to ensure time for adequate self-care and engagement in distraction activities she could lose herself in were discussed. Ms S reported good benefit from this type of behavioural activation.

### Development of hypervigilance – symptom onset quadrant

The last quadrant focuses on the probability that hypervigilance to symptom experience as well as attentional precursors to symptom experience can themselves bring about symptoms. This occurs when patients interpret belly pain as symptom onset rather than hunger; this can cause autonomic arousal that further perpetuates symptom experiences. Teaching patients to be mindful of their own symptom experiences and their relation to normal bodily function or nonpathological patterns is an important step in managing symptom onset and propagation. As an example, Ms S had a tendency to report any abdominal discomfort as a need to have a bowel movement.

To address this quadrant Ms S was instructed about the role of treating visceral hypersensitivity and central sensitization in the treatment of IBS. She was educated about ways that taking psychotropic medication can reduce the body's sensitivity to threatening stimuli from internal and external cues. Additionally, Ms S was instructed on the role of mindfully observing bodily processes in an attempt to become aware of the fact that while her symptom experience is triggered by a variety of causes, not all situations will result in the development of symptoms. Simply becoming aware of times that she was not experiencing symptoms had a direct measurable improvement on Ms S's quality of life.

## Finding and working with a psychologist

The use of psychologists and mental health professionals as a part of GI practice is not common but is clearly needed. While psychological therapies have evidenced some of the most effective treatments for IBS, they are often done out of the context of the clinical setting and this can affect the patient's motivation for treatment. This can be obviated by integrating the psychologist into the clinical practice, although factors including poor reimbursement and lack of training have made this approach more challenging.

Despite limitations, involving a clinical psychologist in patient care can be a particularly effective addition to any practice. Ford *et al.* [68] showed the numbers needed to treat (NNT) with psychological interventions for IBS ranged from 2 to 3.5. The NNT is the number of patients one would need to treat in order to show a 50% improvement in symptoms in one person. This compares with an NNT of 11.3 for a common gut-focused antibiotic treatment [69]. Moreover, other benefits of psychological treatments are that patients continue to do well for extended periods after the treatment has stopped, there are no known side effects, treatments amplify medical treatments and may be cost effective.

Clinical psychology is a state-regulated profession and psychologists belong to corresponding state psychological associations. Many psychological associations and state licensure boards offer searchable databases of practitioners on their websites (a complete list of websites can be found at www.apa.org). A search of one of these databases will be a good place to start looking to find a psychologist or other mental health professional with experience in behavioural medicine or health psychology. Practitioners who have this type of training will be familiar with all of the concepts necessary to effect change and treat patients with IBS. Intermediate level clinicians in counselling or with masters' level training may also be effective at teaching specific relaxation strategies or engaging in mindfulness exercises; however, they may not have the familiarity with medical conditions and may be more wary to work with IBS patients given a lack of understanding of the functional nature of symptom experience.

## Selection of psychological treatment

Appropriate treatment selection by a psychologist depends on the initial assessment and interactions between the patient and clinician. It is a collaborative effort between psychologist, patient and treating clinicians to develop the best treatment plan. During an initial assessment, the psychologist will assess for habits and patterns that maintain symptom experience, look for factors that initiate symptoms and gauge patients levels and abilities to engage in behaviours that are conducive to symptom reduction. Common issues to screen for in this population are a history of trauma or abuse, loss or other severe stressors, current or past substance use and treatment, current adaptations to symptom experiences and costs/benefits of symptom experiences over time. Other factors, such as bodily awareness in the patient and ability to engage outside resources (friends, relatives, work), are also assessed for during the initial visit.

A second area of focus in the initial assessment session is a significant component of psychoeducation. Many patients will not have a familiarity with basic concepts of mind/body integration or ways in which sleep, diet or activity levels can affect symptom experiences. Additionally, just developing a basic understanding of what is/is not related to IBS symptoms can be helpful. Patients may not have been afforded the opportunity to even consider the role of stress or lack of sleep in their lives before the initial session with the psychologist. Allowing time for basic education can go a long way in allaying patient concerns about their symptom experience and may help them feel more able to manage their IBS symptoms.

After the initial assessment, the psychologist will then engage the patient in therapy sessions depending on which area would evidence the greatest effect on symptom improvement. For example, highly anxious patients may benefit from learning how to slow their bodies down and become more in tune with the level of stress and tension they carry at any given point in time. Patients who have difficulty learning to relax may benefit from generalized biofeedback in order to solidify an understanding of how to actively work on decreasing stress and tension. Behavioural activation strategies may be tried with patients who have a more depressive picture presentation.

Once the patient has developed skills for maintaining control of anxious or nervous responses, the therapeutic relationship may move into a phase of examining thoughts and emotional dynamics that are contributing to symptom experiences and maintaining factors. Patients who are able to link their thoughts and feelings to experiences and events may be more responsive to active treatments such as cognitive or interpersonal therapy. It is only in this phase of treatment that patients would begin to focus on aspects of past trauma, as the relationship between clinician and patient is believed to be solid enough and the patient has developed skills of managing with their own reactions in a nonharmful way.

The number of sessions required to evidence benefit in patients will vary depending on the severity and complexity of the symptom experience. A significant proportion of patients may benefit from a single session intervention where they are instructed on the mind/body relationship and what the relationship to symptom experience is. Other patients will be able to develop new skill sets over one to three sessions and evidence significant symptom improvement. Finally, a smaller proportion of patients, usually those with significant personality disorder components or complex abuse histories, may require significantly longer in therapy to make appreciable gains. The strongest predictor of who will benefit from psychotherapy is the relationship with the treatment provider [70].

## Ways to introduce topics related to psychology in IBS with patients

### Introducing psychotherapy services
'Often patients report that they experience difficulties in managing with their symptom experiences or situations around their symptom experiences. Sometimes talking with somebody who has a good understanding of management strategies with IBS can be effective. To be clear, your IBS symptoms are not indicative of psychopathology, but talking with a psychologist may help you manage them more effectively'.

### Taking psychopharmacologic agents
'Many medicines are used for more than one purpose. For instance, aspirin is commonly given out for headache as well as for heart attacks. We all have

nerves that run throughout our body, not just in our brain. Antidepressants work on nerves in your gut, not necessarily just in your brain'.

## Imaging studies for IBS

'There are many conditions for which imaging studies are not necessarily helpful. For instance, migraine headaches do not show up on X-rays because they reside in the soft tissues of the body. IBS symptom experiences are similar in that they do not show up on X-ray. However, we know that your symptoms are real and that they are affecting you'.

## Quick changes in symptom experience

'Do you know how to ride a bicycle? How long did it take you to learn? Isn't it amazing that something you learned so long ago, for such a brief time, is still something you can do today? Your body has learned how to experience IBS symptoms in a similar fashion. Your gut and your brain have incorporated them into your body. Just as you cannot really 'forget' how to ride a bike, you cannot really 'forget' IBS. Rather, you have to take steps to avoid getting on the IBS bicycle. This can take some time to do'.

## Up regulation of CNS activity

'Your gut has become very sensitive over your time living with IBS Symptoms. Things that do not activate symptom experiences in other people do tend to activate your symptom experience. Things that you used to eat and do, nowadays cause symptoms. Your body has learned how to have symptoms and does so with increasing ease as time goes on. In order to get away from this we have to find a way to turn down your gut and bodily sensitivity. Picture a volume knob on a radio that controls how sensitive your gut is. We can turn that sensitivity down by teaching you how to slow your body down, distract yourself and think about your symptoms differently'.

## On not perceiving increased levels of stress, in the presence of stressful events

'An analogy in learning to play a song on an instrument can be drawn here. The first time one plays a song on an instrument it is hard; however, with successive tries, as with successive activations of this pathway, it can occur without conscious thought being applied to it. The first time one is placed in a stressful situation or event it is a novel situation that requires much effort to overcome. As the body gets more and more used to stress it adapts to stressful circumstances as being the norm'.

## On hypervigilance contributing to increased symptom perceptions

'Sometimes when we are dealing with issues related to sensitive areas like bowel control we can have a tendency to focus a lot of attention on that difficulty. That attention can act like a pair of sunglasses that only let you see problems and issues of difficulty related to your IBS. Those glasses make it hard to notice when you are *not* having symptoms. Working with a psychologist is one way of changing your focus back to the way it was before your bowel problems became so hard to deal with, so that you are able to see your symptoms accurately and completely'.

## On avoiding multiple specialists opinions

'Have you ever heard the saying "Too many cooks spoil the broth?" It may be hard to believe but that saying can also be true when dealing with complex medical issues like IBS. Often in medicine it is a good idea to find one provider you trust and can work with rather than constantly seeking new opinions. New opinions can seem comforting at first but after a while the pattern of looking for them can cause stress and anxiety in its own right and contribute to stress you may feel in dealing with IBS'.

## Summary

IBS is a condition of up regulated gut functioning that has predisposing, precipitating and perpetuating factors. Early childhood environment, parental influence, abuse and trauma history and illness history can all predispose somebody to develop gut-focused symptoms. Precipitating factors of psychological distress and illness experience paired with perpetuating factors of high levels of stress, cognitive dysfunction and situational characteristics can maintain symptoms at a level that is difficult for patients to manage.

A range of psychological treatments has been shown to be effective in helping patients learn to manage their IBS symptom experience. Through decreasing autonomic activation, decreasing cognitive dysfunction and teaching patients how to become observant in monitoring their symptom experience a greater level of symptom management can be taught, thereby improving quality of life and symptom severity. Psychological treatments of CBT, interpersonal therapy, hypnosis, relaxation and mindfulness all affect autonomic activation, and therefore can be effective in decreasing symptom experiences that result from such activation.

Finding clinicians to work with can be challenging. However, a number of resources are available to the physician who wishes to join with additional practitioners. Clinical psychologists, hypnosis practitioners and biofeedback practitioners are all certified through their respective accreditation organizations. Working with a properly trained clinician can be a valuable asset and provide a greater sense of ability in working with patients with functional GI disorders.

## Useful web links

- www.iffgd.org – The International Foundation for Functional GI Disorders maintains a list of psychologists and other practitioners who work with functional GI disorders. Additionally, IFFGD creates and publishes patient educational materials and hosts biannual scientific conferences fostering research in this area.
- www.med.unc.edu/ibs – UNC Center for Functional GI & Motility Disorders – The centre sponsors patient and clinician annual conferences and research looking at the most current research.
- www.apa.org – Web site for the American Psychological Association, which maintains a list of state psychological associations as well as links to practitioner databases to find clinicians with experience in behavioural medicine
- www.bcia.org – Biofeedback Certification Institute of America – Web site of the accreditation organization for biofeedback practitioners. This site maintains a searchable listing of biofeedback providers that can assist in teaching patients relaxation strategies.

## References

1 North CS, Downs D, Clouse RE *et al.* The presentation of irritable bowel syndrome in the context of somatization disorder. *Clin Gastroenterol Hepatol* 2004;2:787–795.
2 Dalton CB, Hathaway JM, Bangdiwala SI and Drossman DA. After hours telephone calls from patients with functional or organic diagnoses: Do physician and patient perceptions differ? *Am J Gastroenterol* 2002;122(9):S233–S234.
3 Drossman DA. Presidential Address: Gastrointestinal Illness and Biopsychosocial Model. *Psychosom Med* 1998;60:258–267.
4 Drossman DA. Challenges in the physician-patient relationship: Feeling "drained". *Gastroenterol* 2001;121:1037–1038.
5 Drossman DA, Corazziari E, Delvaux M *et al*. *Rome III: The Functional Gastrointestinal Disorders*. 2006, Degnon Associates Inc., McLean, VA.
6 Longstreth GF, Thompson WG, Chey WD *et al.* Functional Bowel Disorders. In Drossman DA, Corazziari E, Delvaux M et al. (eds), *Rome III: The Functional Gastrointestinal Disorders*, 3rd edn. 2006, Degnon Associates, Inc., McLean, VA: 487–555.
7 Naliboff B. Psychosocial Co-Morbidities. IFFGD World Congress, Psychosocial Comorbidities in Functional GI Disorders, April 2011.
8 Spiller RC. Post infectious irritable bowel syndrome. *Gastroenterol* 2003;124: 1662–1671.
9 Irwin C, Falsetti SA, Lydiard RB *et al.* Comorbidity of posttraumatic stress disorder and irritable bowel syndrome. *J Clin Psychiatry* 1996;57:576–578.
10 Lydiard RB, Fossey MD, Marsh W and Ballenger JC. Prevalence of psychiatric disorders in patients with irritable bowel syndrome. *Psychosomatics* 1993;34:229–234.
11 North CS, Alpers DH, Thompson SJ and Spitznagel EL. Gastrointestinal symptoms and psychiatric disorders in the general population: Findings from NIMH epidemiologic catchment area project. *Dig Dis Sci* 1996;41:633–640.
12 Lydiard RB and Falsetti SA. Experience with anxiety and depression treatment studies: Implications for designing irritable bowel syndrome clinical trials. *Am J Med* 1999; 107:65S–73S.

13 Drossman DA, McKee DC, Sandler RS *et al*. Psychosocial factors in the irritable bowel syndrome. A multivariate study of patients and nonpatients with irritable bowel syndrome. *Gastroenterol* 1988;95:701–708.

14 Drossman DA, Corazziari E, Delvaux M *et al*. Rome III: The Functional Gastrointestinal Disorders. *Gastroenterol* 2006:130(5):1377–1556.

15 Levy RL, Whitehead WE, Walker LS *et al*. Increased somatic complaints and health-care utilization in children: effects of parent IBS status and parent response to gastro-intestinal symptoms. *Am J Gastroenterol* 2004;99:2442–2451.

16 Walker LS and Greene JW. Children with recurrent abdominal pain and their parents: more somatic complaints, anxiety, and depression than other patient families. *J Pediatr Psychol* 1989;14:231–243.

17 Walker LS, Garber J and Greene JW. Somatic complaints in pediatric patients: A prospective study of the role of negative life events, child social and academic competence, and parental somatic symptoms. *J of Consulting and Clinical Psych* 1994;62:1213–1221.

18 Levy RL, Whitehead WE, Von Korff MR *et al*. Intergenerational transmission of GI Illness Behavior. *Am J Gastroenterol* 1998;95:451–456.

19 Lowman BC, Drossman DA, Cramer EM and McKee DC. Recollection of childhood events in adults with irritable bowel syndrome. *J Clin Gastroenterol* 1987;9:324–330.

20 Gwee KA, Leong YL, Graham C *et al*. The role of psychological and biological factors in post- infective gut dysfunction. *Gut* 1999;44:400–406.

21 Drossman DA. Mind over matter in the postinfective irritable bowel. *Gut* 1999;44:306–307.

22 Sperber AD, Morris CB, Greemberg L *et al*. Development of abdominal pain and IBS following gynecological surgery: A prospective, controlled study. *Gastroenterol* 2008;134:75–84.

23 Cooper SJ and Donald O. Hebb's synapse and learning rule: A history and commentary. *Neurosci Biobehav Rev* 2005;28:851–874.

24 Ringel Y, Drossman DA, Leserman JL *et al*. Effect of abuse history on pain reports and brain responses to aversive visceral stimulation: An fMRI study. *Gastroenterol* 2008;134:396–404.

25 Drossman DA. Abuse, trauma and GI illness: Is there a link? *Am J Gastroenterol* 2011;106:14–25.

26 Ringel Y, Drossman DA, Leserman J *et al*. Association between central activation and pain reports in women with IBS. *Gastroenterol* 2006;130(4, Suppl 2):A-77.

27 Drossman DA. Brain imaging and its implications for studying centrally targeted treatments in ibs: a primer for gastroenterologists. *Gut* 2005;54:569–573.

28 Drossman DA, Ringel Y, Vogt B *et al*. Alterations of brain activity associated with resolution of emotional distress and pain in a case of severe IBS. *Gastroenterol* 2003;124:754–761.

29 Drossman DA, Toner BB, Whitehead WE *et al*. Cognitive-behavioral therapy verses education and desipramine verses placebo for moderate to severe functional bowel disorders. *Gastroenterol* 2003;125:19–31.

30 Koloski NA, Talley NJ, Matheson M and Boyce PM. Psychosocial predictors of irritable bowel syndrome (IBS) and functional dyspepsia (FD) in the general population. *Gastroenterol* 2001;120(5, Suppl 1):A-758.

31 Nicholl BI, Halder SL, Macfarlane GJ *et al*. Psychosocial risk markers for new onset irritable bowel syndrome–results of a large prospective population-based study. *Pain* 2008;137:147–155.

32 Spence MJ and Moss-Morris R. The cognitive behavioural model of irritable bowel syndrome: A prospective investigation of patients with gastroenteritis. *Gut* 2007;56:1066–1071.

33 Sostek MB, Jackson S, Linevsky JK *et al*. High prevalence of chronic gastrointestinal symptoms in a National Guard Unit of Persian Gulf veterans. *Am J Gastroenterol* 1996;91:2494–2497.

34 Tuteja AK, Tolman KG, Talley NJ *et al*. Bowel disorders in gulf war veterans. *Gastroenterol* 2008;134(4, Suppl 1):A-31.

35 Institute of Medicine. *Gulf War and health: Update of health effects of serving in the Gulf War: Diseases of the Digestive System*. 2010, The National Academic Press, Washington, DC:155–163.

36 Dickhaus B, Mayer EA, Firooz N *et al*. Irritable bowel syndrome patients show enhanced modulation of visceral perception by auditory stress. *Am J Gastroenterol* 2003;98:135–143.

37 Dickhaus B, Firooz N, Stains J *et al*. Psychological stress increases visceral sensitivity in patients with irritable bowel syndrome (IBS) but not controls. *Gastroenterol* 2001;120(5, Suppl 1):A-67.

38 Murray CD, Flynn J, Ratcliffe L *et al*. Effect of acute physical and psychological stress on gut autonomic innervation in irritable bowel syndrome. *Gastroenterol* 2004;127:1695–1703.

39 Mayberg HS. Limbic-Cortical dysregulation: A proposed model of depression. *J Neuropsychiatry Clin Neurosci* 1997;9:471–481.

40 Drossman DA. Patients with psychogenic abdominal pain: six years' observation in the medical setting. *Am J Psychiatry* 1982;139:1549–1557.

41 Drossman DA, Li Z, Leserman J *et al*. Effects of coping on health outcome among female patients with gastrointestinal disorders. *Psychosom Med* 2000;62:309–317.

42 Lackner JM. No brain, no gain: The role of cognitive processes in irritable bowel syndrome. *J Cogn Psychother* 2005;19:125–136.

43 Blanchard EB, Lackner JM, Sanders K *et al*. A controlled evaluation of group cognitive therapy in the treatment of irritable bowel syndrome. *Behav Res Ther* 2007;45: 633–648.

44 Lackner JM, Coad ML, Mertz HR *et al*. Cognitive therapy for irritable bowel syndrome is associated with reduced limbic activity, GI symptoms, and anxiety. *Behavior Research and Therapy* 2006;44:621–638.

45 Lackner JM, Jaccard J, Krasner SS *et al*. How does cognitive behavior therapy for irritable bowel syndrome work? A mediational analysis of a randomized clinical trial. *Gastroenterol* 2007;133:433–444.

46 Lackner JM, Gudleski GD, Keefer L *et al*. Rapid response to cognitive behavior therapy predicts treatment outcome in patients with irritable bowel syndrome. *Clin Gastroenterol Hepatol* 2010;8:426–432.

47 Lackner JM, Jaccard J, Krasner SS *et al*. Self-administered cognitive behavior therapy for moderate to severe irritable bowel syndrome: Clinical efficacy, tolerability, feasibility. *Clin Gastroenterol Hepatol* 2008;6:899–906.

48 Weaver TL, Nishith P and Resick PA. Prolonged exposure therapy and irritable bowel syndrome: A case study examining the impact of a trauma-focused treatment on a physical condition. *Cogn Behav Pract* 1998;5:103–122.

49 Powers MB, Halpern JM, Ferenschak MP *et al*. A meta-analytic review of prolonged exposure for posttraumatic stress disorder. *Clin Psychol Rev* 2010;30:635–641.

50 Benson H. *The relaxation response*. 1975, William Morrow, New York.

51 Blanchard EB, Greene B, Scharff L and Schwarz-McMorris SP. Relaxation training as a treatment for irritable bowel syndrome. *Biofeedback Self Reg* 1993;18:125–132.

52 Mittal RK, Shaffer HA, Parollisis S and Baggett L. Influence of breathing pattern on the esophagogastric junction pressure and esophageal transit. *Am J Physiol* 1995;269: G577–G583.

53  Chitkara DK, Van TM, Whitehead WE and Talley NJ. Teaching diaphragmatic breathing for rumination syndrome. *Am J Gastroenterol* 2006;101:2449–2452.

54  Bernstein DA and Borkovec TD. *Progressive relaxation training.* 1973, Champaign Illinois Research Press, Champaign, IL.

55  Neff DF and Blanchard EB. A multi-component treatment of irritable bowel syndrome. *Behavior Ther* 1987;18:70–83.

56  Schwarz SP, Blanchard EB and Neff DF. Behavioral treatment of irritable bowel syndrome: a 1-year follow-up study. *Biofeedback Self Regul* 1986;11:189–198.

57  Schwarz SP, Taylor AE, Scharff L and Blanchard EB. Behaviorally treated irritable bowel syndrome patients: A four- year follow-up. *Behav Res Ther* 1990;28:331–335.

58  Shinozaki M, Kanazawa M, Kano M *et al.* Effect of autogenic training on general improvement in patients with irritable bowel syndrome: A randomized controlled trial. *Appl Psychophysiol Biofeedback* 2010;35(3):189–198.

59  Whorwell PJ, Prior A and Colgan SM. Hypnotherapy in severe irritable bowel syndrome: further experience. *Gut* 1987;28:423–425.

60  Palsson OS. Standardized hypnosis treatment for irritable bowel syndrome: the North Carolina protocol. *Int J Clin Exp Hypn* 2006;54:51–64.

61  Palsson OS and Whitehead WE. The growing case for hypnosis as adjunctive therapy for functional gastrointestinal disorders. *Gastroenterol* 2002;123:2132–2135.

62  Miller NE and Dworkin BR. Effects of learning on visceral functions – biofeedback. *New Engl J Med* 1977;296:1274–1278.

63  Health and Public Policy Committee ACoP. Biofeedback for gastrointestinal disorders. *Ann Intern Med* 1985;103:291–293.

64  Latimer PR. Biofeedback and behavioral approaches to disorders of the gastrointestinal tract. *Psychother Psychosom* 1981;36:200–212.

65  Kabat-Zinn J. *Full catastrophe living: Using the wisdom of your body and mind to face stress, pain, and illness.* 1990, Delacorte, New York.

66  Gaylord SA, Palsson OS, Garland EL *et al.* Mindfulness training reduces the severity of irritable bowel syndrome in women: Results of a randomized controlled trial. *Am J Gastroenterol* 2011;106(9):1678–88.

67  Burnett CK and Drossman DA. Irritable bowel syndrome and other funtinal gastrointestinal disorders. In Haas LJ (ed) *Handbook of Primary Care Psychology.* 2004, Oxford University Press, New York:411–424.

68  Ford A, Talley N, Schoenfeld P *et al.* Efficacy of psychological therapies in irritable bowel syndrome: Systematic review and meta-analysis. *Am J Gastroenterol* 2008; 103(S1):S477.

69  Pimentel M, Lembo A, Chey WD *et al.* Rifaximin therapy for patients with irritable bowel syndrome without constipation. *N Engl J Med* 2011;364:22–32.

70  Weinland SR, Morris CB, Dalton C *et al.* Cognitive factors affect treatment response to medical and psychological treatments in functional bowel disorder. *Am J Gastroenterol* 2010;105:1397–1406.

# Case-Based Multiple Choice Questions

1 Ms M, a 37-year-old professional pilot, presents to your clinic with a five-year history of abdominal pain that is associated with diarrhoeal symptoms that is diagnosed as IBS by her primary care physician. She feels frustrated in dealing with her symptoms and in association with this reports difficulty in managing with life stresses, though she does not elaborate. She has had an extensive evaluation that was negative for other diagnoses and notes that she is not able to socialize or go on trips because of these symptoms. Because of impaired daily functioning due to her IBS symptoms and a possible association with life stresses, you feel that obtaining psychological evaluation and treatment may be effective for her. However she states she is not interested.

You choose to:
  A Inform the patient that medical treatments for IBS may be limited and that psychological treatments may really be the best bet for her. You communicate understanding of her reluctance to working with a psychologist but make a referral anyway.
  B Treat the patient' symptoms, give her literature of the use of nonpharmacologic strategies for IBS and suggest that if she wants to pursue this in the future you would be happy to address the topic again in a future session and make a referral for her if she is interested.
  C Attempt during your clinic visit to understand why she does not want to meet with a psychologist. You ask about her current psychological stressors and why she is resisting psychological treatment in an effort to 'get to the heart' of what is going on and convince her to change her mind.

Best Answer: B

Often, recommending psychological treatment can feel strange or even threatening to patients, as they may not initially see a connection between stress and symptoms or believe that the physician is not taking the symptoms seriously or is looking to stop working with the patient for problems considered 'psychological'. When patients initially resist such a recommendation, contradicting their views may set up a negative interaction, either increasing resistance or leading to a poorer outcome if the patient does go to a psychologist. Engaging the patient around the topic of psychological stressors at this time would be difficult, especially given the time constraints of the limited clinic appointment. Answer (B) is the best response because it preserves your relationship with the patient and introduces the topic in ways that permit timely consideration without pressure. Being able to make a decision, rather than feeling coerced into working with a psychologist, will likely improve the clinical outcome.

2 Mrs T presents to your clinic for an initial appointment with a large number of previous medical records, including past diagnostic workups at state inpatient mental health facilities. You were notified of her scheduling the appointment two weeks prior when an office staff person who scheduled the appointment said she was insistent and 'difficult' on the phone. The patient has a four-year history of using narcotics to treat her abdominal pain for longstanding IBS. The records show that her previous gastroenterologist 'fired' her after she frequently phoned his office with requests for additional pain medications and often demanded to speak with the doctor directly. Over the course of your appointment with her she identifies a history of recent physical violence in her relationship with her ex-husband. He has since left the country but the patient still has persistent and intrusive thoughts and emotional distress about that relationship and believes it is making her symptoms worse. Your clinic has access to psychological resources. You agree to treat the patient and she suggests that she also engage in psychological treatment with a colleague. She agrees.

You recommend:
  A Generalized biofeedback therapy to help the patient learn more ways to relax in an effort to reduce the intensity of her emotions and feelings.
  B Referral for substance dependence treatment for detoxification to reduce her 'difficult' behaviour and permit medical treatment.
  C Initial assessment with a psychologist colleague who is trained in behavioural medicine.

Best Answer: C

Mrs T's symptoms and behaviours likely result from many factors that can affect her interactions with you and with others in her life. Therefore, symptom management that excludes a more comprehensive understanding of all of the contributing factors may lead to suboptimal treatment benefit and may impair her interactions with you. A new patient assessment session by a psychologist usually lasts 90 minutes or more, while therapy sessions can occur weekly or bi-weekly and generally last up to 50 minutes. This allows the psychologist to form a good therapeutic relationship with the patient and permits a full and comprehensive assessment of the factors contributing to the patients 'difficult' behaviours, and also leads to management options. In Mrs T's case, given her prolonged history of psychological difficulties, it is likely that more difficult to treat psychological conditions (e.g. personality or 'trait' characteristics) are contributing to her illness behaviour and symptoms. Psychologists can help provide augmentative treatment to that provided by the clinician and can provide a collaborative role in the overall treatment plan.

# CHAPTER 11

# Gut Motility Related Symptoms

*Juan-R. Malagelada and Carolina Malagelada*

Department of Digestive Diseases, Vall d'Hebron University Hospital, Barcelona, Spain

---

**Key points**

- A proportion of IBS patients have significant intestinal motor disturbances.
- Motor abnormalities in IBS patients are not associated with specific symptoms.
- Evidence of abnormal gastrointestinal motor function should be sought for in IBS patients with longstanding severe symptoms.

---

## Introduction

Irritable bowel syndrome (IBS) is a clinical diagnosis applied to patients presenting with symptoms referable to the digestive tract who meet predetermined symptom criteria. There are no patognomonic features and no established biological markers. It is gradually becoming accepted that a diversity of pathophysiologic mechanisms may generate similar symptoms. Thus, at diagnosis, it cannot be anticipated whether an IBS patient has a gut motility disorder or not. Even if motor disturbances are present, it may be unclear whether these are directly responsible for the clinical manifestations or constitute an epiphenomenon signalling disturbed gut control mechanisms. However, there are patients with such a profound impairment of gut motility that it eventually compromises their ability to nourish, manifests as intense pain and/or recurrent abdominal subocclusive crisis. These patients are separately categorized as having chronic intestinal idiopathic pseudo-obstruction (CIIP) or enteric dysmotility.

As our technical means to investigate gut function advance, we are increasingly recognizing that there is a continuum between common IBS cases (a proportion of who have demonstrable motility abnormalities, as described later) and CIIP. In fact, many patients with incapacitating, life threatening CIIP were previously labelled for years as having IBS. The challenge and, to some extent, the duty of the modern gastroenterologist is to identify among the highly prevalent population of IBS patients, those

---

*Irritable Bowel Syndrome: Diagnosis and Clinical Management*, First Edition.
Edited by Anton Emmanuel and Eamonn M.M. Quigley.
© 2013 John Wiley & Sons, Ltd. Published 2013 by John Wiley & Sons, Ltd.

with significant and treatable gut motor disturbances or, at least, susceptible of prognostic assessment.

---

**CASE STUDY 11.1**

*History*: female
Seen first in 2006, age 21, complaining of abdominal pain, alternating constipation and diarrhoea, some bloating and occasional vomiting for three years. The physical examination was normal.

*Diagnostic evaluation*:
- Bloods, endoscopy, CT scan, barium studies: all negative.
- Intestinal manometry (standard and overload): borderline, nondiagnostic, abnormalities.
- Intestinal gas infusion test: markedly abnormal (1021 ml retention, N<400 ml).
- Endoluminal image motility analysis: markedly abnormal.

*Outcome*: Laparoscopic intestinal full thickness biopsy: mastocyte infiltration, absent intestinal cells of Cajal.
   By 2009 she was requiring home parenteral nutrition.

---

## Who and when to investigate

Since IBS is a symptom-based, clinical diagnosis, the first management decision is whether, and to what extent, should the patient be investigated with the technical resources available today. Besides, the investigation must be conceived with a dual purpose: to uncover an unsuspected organic lesion or condition and to gather evidence of a potential gut neuromuscular disorder underlying the clinical picture. The decision and appropriate procedures to elucidate whether or not there is an occult lesion such as cancer or inflammatory bowel disease are beyond the scope of this chapter but are summarized in Boxes 11.1 and 11.2. We will focus instead on the issue of establishing whether the patient's gut is affected by a motor disorder that could explain the symptomatology. In brief, to evolve from a symptom-based diagnosis of suspected IBS towards a possible diagnosis of gut neuromuscular disease, such as enteric dysmotility.

It is necessary to consider the practicality of undertaking such an investigation. This is usually not a simple decision, because the required technical means involve some discomfort and, particularly, monetary cost. There is also a question of availability, since for certain investigations patients may need to be referred to a specialized unit outside the primary medical facility. As a general rule, most patients with IBS may not be

---

**Box 11.1  Common misdiagnoses in severe IBS to consider prior to physiologic testing of gut function**

- Infiltrating colon cancer
- Localized small bowel Crohn's disease or tumour
- Chronic segmental ischemia
- Central nervous system disorder with dysautonomia
- Mitochondrial disease (i.e. MNGIE)
- Autonomic/intrinsic neuropathy of toxic, paraneoplastic or metabolic origin
- Malabsorption syndromes, various enteropathies
- Peptide secreting neuroendocrine tumours
- Other rare conditions, when applicable

---

**Box 11.2  Conventional diagnostic procedures to consider prior to physiologic testing of gut function in severe IBS**

- Biochemical testing for: autoimmune diseases, coeliac serologies, metabolic pack, other.
  - *Key value*: identifying conditions that may distort gut motility and are difficult to recognize by imaging.
- Upper and lower gut endoscopy (complemented by capsule or enteroscopy, if appropriate).
  - *Key value*: recognizing subtle mucosal disease (ulcer, polyposis) syndromes (i.e. Cronkhite–Canada), neurofibromatosis, other infections (i.e. Whipple's), genetic (i.e. coeliac), and so on.
- CT scan thorax and abdomen.
  - *Key value*: identifying possible small cell lung cancer, thymoma, ovarian tumours, pancreatic tumours, occult cirrhosis, retroperitoneal and mesenteric inflammatory diseases, other.
- Magnetic resonance enterography.
  - *Key value*: excluding mid-bowel lesions and anatomic distortions.

---

candidates for such an in-depth investigation for several reasons. Firstly, some patients with symptoms meeting the criteria for IBS may be primarily concerned about a life threatening or disabling condition and, once they have been assured that such is not the case, they may feel relieved enough as to not demand any specific therapy. Furthermore, these patients may be satisfied with simple management measures, including symptomatic treatment of abdominal discomfort and irregular bowel habit. Secondly, some patients may suffer associated prevalent conditions such as fibromyalgia, headaches, back pain, interstitial cystitis or personality disturbances. In these instances, taking into account the whole of the patient's symptomatology, it may be wiser not to focus on any one of the components and directly attempt a behavioural, psychotherapeutic or psychopharmacologic therapeutic approach. Thirdly, the IBS symptomatology may not be intense enough to justify the expenditure of an in-depth pathophysiological investigation. Whilst initially favouring a restrictive diagnostic approach may fail to establish the underlying pathophysiology in many IBS patients, a conservative observation period may indicate whether the IBS symptoms worsen, vary or reinforce patient insistence to take further action.

At the other end of the spectrum there is an important minority of IBS patients whose symptoms at presentation or at the time of the subspecialist consultation are already intense, protracted, substantially reduce the quality of life of the patient or simply prove uncontrollable by conventional management. The clinician may then legitimately wonder whether there is a demonstrable gut neuromuscular disorder underlying the clinical picture. In such instances, it is quite appropriate to consider further investigation, including a sophisticated assessment of gut motility, sensory perception and neural control.

Before deciding the specific diagnostic strategy, it is appropriate to carefully review, once more, the patient's symptoms and associated signs. Since the initial clinical diagnosis was IBS, it should be assumed that the symptomatology conforms to the criteria set forth by the Rome III consensus that constitutes the current gold standard. However, special notice should be taken of other concurrent symptoms, such as inability to feed normally, nausea and vomiting, electrolyte disturbances and autonomic dysfunction. Other central nervous system, bladder, muscular and skin manifestations may also be present. Logically these potentially 'organic' features will have already been considered and investigated by the physician(s) who originally made the diagnosis of IBS, but a sensible review is in order, to avoid costly and embarrassing blunders (Box 11.1).

An additional important axiom to obey concerns the need to exclude other pathological conditions that may influence gut motility. This usually requires a standard but thorough reinvestigation of associated systemic and digestive tract disease. This is a particularly crucial prerequisite with regard to gut motility tests, since their results cannot be appropriately interpreted without prior assurance of the absence of both a mechanical obstruction as well as metabolic, endocrine or systemic neuromuscular disease. To this end, it would be sensible to review again recent imaging tests or perform them *de novo* (Box 11.2). Finally, genetic risk review is also in order, since a number of neuromuscular gut motility disorders have hereditary roots.

# Gathering evidence of gastrointestinal motor abnormalities in patients with a clinical diagnosis of IBS

## Technical resources available

Conventional diagnostic methods, from contrast radiology to endoscopy, serve to recognize gut morphological abnormalities and, as stated earlier, excluding lesions and potential mechanical obstruction is essential prior to physiological investigation of gut motility. However, standard imaging tests as performed in the clinic may sometimes provide indirect evidence of motor disturbances. Substantial amounts of retained food and secretions observed at morning endoscopy after overnight fast, dilated aperistaltic loops of bowel and some other features may indeed indicate a major failure of motility. Unfortunately, these signs are indicative of an advanced disorder, at which stage patients would have been already recognized as suffering from gastroparesis or pseudo-obstruction syndrome rather than IBS. Therefore, to detect more subtle and early signs of dysmotility it is necessary to apply more precise tests that, although not widely available, can usually be obtained by referring the patient to a specialized medical centre. The main techniques that may be used to evaluate gut neuromuscular function in selected patients with an initial IBS diagnosis are described here.

## Small bowel manometry

This technique for the evaluation of intestinal motor disorders was developed several decades ago [1, 2]. Unfortunately, it is invasive, difficult to interpret and expensive, three drawbacks that limit its use. It is performed by placing a multichannel catheter for water perfusion under fluoroscopic control (sometimes aided by endoscopy to get through the stomach) with pressure recording ports located at various levels along the antrum, duodenum and proximal jejunum. These ports register the amplitude and duration of phasic pressure waves produced by the contractions. The water perfusion method implies that the test is static, with the subject remaining either in bed or reclined in special beds. However, there are ambulatory 'solid state' systems taking advantage of electronic pressure sensors and Holter-type recordings [3].

Most diagnostic facilities that make use of intestinal manometry monitor intestinal motility over several hours either fasting or, more commonly, both during fasting and postprandial periods. In some instances, the catheter has been advanced to the distal small bowel, providing data on ileal motor activity [4, 5].

The diagnostic interpretation of small bowel manometry is based on pattern recognition, employing predetermined criteria. Relatively few abnormal patterns have been characterized by the manometric test regardless of whether relatively short stationary manometry or 24-hour ambulatory manometry is conducted. The test has high specificity in detecting a pathologic motor disturbance, but relatively low sensitivity. Consequently, only patients with major motor disturbances are identified by the test and more subtle dysmotility may remain unrecognized. An additional value of intestinal manometry is that it may provide some indication of whether the abnormal pressure wave pattern has been produced by altered neural regulation (neurogenic pattern) or muscle contractile failure (myopathic pattern), although in advanced stages it may be impossible to distinguish which of them has produced the contractile disturbance [6]. Furthermore, although neural control of gut function may be affected at different levels from the brain to the gut, manometric abnormalities are similar, regardless of the level and cause of the neuropathy. The test may indicate abnormality but rarely hints at its origin.

A variation of the standard intestinal manometry test is the chyme overload technique [7]. This technique is analogous to standard intestinal manometry but it incorporates an artificially thickened chyme with 6.5% magnesium aluminium silicate that is infused directly into the proximal duodenum to challenge the intestine during the postprandial period. Chyme overload appears to destabilize the neuropathic gut and, with this approach, patients with a neuropathic bowel disorder are more prone to generate aberrant motor patterns than after a normal meal, thus facilitating their recognition. Furthermore, by delivering the test meal directly into the small bowel, the potentially confounding effect of delayed gastric emptying on the postprandial motor pattern is overcome.

Small bowel manometry in IBS has been the subject of some investigation. The pioneering studies by Kellow, Phillips and others [4, 5] showed that ileal motor activity was abnormal in some IBS patients and some evidence of concurrence between aberrant contractions and symptom occurrence was also obtained [3, 8]. Both ambulatory and stationary manometry have yielded additional evidence of disturbed small bowel motility in IBS [9–12].

### Endoluminal image motility test

This is a novel noninvasive approach to assess small bowel motility, recently developed and validated in our laboratory [13, 14]. Endoluminal image analysis of intestinal motor activity is based on the use of capsule endoscopy to provide continuous visualization of intestinal wall motion, lumen diameter changes that reflect contraction and relaxation sequences as well as the physical character of bowel contents. Computer vision technology yields automatic analysis of series of specific features from sequential image frames. Mathematical analysis of each feature is then conducted using a series of models measuring numerical parameters. The mathematical

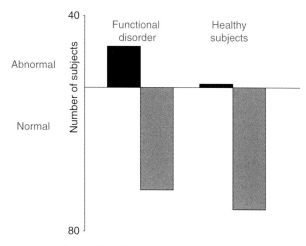

**Figure 11.1** Intestinal dysmotility identified by endoluminal image analysis. 29% of functional patients vs 3% healthy subjects (p=0.000) were identified as abnormal [15].

parameters, each defining one feature, are then processed and machine learning techniques are applied. The computer vision program evaluates contractile events (luminal occlusions and radial wrinkles), noncontractile patterns (open tunnel and smooth wall patterns), type of content (secretions, chyme) and motion of wall and contents. Normality range and discrimination of abnormal cases were established by a machine learning technique that involves an iterative classifier applied randomly to a population of healthy subjects as a training set and to groups of healthy subjects and patients as a test set.

Endoluminal image analysis provides a wider perspective of motor phenomena in the small bowel than intestinal manometry, including contractile and noncontractile activity, as well as motion of gut wall and luminal content. We have validated the new method by performing paired studies in healthy individuals and patients with small bowel abnormalities. We have shown that this noninvasive, operator independent test is at least as specific as and more sensitive than gastrointestinal manometry for diagnosis of severe bowel dysmotility.

Endoluminal motility assessment of patients with irritable bowel syndrome by the new technique has recently yielded some startling results [15]. A group of 80 patients with functional-type intestinal symptoms was recently investigated. The classifier identified 'abnormal' intestinal motility in about one of every three patients. These results suggest that about one-third of patients with functional type intestinal symptoms has abnormal intestinal motility (Figure 11.1). These observations suggest that many patients currently categorized as IBS may in fact suffer from a neuromuscular intestinal motor disorder that may be diagnosed by applying appropriate advanced methodologies, such as endoluminal image analysis. Moreover, IBS patients identified as abnormal clustered in two distinct groups exhibiting either a hyperdynamic or hypodynamic motility pattern. This motor behaviour was unrelated to clinical features and further studies are needed to evaluate its pathophysiological significance.

### Intestinal gas challenge tests

The purpose of this technology, also developed in our laboratory, is to quantify the dynamics of intestinal gas in humans [16, 17]. Therefore, its aim is quite different to that of the pioneering studies by Levitt and associates who used gas washout techniques to determine the content and composition of intraluminal gas in humans [18]. Our method consists of the constant infusion into the proximal jejunum of a gas mixture (88% nitrogen, 6.5% carbon dioxide and 5.5% oxygen) that mimics the partial pressures of venous blood gases to minimize diffusion of infused gas through the intestinal wall. Rectal gas output is quantified via an intrarectal tube connected to a barostat for continuous measurement.

Through an extensive series of studies we have established that, over a broad range of infusion rates, healthy individuals expel as much gas as infused, retaining a maximum of 400 ml inside the gut without experiencing significant symptoms. If healthy individuals (without the rectal cannula) are requested to voluntarily restrain from expelling gas from the rectum during infusion of gas in the upper jejunum, they develop intestinal gas retention with associated abdominal distension and discomfort [19]. In an experimental paradigm, instead of voluntary suppression of flatulence, intravenous glucagon was administered: this agent inhibits peristalsis and relaxes the bowel. Under the influence of glucagon, volunteers developed gas retention and abdominal distension, but without significant discomfort. Thus, the volume of gas retention determines objective abdominal distension but it is the motor and sensory activity of the gut which determines the subjective perception of symptoms.

Most patients with IBS and functional bloating, when challenged with the gas infusion test, show an inability to propulse gas and expel it at the same rate that it is infused into the upper gut [17]. Consequently, over the two-hour test, they retain between 400 and 800 ml of gas inside their bowels. Most importantly, unlike healthy individuals, patients with IBS develop symptoms during the gas infusion test. It is also relevant to point out that the site of gas infusion within the human gut produces different effects in IBS patients. Thus, when gas is infused into the colon, instead of into the jejunum, evacuation occurs at similar rates but symptoms are less prominent with colonic than with jejunal gas infusion. Scintigraphic studies with radiolabelled xenon have shown that gas infused into the proximal small bowel accumulates in the jejunum, suggesting an underlying small bowel

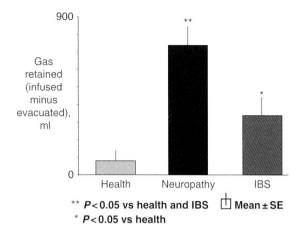

**Figure 11.2** Response to the gas transit test. Healthy subjects did not show gas retention. In patients with intestinal neuropathy, gas retention was significantly greater than in IBS patients.
(Reproduced from Serra *et al.* [21], with permission from Blackwell Publishing.)

motility abnormality [20]. The small bowel dysmotility in IBS patients disclosed by the gas challenge test is rarely picked up by conventional manometry. However, as indicated earlier, the more sensitive endoluminal image motility technique is able to detect it in about one-third of IBS patients.

Patients with documented severe intestinal dysmotility, such as chronic intestinal pseudo-obstruction, also show gas retention during the gas challenge test. Characteristically, however, they retain much larger volumes of infused gas (often more than 800 ml) (Figure 11.2). By contrast, patients with severe intestinal dysmotility develop fewer symptoms than those with IBS or functional bloating [21]. The different response to the gas infusion test suggests that abnormal intestinal reflexes in IBS are associated with visceral hypersensitivity whereas [22] established neuromuscular intestinal disease is associated with greater impairment of propulsive motor function.

Hypersensitivity and dysmotility in IBS may be exacerbated by luminal lipid infusion [23]. Duodenal lipid infusion performed during the gas challenge test increases gas retention and symptoms in IBS patients, whereas it has little or no effect in healthy individuals. Thus, the gas+lipid test raises the specificity and sensitivity of the test to more than 95%, increasing its discriminative power between IBS and normal individuals.

## Tests of colonic motor function

The simplest test of colonic motor function is the measurement of colonic transit by radio-opaque markers [24]. The radio-opaque marker test is most often performed by administering a single capsule containing multiple radio-opaque plastic markers. A plain abdominal X-ray is obtained on day 5 after ingestion of the markers. Gut retention of 20% or more of the markers at that time is considered abnormal. Several other variants of pellet-based measurements of colonic transit also exist. This test helps distinguish slow transit constipation from normal transit in patients claiming to be constipated. Unfortunately, the marker transit studies are often unable to ascertain the cause of impaired colonic function. For instance, the radio-opaque marker test may be abnormal in expulsion defects as well as in colonic inertia. During clinical evaluation the test is usually complemented by an anorectal motility study using manometry, rectal balloon distension and expulsion tests to exclude pelvic floor dyssinergia [25]. In practice, transit markers tests would be deemed indicated only in the context of severe constipation associated to other IBS features.

Two relatively more sophisticated methods for assessing colonic transit are available at specialized centres: scintigraphic measurement of radiolabelled intestinal content and the wireless pressure/pH capsule. Scintigraphic measurements require a suitable gamma camera installation and a nonabsorbable radiolabelled marker that may either be incorporated into a test meal or delivered directly into the distal small bowel/proximal colon via an enteric coated capsule [26]. The scintigraphic images allow assessment of total and segmental transit as well as some estimates of pooling and bowel width changes.

The telemetric capsule (SmartPill) continuously measures pressure, pH and temperature [27]. The device provides a radiation-free technology to measure colonic and whole gut transit, in addition to gastric emptying. Transit measurements obtained with the capsule are usually in good agreement with those obtained with radio-opaque markers. However, the clinical utility of colonic transit measurements remains as yet to be determined. Initially it was, rather optimistically, thought that transit measurements could discriminate patients with colonic inertia from those constipated as a result of pelvic floor dyssynergia (expulsion defects). Unfortunately, as pointed out above, global colonic transit delay is often seen in patients with the latter condition.

The wireless capsule represents a recent innovation valued for its relatively noninvasive capability to assess both small bowel and colonic transit. It does so by measuring the interval between the sharp pH rise that takes place as the capsule enters the duodenum and the change that occurs as it enters the colon, and again when it is eventually evacuated. The capsule provides some information on contractile activity by registering phasic pressure waves as it moves along the small bowel, but this information is very limited (by comparison with multiport manometry) because it only measures point pressure on the single capsule sensor.

The barostat is as instrument initially developed in our laboratory for measuring variations in gastric tone [28, 29]. The conceptual basis of the barostat is simple: by maintaining a constant low pressure inside a flaccid intragastric bag, the barostat records the changes in tonic pressure exerted by the stomach against the bag. The intraluminal component of the barostat consists of an over compliant thin walled plastic bag, connected via a two-way catheter to an external instrument that ensures that the bag is constantly kept at a low pressure by injecting or withdrawing air depending on whether the gut walls relax or contract, respectively. The oscillations provide a continuous measure of tone variations. The barostat has been used in the colon, often in combination with standard manometry to obtain tonic-phasic colonic motility assessments [30, 31]. The barostat may be also employed to measure conscious sensitivity of hollow viscera like the colon, by applying constant distending pressure at the desired level while assessing simultaneously perception via a validated questionnaire/scale. A potential drawback of the barostat as a stimulus to measure perception, however, is that it cannot adjust well for the prevailing visceral tone. Thus, if the organ relaxes, for instance, by administering intravenous glucagon, the perception diminishes and vice versa. To overcome this pitfall we subsequently developed in our laboratory the tensostat, which is a modification of the barostat that applies Laplace's law and automatically corrects for variations in tone when assessing conscious perception in response to intraluminal distension [32]. With the tensostat it is possible to exert constant wall tension at predetermined levels and, consequently, conscious perception of the stimulus truly reflects the stretch of gut walls (that is, tone-independent wall tension).

In the colon, the barostat has proven more accurate than intraluminal manometry to record phasic contractions when the colonic diameter exceeds 5–6 cm. The most useful variables to determine whether colonic motility is disturbed are the detection of high-amplitude propagated contractions (HAPCs) and the measurement of colonic tonic response to a meal [33]. Typically, HAPCs are decreased in chronically constipated patients [34].

### Quantitative imaging of the abdomen and its contents

There are two methodologies applicable to such measurements: modified CT imaging and abdominal magnetic resonance imaging (MRI).

The CT methodology was developed and validated in our laboratory with the collaboration of a team of specialized radiologists [35]. It takes advantage of CT hardware capabilities to introduce novel software programs that acquire digitalized image data from the instrument and transforms it into precise estimates of intra-abdominal shape, volume and physical components, specifically gas.

The computing process, although relatively complex, is automated. It includes the following steps: change the format, delete extra-abdominal features, identify pure and mixed gas, and perform gas volume reconstruction and quantification. This morpho-volumetric image analysis program yields gas volumes contained within various segments of abdominal gut, including stomach, small bowel, right colon, transverse colon, left colon and pelvic colon. At the same time, the program establishes the exact position of the diaphragm, the distance between the spine and the anterior abdominal wall, and the total volume inside the peritoneal cavity. With these elements, it is possible not only to measure intra-abdominal gas volumes but also to determine variations in abdominal shape and diaphragmatic motion.

Patients with functional bloating characteristically report that the bloating sensation fluctuates. Using the above technique for morpho-volumetric analysis of the abdomen, we recently compared abdominal CT scans taken during basal conditions with absent or mild bloating sensation and scans taken during an episode of spontaneous bloating. When compared with that in basal conditions, anterior wall protrusion during bloating was associated with significant diaphragmatic descent [36].

Applying this new methodology to patients with bloating has proven quite useful to discriminate functional bloating from bloating associated with severe intestinal dysmotility, as may occur in patients with gut neuropathies and/or myopathies. In patients with functional bloating, abdominal distension is associated with normal or only minimal increases in intra-abdominal gas, but marked diaphragmatic descent and relaxation of the oblique abdominal wall muscles. The result is protuberance of the anterior lower abdomen without actual change in total intra-abdominal volume. By contrast, patients with neuromuscular gut disorders demonstrate marked increase in intestinal gas volume, diaphragmatic relaxation and ascent, and anterior abdominal protrusion from inflated intestines [21]. Consequently, this methodology provides objective discrimination between bloating caused by gut motility disorders and bloating produced by viscero-somatic dysreflexia.

The MRI technology has been mainly directed towards estimation of gastric emptying and small bowel water content. The latter, which may be more relevant to assessment of diarrhoea-predominant IBS, is performed by obtaining a single shot, fast spin echo sequence similar to that used for magnetic resonance cholangiopancreatography [37]. Study individuals must remain for about six minutes inside the magnet for each time point and scans are obtained at various intervals over 4–5 hours. Results show a smaller calibre ileum in IBS patients and accelerated transit [38, 39]. However, it remains unclear whether these features reflect a primary disturbance of gut motility or they are secondary to higher anxiety and exaggerated intestinal response to central neurohormonal discharge.

### Assessment of viscero-somatic reflexes and abdominal wall muscle activity

This technology is based on the use of electromyography (EMG) to measure diaphragmatic and anterior abdominal myoelectrical activity during certain manoeuvers, including gas distension of the colon [40, 41]. The abdominal EMG electrodes are attached to the anterior abdomen, placing them over the rectus and oblique muscle groups. Trans-oesophageal diaphragmatic EMG recording is also performed by a probe with five ring electrodes, 5 mm wide at 15 mm intervals, connected by insulated copper wires. The radio-opaque electrodes are positioned, under fluoroscopic control, across the diaphragmatic hiatus and the position of the electrodes is controlled periodically by performing the Valsalva manoeuver.

A gas mixture similar to that employed for jejunal gas infusion test is pumped into the colon via a rectal catheter at 24 ml/min (final volume 240 ml at 10 min). The test is conducted with patients sitting on an ergonomic chair with the trunk erect. The abdomino-phrenic responses to the gas load are assessed before and during infusion of gas into the colon for one hour. Abdominal sensations (by perception scales) and abdominal girth (by tape measure) are assessed simultaneously. In patients with functional bloating, colonic gas loads [which are normally accommodated by the colon [42]] induce diaphragmatic contraction and anterior abdominal wall relaxation (mostly the internal oblique muscles). This is a paradoxical abdomino-phrenic response by comparison to the normal response shown by healthy individuals that consists of diaphragmatic relaxation and anterior muscle contraction [43]. It appears that abnormal abdomino-phrenic adaptation to intraluminal content in patients with bloating may be a behavioural response triggered by uncomfortable abdominal sensations. The abnormal response observed in patients with IBS and functional bloating may be a surrogate for the clinical situation when even a modest retention of gas produced by the impaired propulsion and the characteristic hypersensitivity of the IBS gut may induce discomfort and the abnormal viscero-somatic reflex response.

## Practical application of available tests to the evaluation of IBS patients

---

### Common problems
- Patients with IBS, even with significant lifestyle impairment, remain uninvestigated for possible underlying motility abnormalities.
- Where and how to investigate selected IBS patients? Refer to specialized groups with interest and diagnostic tools in neurogastroenterology.

---

Two pathophysiological elements underline the main clinical manifestations of IBS: conscious hypersensitivity and dysmotility. Since abdominal pain and altered bowel function are the key IBS symptoms, it seems logical that sensory and motor disturbances are pathogenetically implicated, albeit in variable proportions in individual cases. In clinical practice, however, the main reason for investigating sensory and motor abnormalities is not so much to establish a biomarker for IBS (symptom criteria currently suffice for this purpose) but to uncover a hidden enteric neuropathy or myopathy that may change the prognosis and require a different management approach. Patients with a clinical picture of chronic intestinal pseudo-obstruction (subocclusive crisis with radiologically apparent dilated bowel and enteric pooling of content) are relatively obvious and, with a full blown clinical picture, unlikely to be mixed with IBS. But some patients presenting with what appears to be severe IBS may, if appropriately investigated, show evidence of gut dysmotility, which may in turn provide evidence of gastrointestinal neuromuscular disease. It may be difficult, if not impossible, to gather evidence of such pathological alterations. Thus, it may be of substantial practical value to actively seek evidence of abnormal gastrointestinal motor function.

When the clinician makes the decision to investigate a patient with severe IBS by physiologic tests, the key goal is to establish the presence or absence of intestinal sensory and motor disturbance. However, the former is of reduced practical value, since most IBS patients show evidence of visceral hypersensitivity. Indeed, there has been some debate on the possibility that abnormal perception could become a biological marker. Identifying a significant motor abnormality, on the other hand, may be of prognostic and therapeutic value, in many instances.

How do we go about searching for such pathophysiological disturbance? The easiest way is to take a three-step approach (Figure 11.3). Firstly, decide which patients to investigate. As described previously, severity and duration of IBS symptoms is a prerequisite, since physiological tests tend to be invasive, uncomfortable and/or expensive. The second step is to anticipate the practical use of the information that may be obtained in the overall management of the patient. For instance, is the patient too old? Are there other significant associated diseases that would preclude intestinal biopsy? Is the nutritional status such that active nourishment via enteral (if tolerated) or parenteral, needs to come first? and so on. Keep in mind that further testing makes no sense if unlikely to improve the patient. The third step is to guess, on the basis of the clinical manifestations, which part of the gut is more likely to show an abnormality. Generally speaking, for IBS, the small bowel should come first [44–46], but colonic evaluation may be required [47] if protracted constipation is prominent associated feature and colonic inertia is a reasonable diagnostic

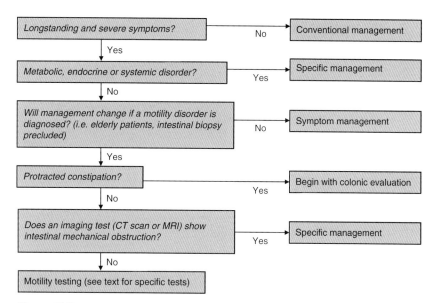

**Figure 11.3** Management algorithm.

possibility. (Note, however, that in any case, prior to moving towards subtotal colectomy it will be imperative to first exclude small bowel dysmotility.) For patients with associated severe dyspepsia and/or bloating, special tests may also need to be performed to evaluate these associated conditions and to enable the attending gastroenterologist to interpret the whole clinical picture [48].

As detailed, there are several advanced methodologies that facilitate evaluation of human small bowel motility with substantial degree of accuracy. To determine how to best use them in clinical practice, these technologies may be broadly divided into two general categories: methods that assess small bowel transit, and hence provide indirect assessment of its propulsive capacity, and methods that evaluate intestinal contractile activity. Transit tests encompass a broad range of sophistication. Imaging tests based on barium, CT scan or magnetic resonance only register relatively major disturbances in transit but, as indicated earlier, they are valuable tools to inform on potential mechanical impediments to transit from neoplastic, inflammatory, ischemic or even adhesive disorders that would distort motor patterns and confuse the interpretation of manometric and other motility tests. They should, therefore, be performed first (Box 11.2). If major motility alterations are uncovered by these imaging tests, even in the absence of lesions or mechanical problems, it may not be necessary to proceed with physiological testing, since the motor disturbance is likely major and transmural biopsy and/or long-term parenteral nutritional support may be warranted anyway.

The second group of transit studies to consider performing is those based on breath tests (usually recording the interval between ingestion of a non-absorbable sugar and peak breath hydrogen excretion resulting from arrival to the colon and local fermentation). We usually do not perform these tests for they are fraught with problems such as bacterial overgrowth (likely in a small bowel motor disorder) and other pitfalls. Another relatively simple and noninvasive approach is to use the SmartPill, a device that indirectly measures transit by recording abrupt pH changes along the gut, as detailed earlier. Unfortunately, simply measuring small bowel transit is unlikely to reliably pinpoint a subtle small bowel disorder because of the variability and broad normal range of intestinal transit times. A third approach – to measure intestinal transit based on radioscintigraphic labelling of a test meal – merits special consideration, as it provides additional information on regional pooling, bowel diameter and so on. However, it is an expensive and cumbersome test for nuclear medicine hospital facilities (unless a dedicated gamma camera and team are available).

Thus, after completing a thorough conventional imaging evaluation to exclude obstruction, our group favours to move directly to assessment of intestinal contractile patterns and function. The standard method for such a purpose is intestinal manometry but, as previously stated, intestinal manometry is only particularly useful if clearly abnormal. A pathological manometry tracing may even provide some indication about whether the disorder involves primarily a myopatic failure or aberrant neural control of gut motility, although the practical accuracy of manometry to distinguish myopatic and neuropathic dysmotility has been recently challenged. The problem with intestinal manometry is its relatively low sensitivity and the fact that a substantial number of tracings may show uncertain patterns, that is, appear to show abnormalities but not consistent enough to be certain. At present, in our laboratory we are gradually shifting from conventional perfused pressure catheter manometry to evaluation by the endoluminal capsule method. We have shown that the latter, besides being less invasive and uncomfortable for the patient, is at least equal to intestinal manometry in its potential to detect intestinal dysmotility. It is probably more sensitive too. In a recent study involving patients with the diagnosis of IBS and functional bloating the endoluminal capsule method picked up one-third of patients with disturbed small bowel motility, suggesting that such abnormality is more prevalent in IBS patients than previously anticipated.

Regardless whether intestinal dysmotility is evidenced by the manometric or by the endoluminal imaging methods, performance of a gas infusion or gas+lipid test may be an appropriate next step [21]. Patients with abnormal intestinal motility and marked (>800 ml) gas retention (particularly if associated with a low perception score) are likely to suffer from a gut neuromuscular disorder and may be candidates for a full thickness biopsy to further ascertain the nature of their bowel disease.

The applicability of colonic tests in the context of IBS clinical manifestations is more restricted. The main target group would be patients with constipation-predominant IBS. In these patients it may be of interest to determine the presence of colonic inertia that may benefit from surgical or device treatment. However, unlike patients with severe constipation without IBS, the abdominal pain component should introduce an element of caution to move towards subtotal colectomy, since pain is less likely to be relieved by removing the colon. Therefore, the practical need to ascertain colonic motility is not so imperative and empiric medical treatment should be tried first.

## IBS associated with other functional-type syndromes

There is a great deal of overlap among functional syndromes. Thus, in clinical practice it is quite common to encounter patients with IBS who share features of functional dyspepsia, bloating and even oesophageal manifestations. These mixed clinical pictures may be the expression of significant motor disturbances arising from an underlying neuromuscular dysfunction. These special situations require specific tests that may serve to identify the abnormalities and to direct appropriate management [49, 50].

Functional dyspepsia is characterized by abnormal hypersensitivity to gastric distension, abnormal viscero-visceral reflex regulation (resulting in impaired accommodation of the proximal stomach and a dilated antrum after meals). About one-third of these patients have abnormally delayed gastric emptying and a lesser, but significant proportion, accelerated emptying [51, 52]. In the context of severe IBS symptomatology, the concurrence of features of functional dyspepsia may warrant physiological testing to establish whether the upper gut is involved by a neuromuscular disorder. In such instances the issue is to determine whether gastroparesis or functional dyspepsia is present. Gastric emptying tests are usually performed, as a starting point, but there is a grey zone of mild to moderately delayed gastric emptying where gastroparesis and functional dyspepsia overlap. Therefore, performing a gastric emptying test, unless it shows a profound delay, will have limited practical value.

To evaluate upper gut motility we favour gastric barostat evaluation, a technique that enables quantification of gastric compliance and gastric tone. At the same time we can measure the conscious perception of gastric stretch by applying stepwise tension increments with the tensostat and simultaneously assess the symptomatic response by questionnaire [31, 48]. The test also allows evaluation of the proximal gastric response to duodenal infusion of nutrients (the normal relaxatory duodeno-gastric reflex is blunted in dyspepsia). The test is completed by evaluation of the effects of erythromycin, infused intravenously, to ascertain the capacity of gastric muscle to contract by direct stimulation of motilin receptors present in the smooth muscle.

Application of the tests described above may produce two distinct sets of results. Firstly, the patient may show both delayed gastric emptying and increased compliance, without increased conscious perception of gastric distension. Such a combination would be more characteristic of gastroparesis. If the gastric motor abnormality results from an alteration in neural regulation, erythromycin should be able to elicit gastric contraction. By contrast, if the abnormality is secondary to smooth muscle impairment, abnormal interstitial cell of Cajal's function or to certain forms of advanced intrinsic neuropathy, the response to erythromycin may be absent.

The second possible set of results would consist of mild or no delay in gastric emptying, normal compliance, hypersensitivity to gastric wall tension increments and impaired entero-gastric reflexes elicited by nutrient infusion into the duodenum. Moreover, the relaxatory response of the proximal stomach to antral distension may be impaired, provided that this less habitual part of the test is also performed. Such a combination of results would fit best with the diagnosis of functional dyspepsia and argue against an underlying neuromuscular disorder.

In patients with severe IBS and prominent bloating it may be advisable to perform a separate evaluation of abdominal volume, shape and viscerosomatic reflexes, to ascertain the origin of the abdominal distension. To this end we would employ two key tests: the adapted CT scan method and EMG of diaphragm and/or abdominal muscles, which will help us sort out the origin of bloating in individual cases. One category of patients with bloating is those who complain of uncomfortable bloating but without objective abdominal distension (with the important proviso that distension may be present during bloating episodes that may occur at times other than when the physical examination is performed). Another group of patients is those with both a bloating sensation and an obvious distension of the abdomen. This latter group is more likely to present identifiable abnormalities in gut motility, although it should be clear that the distension in itself is not necessarily directly related to abnormal intestinal motor performance.

The CT scan test will aim at discriminating between two separate groups: functional bloaters and patients with luminal gas/liquid retention as the physical cause of distension. In patients with functional bloating, intra-abdominal volume is not or is only minimally expanded, but the appearance of distension results from active reshaping of the abdomen by the dual action of diaphragmatic descent and anterior oblique muscle relaxation. CT images will show little or no intraluminal gas increment and, instead, a reshaped abdominal cavity with a descended diaphragm and relaxed oblique abdominal muscles [36, 53]. To reaffirm the paradoxical diaphragmatic and abdominal muscle activities the EMG test will also be of use in these patients.

Some patients with gut neuromuscular disorders show oesophageal involvement and it may be appropriate to obtain oesophageal motor evaluation as part of the overall examination, particularly if the patient complains of chest pain or dysphagia. The modern electronic sensor probes allowing high resolution esophageal manometry have greatly facilitated and expanded the diagnostic yield of esophageal motility investigation.

## Useful web links

- European Society of Neurogastroenterology and Motility: www.esnm.eu
- American Neurogastroenterology and Motility Society: www.motilitysociety.org

## References

1 Malagelada, J-R., Camilleri, M. and Stanghellini, V. *Manometric diagnosis of gastrointestinal motility disorders*. 1986, Thieme-Stratton, New York.
2 Stanghellini V, Camilleri M and Malagelada JR. Chronic idiopathic intestinal pseudo-obstruction: clinical and intestinal manometric findings. *Gut* 1987;28(1):5–12.
3 Kumar D and Wingate DL. The irritable bowel syndrome: a paroxysmal motor disorder. *Lancet* 1985;2:973–977.
4 Kellow JE and Phillips SF. Altered small bowel motility in irritable bowel syndrome is correlated with symptoms. *Gastroenterology* 1987;92:1885–1893.
5 Kellow JE, Phillips SF, Miller LJ *et al*. Dysmotility of the small intestine in irritable bowel syndrome. *Gut* 1988;29:1236–1243.
6 Lindberg G, Törnblom H, Iwarzon M *et al*. Full-thickness biopsy findings in chronic intestinal pseudo-obstruction and enteric dysmotility. *Gut* 2009;58:1084–1090.
7 Arcos E, Accarino A, Azpiroz F and Malagelada J-R. Chyme overload improves manometric evaluation of the small bowel. *Gastroenterology* 2007;132:A462.
8 Clemens CH, Samsom M, Roelofs JM *et al*. Association between pain episodes and high amplitude propagated pressure waves in patients with irritable bowel syndrome. *Am J Gastroenterol* 2003;98:1838–1843.
9 Schmidt T, Hackelsberger N, Widmer R *et al*. Ambulatory 24-hour jejunal motility in diarrhea-predominant irritable bowel syndrome. *Scand J Gastroenterol* 1996;31:581–589.
10 Simren M, Castedal M, Svedlund J *et al*. Abnormal propagation pattern of duodenal pressure waves in the irritable bowel syndrome (IBS) [correction of (IBD)]. *Dig Dis Sci* 2000;45:2151–2161.
11 Small PK, Loudon MA, Hau CM *et al*. Large-scale ambulatory study of postprandial jejunal motility in irritable bowel syndrome. *Scand J Gastroenterol* 1997;32:39–47.

12 Wackerbauer R, Schmidt T, Widmer R *et al*. Discrimination of irritable bowel syndrome by non-linear analysis of 24-h jejunal motility. *Neurogastroenterol Motil* 1998;10:331–337.

13 Malagelada C, De Iorio F, Azpiroz F *et al*. New insight into intestinal motor function via non-invasive endoluminal image analysis. *Gastroenterology* 2008;135:1155–1162.

14 De Iorio F, Malagelada C, Azpiroz F *et al*. Intestinal motor activity, endoluminal motion and transit. *Neurogastroenterol Motil* 2009;21:1264–1270.

15 Malagelada C, De Iorio F, Segui S *et al*. Functional gut disorders or disordered gut function? Small bowel dysmotility evidenced by an original technique. *Neurogastroenterol Motil* 2012;24: 223–228.

16 Serra J, Azpiroz F and Malagelada J-R. Intestinal gas dynamics and tolerance in humans. *Gastroenterology* 1998;115: 542–550.

17 Serra J, Azpiroz F and Malagelada J-R. Impaired transit and tolerance of intestinal gas in the irritable bowel syndrome. *Gut* 2000;48: 14–19.

18 Levitt MD. Volume and composition of human intestinal gas determined by means of an intestinal washout technique. *N Engl J Med* 1971;284(25):1394–1398.

19 Serra J, Azpiroz F and Malagelada J-R. Mechanisms of intestinal gas retention in humans: impaired propulsion versus obstructed evacuation. *Am J Physiol (Gastrointest Liver Physiol)* 2001;281:G138–G143.

20 Hernando-Harder AC, Serra J, Azpiroz F and Malagelada J-R. Sites of symptomatic gas retention during intestinal lipid perfusion in healthy subjects. *Gut* 2004;53: 661–665.

21 Serra J, Villoria A, Azpiroz F *et al*. Impaired intestinal gas propulsion in manometrically proven dysmotility and in irritable bowel syndrome. *Neurogastroenterol Motil* 2010;22:401–408.

22 Accarino A, Azpiroz F and Malagelada J-R. Selective dysfunction of mechanosensitive intestinal afferents in the irritable bowel syndrome. *Gastroenterology* 1995;108:636–643.

23 Serra J, Salvioli B, Azpiroz F and Malagelada J-R. Lipid-induced intestinal gas retention in the irritable bowel syndrome. *Gastroenterology* 2002;123:700–706.

24 Metcalf AM, Phillips SF, Zinsmeister AR *et al*. Simplified assessment of segmental colonic transit. *Gastroenterology* 1987;92(1):40–47.

25 Azpiroz F, Enck P and Whitehead WE. Anorectal functional testing. Review of a collective experience. *Am J Gastroenterol* 2002;97:232–240.

26 Stiuland T, Camilleri M, Vassallo M *et al*. Scintigraphic measurement of regional gut transit in idiopathic constipation. *Gastroenterology* 1991;101:107–115.

27 Rao SS, Kuo B, McCallum RW *et al*. Investigation of colonic and whole-gut transit with wireless motility capsule and radiopaque markers in constipation. *Clin Gastroenterol Hepatol* 2009;7(5):537–544.

28 Azpiroz F and Malagelada JR. Gastric tone measured by an electronic barostat in health and postsurgical gastroparesis. *Gastroenterology* 1987;92(4):934–943.

29 Castro A., Mearin F and Malagelada J-R. Gastric fundus relaxation and emetic sequences induced by apomorphine and intragastric lipid infusion in healthy humans. *Am J Gastroenterol* 2000;95: 3404–3411.

30 Von der Ohe MR, Hanson RM and Camilleri M. Comparison of simultaneous recordings of human colonic contractions by manometry and a barostat. *Neurogastroenterol Motil* 1994;6(3):213–222.

31 Ford MJ, Camilleri M and Wiste JA. Differences in colonic tone and phasic response to a meal in the transverse and sigmoid human colon. *Gut* 1995;37;264–269.

32  Distrutti E, Azpiroz F, Soldevilla A and Malagelada J-R. Gastric wall tension determines perception of gastric distension. *Gastroenterology* 1999;116:1035–1042.

33  Rao SS, Sadaghi P, Beaty J *et al.* Ambulatory 24-h colonic manometry in healthy humans. *Am J Physiol (Gastrointest Liver Physiol)* 2001;280:G629–G639.

34  Rao SS, Sadaghi P, Beaty J *et al.* Ambulatory 24-h colonic manometry in slow transit constyipation. *Am J Gastroenterol* 2004;99: 2405–2416, .

35  Pérez F, Accarino A, Azpiroz F *et al.* Gas distribution within the human gut: effect of meals. *Am J Gastroentol* 2007;102(4): 842–849.

36  Accarino, A., Perez, F., Azpiroz, F. *et al.* Abdominal distension results from caudoventral redistribution of contents. *Gastroenterology* 2009;136:1544–1551.

37  Hoad CL, Marciani L, Foley S *et al.* Non-invasive quantification of small bowel wáter content by MRI: a validation study. *Phys Med Biol* 2007;52:6909–6922.

38  Marciani L, Cox EF, Hoad CL *et al.* Postprandial changes in small bosel water content in healthy subjects and patients with irritable bowel syndrome. *Gastroenterology* 2010;138: 469–477.

39  Marciani L, Wright J, Foley S *et al.* Effects of a 5HT$_3$ antagonist, odansetron, on fasting and postprandial small bowel water content assessed by magnetic resonance imaging. *Alimn Pharmacol and Therap* 2010;32: 655–663.

40  Tremolaterra F, Villoria A, Azpiroz F *et al.* Impaired viscerosomatic reflexes and abdominal-wall dystony associated with bloating. *Gastroenterology* 2006;130: 1062–1068.

41  Villoria A, Azpiroz F, Soldevilla A *et al.* Abdominal accommodation: a coordinated adaptation of the abdominal walls to its content. *Am J Gastroenterol* 2008;103: 2807–2815.

42  Hernando Harder AC, Serra J, Azpiroz F *et al.* Colonic responses to gas loads in subgroups of patients with abdominal bloating. *Am J Gastroenterol* 2010;105: 876–882.

43  Villoria A, Azpiroz F, Burri E *et al.* Abdomino-phrenic dyssynergia in patients with abdominal bloating and distension. *Am J Gastroenterol* 106:815–819, 2011.

44  Salvioli B, Serra J, Azpiroz F and Malagelada J-R. Impaired small bowel gas propulsion in patients with bloating during intestinal lipid infusion. *Am J Gastroenterol* 2006;101:1853–1857.

45  Harder H, Serra J, Azpiroz F *et al.* Intestinal gas distribution determines abdominal symptoms. *Gut* 2003;52:1708–1713.

46  Passos MC, Tremolaterra F, Serra J *et al.* Impaired reflex control of intestinal gas transit in patients with abdominal bloating. *Gut* 2005;54:344–348.

47  Distrutti E, Salvioli B, Azpiroz F and Malagelada J-R. Rectal function and bowel habit in irritable bowel syndrome. *Am J Gastroenterol* 2004;99:131–137.

48  Caldarella MP, Azpiroz F and Malagelada J-R. Antro-fundic dysfunctions in functional dyspepsia. *Gastroenterology* 2003;124:1220–1229.

49  Notivol R, Saperas E, Coffin B *et al.* Gastric tone determines the sensitivity of the stomach to distension. *Gastroenterology* 1995;108:330–336.

50  Salvioli B, Serra J, Azpiroz F *et al.* Origin of gas retention and symptoms in patients with bloating. *Gastroenterology* 2005;128:574–579.

51  Tack J. Gastric motor and sensory function. *Curr Opin Gastroenterol* 2009;25:557–565.

52  Sarnelli G, Caenepeel P, Geypens B *et al.* Symptoms associated with impaired gastric emptying of solids and liquids in functional dyspepsia. *Am J Gastroenterol* 2003; 98:783–788.

53  Accarino A, Perez F, Azpiroz F *et al.* Intestinal gas and bloating: effect of prokinetic stimulation. *Am J Gastroenterol* 2008;103:2036–2042.

# Multiple Choice Questions

1 Irritable bowel syndrome is a condition:
   **A** Defined by specific symptom criteria.
   **B** An expression of chronic depression-anxiety.
   **C** Never associated with gut motor disturbances.
   **D** Commonly has an iatrogenic basis.
   **E** Psychopharmacologic treatment is mandatory.

Answer: A

2 Patients with irritable bowel syndrome who deserve in-depth pathophysiological investigation are:
   **A** Without appreciable psychopathological features.
   **B** Females only.
   **C** With chronic, severe symptoms unresponsive to conventional therapeutic measures.
   **D** Only if abnormal abdominal features are detected by imaging tests.
   **E** Only if nutritionally compromised.

Answer: C

3 Potentially useful diagnostic tests to investigate potential gut motor, disturbances in patients with irritable bowel syndrome include:
   **A** Intestinal manometric study.
   **B** Gammagraphic gastrointestinal transit study.
   **C** Quantitative CT imaging of abdominal contents and shape variations.
   **D** Gas challenge study.
   **E** All of the above.

Answer: E

## CHAPTER 12

# Gut Hypersensitivity Related Symptoms

*Adam D. Farmer, Madusha Peiris and Qasim Aziz*

Centre for Digestive Diseases, Blizard Institute, Wingate Institute of Neurogastroenterology, Barts and the London School of Medicine & Dentistry, Queen Mary University of London, London, UK

---

**Key points**
- Visceral hypersensitivity is a common feature of IBS, but is not pathognomonic.
- Visceral hypersensitivity often manifests clinically as chronic abdominal pain.
- A number of peripheral and central molecular mechanisms have been proposed to account for this epiphenomenon.
- A graduated stepwise approach to the treatment of visceral hypersensitivity is advocated.
- Treatments include psychological and pharmacological approaches.
- Psychological treatments include CBT and gut-focused hypnotherapy, although availability of these can be limited.
- Pharmacological therapies include antispasmodics, TCAs, SSRIs, neuropathic agents, nonabsorbable antibiotics and probiotics.
- Improvements in understanding the pathophysiological mechanisms that are proposed to underlie the cause of visceral hypersensitivity are facilitating the development of new treatments.

---

## Introduction

Functional gastrointestinal disorders (FGIDs) are a group of prevalent syndromes of which irritable bowel syndrome (IBS) is the most common. IBS is defined as symptoms of recurrent abdominal pain or discomfort associated with a marked change in bowel habit for at least six months, with symptoms experienced on at least three days of at least three months [1]. Furthermore, untreated abdominal pain is the symptom that is most likely to prompt a sufferer to seek medical advice and is often the most difficult for the clinician to successfully treat [2].

IBS has an estimated population prevalence of about 40% in the western world, accounting for between 40 and 60% of outpatient referral to

---

*Irritable Bowel Syndrome: Diagnosis and Clinical Management*, First Edition.
Edited by Anton Emmanuel and Eamonn M.M. Quigley.
© 2013 John Wiley & Sons, Ltd. Published 2013 by John Wiley & Sons, Ltd.

the gastroenterology clinic [3, 4]. Currently, there is no uniform investigational or treatment protocol for patients with FGID. FGIDs cause significant morbidity through a reduction in quality of life [1, 5]. Thus, with such a huge burden of disease the development of a complete understanding of the underlying pathophysiology of this complex disorder remains the prerequisite step on the road to the development of efficacious treatments. The aim of this chapter is to provide the reader with a succinct, yet comprehensive, review of the pathophysiological mechanisms that have been proposed to account for visceral hypersensitivity, the main hypothesis in accounting for IBS. In addition, the evidence base for treatments currently used specifically for the management of visceral pain in IBS is reviewed.

## Visceral hypersensitivity

Visceral pain is a common presenting symptom indicative of demonstrable pathology in wide range of different medical specialities. Many hypotheses have been proposed to explain the origin of this symptom in IBS but no single factor has achieved primacy in the literature, largely due to the significant heterogeneity of these disorders. However, a common feature of FGID is that patients often display a heightened sensitivity to experimental gut stimulation, termed visceral hypersensitivity. First reported in 1973, Ritchie, and subsequently others, observed in patients rectal hyperalgesia to mechanical distension of their sigmoid colon using an inflatable balloon [6]. Indeed rectal hypersensitivity to mechanical distension has been proposed to be a clinically useful discriminatory feature between IBS and other GI disorders [7, 8]. However, visceral hypersensitivity is not a *sine non qua* facet of IBS with a number of studies not reproducing these initial observations. Whilst the evidence for the role of visceral hypersensitivity in IBS is often conflicting it should be noted that the positive association between functional symptoms and rectal hypersensitivity were found in the studies with the largest number of patients [9, 10].

The observation of visceral hypersensitivity has spawned a considerable research effort from academia and the pharmaceutical industry alike in the attempt to identify the culpable molecular mechanisms that are responsible for this epiphenomenon. Therefore, the pathophysiology of visceral hypersensitivity may be conceptualized as being due to aberrant processes that may arise at any level of the visceral nociceptive pathway. Although the pathophysiology of visceral hypersensitivity has not been completely elucidated, several mechanisms have been proposed. These include subtle (low-grade) inflammation, psychosocial factors and changes in the sensorimotor function of the gastrointestinal (GI) tract, including both peripheral and central sensitization of the visceral afferent neuronal pathways.

## Visceral innervation

The GI tract receives dual innervation from spinal afferent neurones and the vagus nerve. This extrinsic innervation is complemented by intrinsic innervation, which comprises the enteric nervous system (ENS), which is separated into neurons including intrinsic primary afferent neurones (IPANs), which are primarily responsible for GI motility, as well as enteric glial cells that make up the majority of the cell population [11]. Three types of neurones are represented in this system. Firstly, Aβ fibres, which are large myelinated and thus conduct rapidly, which detect non-noxious stimuli. Secondly, small myelinated Aδ fibres and, finally, unmyelinated C-fibres, both of which detect and transmit noxious stimuli to the central nervous system (Table 12.1).

These primary sensory afferents display a degree of neuronal plasticity, referring to their ability to adapt in response to changes the internal milieu, thereby altering their transduction thresholds. For instance, in the process of peripheral sensitization, nociceptor activation thresholds are decreased and their excitability is increased. A nociceptor may be defined as '...*a primary sensory neuron that is activated in response to a* (noxious) *stimuli that is capable of causing damage...*' [12]. To achieve this function, a nociceptor requires a receptor, which is located at its peripheral terminus. When activated, the receptor triggers neuronal depolarization, ultimately culminating in the conscious awareness of pain. Nociceptors may be classified based on their physical characteristics, such as size, myelination and their responsiveness to specific stimuli, such as acid, heat or mechanical deformation. Some nociceptors may respond to more than one form of stimuli and are thus known as polymodal, whereas others may normally be silent but recruited in response to prolonged inflammation. Altered signalling may be mediated by neuronal ion channels, themselves activated through the release of inflammatory mediators, recruitment of previous silent nociceptors, or nerve damage/immunological mechanisms. Additionally, novel interstitial

**Table 12.1** A comparison of the different types of nociceptors within the gastrointestinal tract.

| Fibre type | Fibre diameter (µM) | Conduction velocity (m/s) | Myelination | Distribution | Type of pain experienced |
|---|---|---|---|---|---|
| Aδ | 2–5 | 5–15 | ++ | Skin surface, muscles, joints | Rapid, severe, localized |
| A/αβ | 5–20 | 70–120 | +++ | Spinal cord | Cutaneous touch and pressure |
| C | <2 | 0.5–2 | – | All tissues | Slow, diffuse, dull, aching |

cells, such as fibroblast-like cells, have also been implicated as class of excitable cells responsive to purine (ATP) stimulation in GI smooth muscle, thus demonstrating visceral hypersensitivity is modulated by both neuronal and non-neuronal cells [13].

Recent evidence has thrust enteric glial cells (EGC) into the spotlight and suggests they possess a more significant role than mere neuronal support structures. Indeed, they appear to be involved in GI motility as well as inflammation-induced IBS and, importantly, may act as neuronal precursors [14]. Laranjeira *et al.* recently demonstrated that EGC are multilineage progenitors of adult enteric neurones in response to altered microenvironment, such as in the case of injury to enteric glia. Increased gliogenesis was also observed in response to a gut inflammation and infection in a rodent model [15]. In IBS, EGC have been observed to be closely associated with immune infiltrates and mucosal activation of the immune system [16]. Taken together, these studies suggest that EGC may contribute to hypersensitivity induced by both inflammation and nerve injury by promoting neurogenesis, thereby increasing the population of responsive neurons.

## Peripheral visceral nociceptive afferent pathways

Noxious stimuli may cause the peripheral release of several inflammatory mediators such as $K^+$, $H^+$, adenosine triphosphate (ATP), 5-hydroxytryptamine (5-HT), bradykinins and prostaglandins [17, 18]. These may elicit a number of effects, including the activation and peripheral sensitization of nociceptive afferent nerves, by reducing their transduction thresholds and by inducing the expression and recruitment of previously silent nociceptors. The main consequence of these inflammatory mediators is an increase in pain sensitivity at the site of injury, known as primary hyperalgesia [19]. A number of ion channels, neurotransmitter receptors and trophic factors have been implicated in the development of peripheral sensitization. Whilst it is beyond the scope of this chapter to examine all of the possible mechanisms previously studied in the literature, some of the more important advances in our understanding of the molecular mechanisms of peripheral sensitisation are highlighted.

### Transient receptor potential vallinoid receptors

Transient receptor potential vallinoid (TRPV) receptors1 and 4 are members of a larger family of TRPV channels that serve many sensory functions ranging from hearing to mechanosensory transduction [20, 21]. The TRPV 1 receptor was first identified and cloned by Caterina *et al.* in 1997; it is expressed on small-to-medium-sized nerve fibres throughout the nervous system and is a nonselective cation channel [22]. The TRPV1 receptor may be activated by capsaicin and its analogues as well as noxious heat and is thought to play an important role in mechanotransduction in the GI tract and to the development and maintenance of visceral hypersensitivity [20, 23]. When activated, the TRPV1 receptor evokes a sensation of burning pain and with concomitant release of substance P (SP) neurogenic inflammation may ensue. Hydrogen ions strongly potentiate activation of the TRPV1 channel [24]. Thus, TRPV1 is considered to mediate the process of peripheral sensitization and several inflammatory mediators have been demonstrated to reduce the threshold for TRPV1 activation, including bradykinin, adenosine and ATP.

In humans there is a wealth of evidence linking TRPV1 with visceral hypersensitivity. For instance, a recent study by Akbar *et al.* demonstrated a 3.5-fold increase in the density of TRPV1 immuno-reactive fibres in the colonic biopsies of patients with IBS compared to healthy controls [25]. Furthermore, in rat models, TRPV1 receptor antagonists have been found to ameliorate visceral hypersensitivity [26]. These observations have led to considerable interest in the research and development of orally bioavailable agents that may modulate the TRPV1 receptor. Both TRPV1 agonists, which are postulated to desensitize the receptor, and TRPV1 antagonists are currently being evaluated. Early results from human studies evaluating this novel class of analgesic have yielded promising results [27, 28]. However, early phase 1 studies of the TRPV1 antagonist AMG517 have raised safety concerns as they have caused hyperthermia in some patients [29].

TRPV4 is a mechanotransductive, osmosensitive channel that has been recently associated with visceral hypersensitivity [30]. Further evidence for TRPV4's role in visceral hypersensitivity comes from an elegant study recently reported by Cenac *et al.*, where a TRPV4 agonist induced visceral hypersensitivity in response to colorectal distension in mice, although this effect was lost in TRPV4-/- knockouts [31].

## Protease activated receptors

Four types of protease activated receptors (PAR) have been described, of which PAR-1 and PAR-2 are expressed on spinal afferents and contain calcitonin gene related peptide (CGRP) [32]. PAR-2 receptors are activated by mast cell tryptase and are G-protein coupled receptors [33]. PAR-1 is activated by a number of mediators, including thrombin and trypsin, and are ubiquitously expressed throughout the GI tract [34]. Interestingly, increased expression of PAR-1 has been demonstrated in patients with inflammatory bowel disease, although this expression was higher in patients with Crohn's disease compared to those with ulcerative colitis [35]. This study provides a mechanistic rationale for inflammation-induced sensitization with the GI tract. Whilst the traditional definition of IBS has precluded it being an (occult) disorder of inflammation within the GI tract, recent evidence presented by Cenac *et al.* observed an increase in proteolytic enzyme activity from colonic biopsies of patients with IBS compared to controls [36]. The supernatant from IBS patients, but not controls, released mediators that sensitized cultured murine sensory neurons. This sensitization was prevented by a serine protease inhibitor and in those mice lacking functional PAR-2. In addition, supernatants from IBS patients, when administered intra-colonically to mice, caused somatic and visceral hyperalgesia; such effects were inhibited by serine protease inhibitors, a PAR-2 antagonist, and were absent in PAR-2-deficient mice. It is interesting to note that PAR-2 closely interacts with the TRPV4 receptor, potentially providing a link between these molecular mechanisms in causing visceral hyperalgesia [37]. Human studies examining the efficacy of PAR-2 receptor antagonists are eagerly awaited as they represent an attractive therapeutic target.

## The nitric oxide pathway

Three nitric oxide (NO) synthase isoforms (inducible, neurogenic and endothelial) catalyse the formation of endogenous NO. Inducible NO (NOS2) and neurogenic NO (NOS1) are ubiquitously present within the nervous system and the endothelium, and endogenous NO may modulate the efficacy and tolerability of opioid analgesics [38]. The NO pathway also aids in the regulation of GI motility and mucosal integrity [39]. Lithium, widely used in the treatment of bipolar disorder, mediates some of its actions through the NO pathway, and it has been recently shown by Shamshiri *et al.* that chronic lithium administration attenuates sensitivity to colonic distension, increasing nociceptive thresholds and decreasing stool frequency in a visceral hypersensitivity rat model [40]. A number of studies exploring the role of NO in visceral sensation have shown increased levels of NO synthase in the spinal cord of animal models of colitis as well as increased levels of NO synthase positive neurons within the rostral ventromedial medulla [41]. In addition, Tjong *et al.* demonstrated increased expression of NO in a neonatal maternal separation (NMS) model of IBS where L-NAME (non-selective inhibitor) and L-NINA (selective neuronal NOS inhibitor) attenuated visceral hyperalgesia [42]. Further evidence of the role of NO in pain sensation is provided from human trials where the nitric oxide synthase inhibitor L-NMMA increased the discomfort threshold in IBS patients, while there was no difference between treatment and placebo group in healthy volunteers [43]. Taken together, these studies suggest that the NO pathway is a potential therapeutic target.

## Mast cells, enterochromaffin cells and 5-hydroxytriptamine

Up to 20% of patients with IBS report that their symptoms are initiated following an episode of acute infection, which may be GI or non-GI; a phenomenon known as post-infectious IBS (PI-IBS) [44]. In this group, increased numbers of enterochromaffin cells (EC), mast cells and T-lymphocytes may be observed in the lamina propria of colonic biopsies, suggesting the presence of a low-grade inflammatory infiltrate [45]. Piche *et al.* have shown that the degree of mast cell infiltration is positively associated with the degree of fatigue and depression in IBS patients [46]. Mast cells *per se* have been shown not to modulate visceral nociception but are, nevertheless, essential in the development of visceral hypersensitivity; in mast cell deficient rats, the development of visceral hypersensitivity can be ameliorated with mast cell stabilizers in a dose-dependent manner [47, 48]. Interestingly, treatment with the mast cell stabilizer, disodium cromoglycate, in conjunction with exclusion diets may be of some symptomatic benefit in a small percentage of patients with diarrhoea-predominant IBS [49]. Recent interest has focused on another mast cell stabilizer, ketotifen. A recent study by Klooker *et al.* examined rectal sensitivity in a group of IBS patients before and after treatment with ketotifen or placebo [50]. Ketotifen, but not placebo, reduced rectal sensitivity, significantly decreased abdominal pain and improved quality of life. Further larger scale trials are now underway to substantiate these initial findings.

EC and mast cells contain serotonin (5-HT), one of the major neurotransmitters of the ENS, which is involved in signal transduction of visceral stimuli, in addition to effecting changes in GI motility [51]. Increases in 5-HT bioavailability, through increased availability and reduced uptake, have been observed in models of post-inflammatory visceral hypersensitivity and may manifest as changes in gut sensorimotor function. Pharmacotherapeutic interventions directed towards the 5-HT pathway, most notably 5-HT$_3$ antagonists, 5-HT$_4$ agonists and most recently 5-HT$_{1A}$ antagonists, have had, at best, only a modest effect in the modulation of visceral pain and the restoration of abnormal bowel habit to normal. However, a number of drugs targeting this system in the treatment of IBS have made it to market. For example, the 5-HT$_4$ agonist, tegaserod, was shown to have a beneficial effect on symptom relief in patients with constipation-predominant IBS, and was approved by the Food and Drug Administration (FDA) in 2002 [52]. In addition, the 5-HT$_3$ antagonist alosetron, was demonstrated to improve abdominal pain and stool patterns in diarrhoea-predominant IBS patients, being approved by the FDA in 2000 [53]. Whilst initially these new treatments offered new therapeutic avenues for patients, evidence emerged for the existence of serious adverse side effects. Both tegaserod and alosetron were withdrawn due to increased cardiovascular side effects and ischaemic colitis respectively [54–56]. Subsequently, however, alosetron has been re-introduced in the USA albeit with a restricted license.

### Cannabinoid receptors

Cannabinoid receptor 1 (CB1) is expressed within cholinergic nerves and sensory afferents in the human ileum and colon, with their activation inhibiting activation of cholinergic-induced smooth muscle contraction, while cannabinoid receptor 2 (CB2) is present in neurons within the rat ileum [57]. Indeed, a rodent study using colorectal distension demonstrated that agonists of both receptor types decreased visceromotor (VMR) responses while antagonist treatment resulted in colitis-induced hyperalgesia [58]. *In vitro* studies have demonstrated that the CB1 receptor plays a key role in reducing motility in human ileum and colon [59, 60]. However, a recent randomized, double-blind study reported that in both IBS patients and healthy volunteers groups, there was no significant difference between placebo and delta-9-tetrahydrocannabinol (a mixed CB1/CB2 receptor agonist) treated subjects when subjects were asked to rate discomfort in response to graded rectal distension [61]. These results suggest that further investigation is required to clarify the role of CB receptors in human visceral pain sensation. Nevertheless, CB receptors may affect other visceral pain mechanisms by, for example, regulating colonic inflammation. Activation of both CB1 and CB2 receptors appears to confer protection in experimental models of colitis, with increased CB1 receptor expression also observed in diseased animals [62]. A further study showed that a CB2 agonist protected against inflammatory processes in a mustard oil model of colitis, which involves neurogenic mechanisms [63]. Therefore, there is evidence to suggest that the cannabinoid receptor family may be involved in visceral pain mechanisms. However, there are many unanswered questions and further studies are required to conclusively define a role for these receptors in gut hypersensitivity.

### Prostaglandin receptors

Prostanoids are key molecules involved in mediating hyperalgesia; they include PG, leukotrienes and thromboxanes. All three are synthesized from arachandonic acid using either the cyclo-oxygenase (PG D, E and F and thromboxane) or lipo-oxygenase (leukotriene $A_4$, $B_4$, $C_4$ and $D_4$) pathways. $PGE_2$ is an important mediator of both peripheral and central sensitization and acts via four g-protein coupled receptors EP-1–4, which are all expressed in the nervous system; however, the EP-1 receptor appears to play the most significant role of the four [64].

In the periphery, the process of inflammation releases prostaglandins from activated immune cells and sympathetic nerve terminals which act on prostaglandin EP receptors expressed on vagal and spinal afferent endings, resulting in the sensitization of sensory nerves [65]. Studies on rodent mesenteric afferents show $PGE_2$ increases neuronal discharge in a dose-dependent manner [65]. Furthermore, increased activation of mesenteric afferents by bradykinin has been shown to be dependent on $PGE_2$ [66]. A study by Sarkar *et al.*, which examined the effect of EP-1 receptor antagonist ZD6416 in healthy volunteers who received a dose of hydrochloric acid or saline into the lower oesophagus, revealed that secondary hyperalgesia was reduced in the group pre-treated with the antagonist [67]. Therefore, it is clear that prostaglandins have an important role both in peripheral and central sensitization mechanisms involved in visceral hypersensitivity.

## Voltage gated sodium channels

There are ten functional subtypes of the voltage gated sodium channels (VGSCs), which gives VGSCs a central role in the genesis of nerve impulse conduction and makes them, therefore, targets for clinically efficacious analgesics such as lignocaine. Data from the last decade have shown that certain VGSC isoforms ($Na_v$1.3–1.9) are predominantly expressed in peripheral sensory afferent neurones, that the expression and functional properties of these isoforms can be dynamically regulated *in vivo* in response to axonal injury or inflammation and that they may play an important role in the generation of peripheral sensitization [68]. Arguably some of the most observations have emanated from genetic studies that have identifying rare mutations of the sodium channel gene SCN9A that encodes $Na_v$ 1.7. Gain of function missense mutations have been found to cause primary erythermalgia and paroxysmal extreme pain disorder [69] whilst nonsense mutations result in loss of function leading to conditions known as channelopathy-associated insensitivity to pain [70]. Recent studies have implicated VGSC in the pathophysiology of IBS. For instance, Yiangou *et al.* demonstrated an increase in the immunoreactivity of $Na_v$ 1.7 fibres in IBS patients with rectal hypersensitivity in comparison to healthy controls [71]. Furthermore, in a double-blind crossover design, Verne *et al.* observed that the introduction of rectal lignocaine reduced both rectal sensitivity and abdominal pain [72]. Whilst these studies provide direct and indirect evidence for the role of VGSC in the pathophysiology, one must interpret these data with a degree of caution due to the relatively small numbers of participants in these studies. Nevertheless, these findings suggest that VGSCs are intimately involved in pain transduction and they potentially present an exciting and novel therapeutic target for the analgesics of the future [73].

## Acid sensing ion channels

Tissue damage causes a complex cascade of effects causing local tissue acidosis and, ultimately, pain. Sensory manifestation of this pain may be caused, as we have outlined, by receptors such as TRPV1 in response to acidosis. In addition, acid sensing ion channels (ASICs), of which there are three functional subclasses, are proton gated cation channels ubiquitously expressed throughout the enteric nervous system [74]. An ASIC comprises two transmembrane domains and is a nonvoltage gated sodium selective channel on sensory neurones; it is closed at a pH of 7.4 but is activated below a pH of 7.0. Whilst ASICs are likely to play a role in nociception, and thus visceral hypersensitivity, human experimental evidence is, at the current time, lacking. However, murine models of ASIC knockout mice have demonstrated reduced visceral sensitivity to mechanical distension in comparison to controls [75]. In addition, ASICs have been shown to contribute to visceral sensitivity in a zymogen induced murine model of IBS [76]. In relation to human FGID, ASICs may represent particularly attractive potential therapeutic candidates in visceral hypersensitivity emanating from the foregut pathologies such as gastro-oesophageal reflux and nonerosive reflux disease, as gastric acid has been implicated in the pathophysiology of these disorders [77].

## Tachykinin receptors

Tachykinins are a family of neuropeptides that includes SP, neurokinin A (NKA) and B (NKB), and are well-characterized excitatory neurotransmitters. Tachykinins exert their biological effects by acting on the NK1, NK2 and NK3 g-coupled protein receptors. SP and NKA are released by primary sensory afferent endings both centrally and peripherally, while NKB is found in the spinal cord and CNS. Studies in rats show SP to be present primarily in neurovascular bundles innervating the upper jejunum, while there is less innervation to the terminal ileum [78] and release of SP facilitates the activation of further prostaglandins and histamine from mast cells. In two animal models of colonic hypersensitivity, the NK1 receptor antagonist TAK-637 returned VMR responses to basal level in animals with colonic inflammation but had no effect on animals with normosensitive colons [79]. However, in a human pilot study, the NK1 receptor antagonist CJ-11974 did not demonstrate a significant decrease in discomfort ratings to colorectal distension in IBS patients [80], although there was a decrease in negative emotional response suggesting that CJ-11974 may exert central effects.

There is conflicting evidence on the role of NK2 receptors in visceral hypersensitivity. While some groups show central as well as peripheral administration of NK2 receptor antagonists reduce visceral pain responses in hypersensitive animals [81, 82], there are others who have found no effect [83]. It is likely that this is due to differences in study design. However, further studies are required to clarify the role NK2 plays in modulating visceral pain sensation.

Rats treated with the NK3 receptor antagonist SR 142, 801 had decreased VMR responses to colorectal distension (CRD) and decreased neuronal firing in electrophysiology experiments, while the agonist, senkatide, increased sensitivity [81]. Similar to the human NK1 antagonist study, the NK3 antagonist Talnetant SB223412 does not significantly alter rectal sensation in healthy volunteers or IBS patients [84]. Overall, the complex role of tachykinins in inflammation-induced pain mechanisms within the GI tract warrants further investigation both in human *in vivo* and *in vitro* studies in order to clearly identify a role for these receptors as therapeutic targets.

## Cholecystokinin receptors

Choleycystokinin (CCK) is released from enteroendocrine (EEC) cells following ingestion of meals rich in protein or fat. Thus, its primary actions are to inhibit gastric emptying and food intake, and stimulate pancreatic enzyme secretion, both of which are induced by stimulation of vagal afferents. Indeed, vagal afferent activation by CCK increases intracellular calcium levels and afferents have been shown to express CCK1 receptor [85]. Collective studies show that CCK regulates vagal afferent activity by post-prandial stimulation of afferents signalling satiety, while low levels of CCK signal for appetite stimulation [86]. In IBS patient studies, the level of CCK is significantly elevated compared to controls following lipid infusion, and post-infectious IBS patients also had increased levels of CCK compared to controls, suggesting that CCK release activates sensory nerves [87]. The agonist effect of CCK has been demonstrated by the use of CCK-octapeptide where sensory thresholds are decreased to rectal distension [88]. Studies using the CCK antagonist loxiglumide demonstrated that IBS patients had improved symptoms with less abdominal pain and restoration of normal bowel habit [89]. However, results from large clinical trials have been conflicting, with some reporting that dexloxiglumide (a competitive antagonist of $CCK_1$) has limited efficacy in C-IBS with no significant improvement of symptoms while others have shown improvement of symptoms although only 48% of participants were responders [90]. Therefore, collective results from these studies show a degree of promise for this class of receptor. However, further trials are required to determine its potential as a viable treatment for visceral hypersensitivity.

## Kappa opioid receptor

All three opioid receptor types, κ, μ, δ, have a role in visceral sensation and are found in the CNS as well as peripheral nerves. While μ opioid agonists relieve pain, their many side effects, including constipation, often prevent them from being clinically useful in the treatment of IBS. The κ receptor, however, does not have these effects and has therefore become a target for IBS pain relief. The κ receptors are found in the myenteric plexus within the stomach and proximal colon and appear to reduce activity of visceral afferents which modulate gut motility in the rat [91]. Fedotozine, a κ receptor agonist is effective in increasing the discomfort and pain perception threshold in healthy volunteers and IBS patients, respectively, and a large multicentre study reported decreased abdominal pain and bloating [92–94]. Asimodaline, another κ receptor agonist is also effective in treating patients with diarrhoea-predominant IBS as well as those with altered bowel habits, following a chronic dosing schedule [95]. This group of receptors hold great promise for the treatment of symptoms associated with visceral hypersensitivity and future studies shall evaluate the use of these drugs in the clinic.

## Central sensitization

Sensitization is not solely confined to the periphery. When a noxious stimuli is transmitted from the periphery, it induces a constellation of changes at the spinal dorsal horn by the activation of intracellular signalling cascades (comprehensively reviewed by Anand *et al.* [96]). This may lead to central sensitization and amplification of the nociceptive response to the stimuli (secondary hyperalgesia), and previously innocuous stimuli may provoke a nociceptive response (allodynia). Whilst these observations have long been recognized in somatic pain, increasingly central sensitization is thought to play a central role in the development and maintenance of visceral hypersensitivity [97, 98]. In a landmark paper, Sarkar *et al.* demonstrated the concept of central sensitization in a reproducible oesophageal model in humans, in which hydrochloric acid was infused into the healthy distal oesophagus [97]. Pain thresholds were not only reduced in the acid-exposed distal region but also in the adjacent proximal unexposed region. This effect of central sensitization was prolonged, lasting up to five hours after 30 minutes of acid exposure, suggesting that the duration and magnitude of central sensitization of the nonexposed proximal oesophagus was related directly to the intensity of acid exposure in the distal oesophagus.

$PGE_2$ and the n-methyl d-aspartate (NMDA) receptor have been elucidated as the most important molecular factors in the development of central sensitization at the spinal dorsal horn [99]. Human pharmacological studies have demonstrated that antagonism of the $PGE_2$ or the NMDA receptor prevents the development of central sensitization within the oesophagus, and antagonism of the NMDA receptor with ketamine may even reverse established visceral hypersensitivity [67, 100]. Central sensitization may also occur after a noxious stimulus is applied to an anatomically distant site. For instance, oesophageal sensitization may occur after a noxious stimulus is applied to the duodenum and balloon distension in the left colon may result in rectal sensitization [101, 102]. In patients with IBS, following repetitive distension of the sigmoid colon, central sensitization may ensue, as manifested by rectal hyperalgesia and increased viscerosomatic referral to experimental rectal distension [10].

## Treatment of visceral hypersensitivity

The most common symptomalogical sequelae of visceral hypersensitivity, and one that most readily provokes a patient to seek medical help, is abdominal pain. Indeed, evidence suggests that the symptom of abdominal pain is often the most bothersome with the greatest negative impact on quality of life [103]. Whilst central to the definition of IBS, it can often be the most challenging symptom to treat effectively. Despite a number of evidence-based guidelines from national societies such as the British Society of Gastroenterology and the American College of Gastroenterology, there remains controversy over the most effective method of managing IBS [104]. It is interesting that Khan and Chang have recently proposed a *'graduated treatment approach with a palliative coping strategy'*, whereby treatment is escalated from education, to dietary manipulation, to behavioural therapies and, finally, pharmacotherapy dependant on, and titrated to, symptoms [105]. We would entirely concur with these sentiments from our experience that the therapeutic potential of the doctor–patient relationship should not be underestimated in exchanging information and planning management. The focus of the next part of this chapter is, however, on effective evidence-based therapies for visceral pain. In this section, the evidence for established treatments for visceral pain in IBS, which include pharmacotherapy, behavioural and alternative therapies, is examined.

## Antispasmodics

The visceral pain suffered by patients with IBS has been suggested to be partially due to intracolonic smooth muscle, and hence the rationale for the older terminology of 'spastic colon'. Therefore, it is not surprising that smooth muscle relaxants, and hence anticholinergic agents, have been used in the treatment of IBS with some success. For instance, a meta-analysis by Ford *et al.* demonstrated the efficacy of antispasmodics *per se* in a global reduction in pain and symptoms. Specifically, 39% patients treated with antispasmodics had persistent symptoms after treatment compared 56% of those treated with placebo (relative risk 0.68, 95% confidence interval 0.57 to 0.81). However, it must be noted that there was statistically significant heterogeneity detected between studies, thus suggesting a degree of publication bias. Interestingly, the overall number needed to treat to prevent symptoms persisting in one patient was five (95% confidence interval 4–9). In addition, the same study found that specific antispasmodics such as hyoscine, cimetropium, otilonium, trimebutine and pinaverium showed a reduction in abdominal pain in comparison to placebo. Of particular interest was that mebeverine did not exhibit any benefit over placebo, despite its widespread use in UK practice. Whilst long-term safety data are lacking, antispasmodics are generally well tolerated although anticholinergic side effects are occasionally observed, such as blurred vision and dry mouth.

## Tricyclic antidepressants

The exact mechanisms by which tricylic antidepressants (TCAs) exert their analgesic effects are yet to be completely understood. TCAs inhibit reuptake of noradrenaline and 5-HT as well as influence both histaminergic and cholinergic transmission. It has been postulated that the analgesic mechanism of action of TCAs is by retarding GI transit, treating comorbid anxiety and depression and modulating ascending visceral afferent sensory and central transmission [106]. Morgan *et al.*, using functional brain imaging techniques, evaluated the central effects of TCAs on pain perception in females with IBS in response to auditory stress and rectal distension [107]. They found that in patients treated with amitriptylline there was a reduction in brain activity in areas such as the anterior cingulate cortex, an area which has been demonstrated to play a role in the affective motivational component of pain [108].

However, these data should be interpreted in the context of the findings reported Gorelick *et al.* [109]. In a double-blind study, they evaluated the pain thresholds to somatic and visceral pain in a small number of healthy volunteers, before and after 21 days of double-blind 50 mg amitriptyline. They found amitriptyline had no effect on perception of rectal and oesophageal distension in the absence of change in luminal compliance; thus suggesting that lack of effect on perception is not due to altered biomechanics of the visceral wall. However, pain thresholds to electrical somatic stimulation increased suggesting a differential effect of TCA on pain perception. Nevertheless, it must be noted that this study was only performed in a small group of healthy volunteers and the run in period for the group treated with amitriptylline was relatively short. More recently, Thoua *et al.* examined whether amitriptyline, in an open label study, altered the response to acute stress in IBS patients which included rectal electrosensitivity [110]. This study observed that patients treated with amitriptyline had a reduction in stress-induced rectal sensitivity that was independent of autonomic tone.

Other TCAs evaluated in clinical trials include imipramine, clomipramine, trimepramine, desipramine and nortriptylline. Two recent meta-analyses have addressed the question of whether TCAs are helpful in treating abdominal pain in IBS. Ford *et al.* identified nine clinical trials, which had studied 575 patients [111]. Of the 319 patients who had received active treatment, 41.4% had continued symptoms compared to 59.8% of those treated with placebo. This equated to a relative risk (reduction) of IBS symptoms persisting of 0.68 (95% confidence interval 0.56–0.83) in those treated with TCA. Interestingly, Rahimi *et al.* performed a meta-analysis of seven trials of TCAs in IBS and reported a pooled relative risk for treatment response was 1.93 (95% confidence interval 1.34–2) [112]. This meta-analysis noted the different dosages of TCAs across the included studies and that side effects were often a limiting factor. We concur with the authors suggestions that commencing with a low dose, titrating it up to the desired therapeutic dose may minimize troublesome side effects for patients, the most notable being somnolence, dry mouth and constipation.

## Selective serotonin reuptake inhibitors

Selective serotonin reuptake inhibitors' (SSRIs) mechanism of action is through the selective pre-synaptic blockade of the serotonin reuptake transporter, thereby increasing the quantity of serotonin within the synaptic space. Whilst evidence is somewhat lacking concerning the efficacy of SSRIs in the treatment of visceral pain, it has been demonstrated that they do improve well-being with their effect being adjunctive with TCAs [111]. Tack *et al.* evaluated the effect of the SSRI citalopram in 23 IBS patients in a crossover design that compared six weeks of treatment with placebo [113]. Citalopram was found to significantly improve abdominal pain compared with placebo. This therapeutic effect was independent of effects on anxiety and depression. These promising initial results need replicating a larger cohort of patients with IBS but do confirm that SSRIs have efficacy in treating visceral pain associated with IBS.

## Neuropathic agents

Pregabalin is a novel second-generation $\alpha 2\delta$ ligand that is structurally related to $\gamma$-aminobutyric acid (GABA). Pregabalin binds to the $\alpha 2\delta$ subunit of CNS voltage-dependent calcium channel in the CNS. Pregabalin decreases the release of neurotransmitters, including glutamate, noradrenaline and SP, and increases neuronal GABA levels by producing a dose-dependent increase in glutamic acid decarboxylase activity [114]. A recent study by Ravnefjord *et al.* evaluated the effects of oral pregabalin on the visceral pain related viscerosomatic and autonomic cardiovascular responses to CRD and colonic compliance in rats [115]. They demonstrated that pregabalin reduced the viscerosomatic and autonomic responses associated with distension-induced visceral pain. Houghton *et al.* performed a randomized, double-blind, placebo-controlled, parallel-group study in which 26 patients with IBS received three weeks titrated oral pregabalin or placebo control [116]. Rectal sensitivity, using a barostat, was assessed both before and after treatment. They found that pregabalin increased sensory thresholds to colorectal distension to normal levels in patients, thus confirming the role for pregabalin in the management of visceral hypersensitivity. However, it must be noted that this paper only evaluated those who had rectal hypersensitivity in a relatively small number of patients with IBS, so further studies confirming and replicating these findings are now needed.

## Behavioural therapies

Behavioural therapies, including cognitive behavioural therapy (CBT), dynamic psychotherapy and hypnotherapy all alleviate the symptoms associated with IBS to a variable degree [111]. The role of CBT was specifically addressed by Lackner *et al.* where patients with moderate to severe IBS were randomized to receive psychotherapist-delivered CBT, self-administered CBT or usual care [117]. Those who received therapist-administered CBT and self-administered CBT had superior rates of reporting of adequate relief from abdominal pain in comparison to those receiving usual care (60.9% and 72% vs 7.4%, respectively). Gut-focused hypnotherapy, where the aim is to reassure the patient regarding their symptoms and with the aid of hypnosis improve gut-related symptoms through changes in function, influencing sensitivity, spasm or section, has been evaluated in a number of studies. Whorwell *et al.* demonstrated significant improvement in abdominal pain in a cohort of patient with refractory IBS with a recent Cochrane review of concluding that hypnotherapy was more efficacious than usual therapy [118, 119]. Given the absence of side effects associated with more traditional pharmacological therapies, hypnotherapy represents an excellent treatment option. However, limited therapist availability often limits accessibility for patients. Overall, psychological therapies can be extremely useful, although patient selection is key. In particular, therapy should be specifically directly at those patients who are open and amenable to receive such treatment, such as those who are willing to acquiesce to the notion that there is a significant psychological component to their symptoms, as psychological treatments are more likely to be successful.

## Probiotics/antibiotics

Probiotics are live microorganisms which when administered in adequate amounts confer a health benefit to the host and, particularly in IBS, positively influence digestive health. The most studied probiotics in relation to IBS belong to the geni *Lactobacillus* and *Bifidobacteria*. Whilst the mechanism of action of probiotics is incompletely understood, it has been suggested that probiotics can enhance gut barrier function, by inhibiting pathogen binding and through the modulation of gut inflammatory response. Probiotics also reduce visceral hypersensitivity associated with both inflammation and psychological stress and can alter colonic fermentation and stabilize the colonic microbiota [120].

Probiotics can vary in terms of their species, strains, doses and preparation, thereby making direct comparisons between studies difficult. For instance, a recent study by Brenner *et al.* undertook a systematic review of the randomized controlled trials that evaluated the role of probiotics in the treatment of IBS [121]. Of the 16 trials that met their selection criteria for inclusion in the review, 11 studies showed poor study design with inadequate blinding, insufficient trial length, small sample size and/or lack of intention to treat analysis. In this review the authors found that *Bifidobacterium infantis 35624* improved abdominal pain/discomfort, bloating/distension and/or bowel movement difficulty compared with placebo. Recent interest has focused on the use of rifaximin semi-synthetic, rifamycin-based antibiotic that has minimal absorption from the GI tract. A recent phase 3, double-blind, placebo-controlled study by Pimentel *et al.* showed that two weeks treatment with rifaximin reduced abdominal pain at four weeks and ten weeks post treatment [122]. Side effects were similar in both treatment and placebo arm suggesting an excellent safety profile.

## Conclusions

The clinical observation that patients with FGID may be hypersensitive to experimental visceral stimulation has had a considerable influence on the direction of research in the field for the last three decades. This breadth of knowledge has been achieved through convergent and complementary research strategies from a number of academic disciplines that include neurogastroenterology, molecular pharmacology, neurophysiology and psychology, to name but a few. However, if the scientific community is to further unravel the mysteries of visceral hypersensitivity in FGID, we need to adopt a tailored, individualistic approach by characterizing our patients in terms of their clinical phenotype, genetics and visceral nociceptive physiology. In conjunction with advances being made in our understanding of the molecular mechanisms that underlie visceral hypersensitivity, including therapeutic agents that target these, this may revolutionise the management of IBS in the future.

---

### CASE STUDY 12.1

Mrs Mary Russell is a 38-year-old nurse with a recent physician confirmed diagnosis of irritable bowel syndrome. She has been extensively investigated and results have shown normal haematological, biochemical and hormonal profiles, normal upper endoscopy with histology, normal coeliac serology and two negative lactose hydrogen breath tests. She has been referred from secondary care with continued symptoms of abdominal discomfort without alteration of bowel habit and is requesting further investigations. She has been having a stressful time at work and feels this has exacerbated her symptoms. She describes anhedonia.

Initially, the first consultation was extremely confrontational from the patient's point of view as she felt that an important diagnosis was being missed. After a lengthy discussion, and explanation in simple terms, she began to understand that the underlying diagnosis was visceral hypersensitivity due to IBS. After careful and empathetic explanations she also accepted she was depressed. Treatment options, both psychological and pharmacological, were discussed but Mrs Russell did not want to pursue the former as she did not feel that these would be helpful. She was initially commenced on buscopan and low dose amitriptylline and was counselled as to the potential side effects of the latter. At an early follow-up appointment, her symptoms had eased but not completely and she was keen to escalate her drug treatment; she was thus commenced on fluoxetine. At review, six months later, she felt significantly better, she was no longer troubled with abdominal pain and had started to enjoy life again and was discharged back to her primary care physician.

**Comment**
This case illustrates the importance of the diagnosis of IBS being made without retorting to overinvestigation. Taking time over simple discussions regarding the pathophysiology of IBS and building the doctor–patient relationship is, in our experience, time well spent. Involving the patient in treatment decisions helps give them a sense of control over their illness. Adopting a stepwise, escalating treatment strategy, including treatment of the comorbid depression, was, in this case, the key to a successful outcome.

## Useful web sites

- Wellcome Institute: http://www.wellcome.ac.uk/en/pain/microsite/index.html
- BSG Guidelines on the Management of IBS: gut.bmj.com/content/56/12/1770.full.pdf
- American Neurogastroenterology & Motility Society: http://www.motilitysociety.org/clinician/manuscripts.php
- National Health Service: www.nhs.uk/conditions/irritable-bowel-syndrome
- Wingate Institute of Neurogastroenterology: www.icms.qmul.ac.uk/neurogastro

## References

1  Drossman DA. *Rome III: the functional gastrointestinal disorders.* 2006, Degnon Associates, McLean, VA.

2  Sandler RS, Drossman DA, Nathan HP and McKee DC. Symptom complaints and health care seeking behavior in subjects with bowel dysfunction. *Gastroenterology* 1984;87:314–318.

3  Jones R and Lydeard S. Irritable bowel syndrome in the general population. *BMJ* 1992;304:87–90.

4  Talley NJ, Zinsmeister AR, Van Dyke C and Melton LJ, 3rd. Epidemiology of colonic symptoms and the irritable bowel syndrome. *Gastroenterology* 1991;101:927–934.

5  Drossman DA, Li Z, Andruzzi E *et al*. U.S. householder survey of functional gastrointestinal disorders. Prevalence, sociodemography, and health impact. *Dig Dis Sci* 1993;38: 1569–1580.

6  Ritchie J. Pain from distension of the pelvic colon by inflating a balloon in the irritable colon syndrome. *Gut* 1973;14:125–132.

7  Wingate DL. The irritable bowel syndrome. *Gastroenterol Clin North Am* 1991;20: 351–362.

8  Bouin M, Plourde V, Boivin M *et al*. Rectal distention testing in patients with irritable bowel syndrome: sensitivity, specificity, and predictive values of pain sensory thresholds. *Gastroenterology* 2002;122:1771–1777.

9  Mertz H, Naliboff B, Munakata J *et al*. Altered rectal perception is a biological marker of patients with irritable bowel syndrome. *Gastroenterology* 1995;109:40–52.

10  Munakata J, Naliboff B, Harraf F *et al*. Repetitive sigmoid stimulation induces rectal hyperalgesia in patients with irritable bowel syndrome. *Gastroenterology* 1997;112: 55–63.

11  Jessen KR. Glial cells. *Int J Biochem Cell Biol* 2004;36:1861–1867.

12  Kumazawa T, Mizumura K, Minagawa M and Tsujii Y. Sensitizing effects of bradykinin on the heat responses of the visceral nociceptor. *J Neurophysiol* 1991;66:1819–1824.

13  Kurahashi M, Zheng H, Dwyer L *et al*. A functional role for the 'fibroblast-like cells' in gastrointestinal smooth muscles. *J Physiol* 2011;589:697–710.

14  Joseph NM, He S, Quintana E *et al*. Enteric glia are multipotent in culture but primarily form glia in the adult rodent gut. *J Clin Invest* 2011;121:3398–3411.

15  Laranjeira C, Sandgren K, Kessaris N *et al*. Glial cells in the mouse enteric nervous system can undergo neurogenesis in response to injury. *J Clin Invest* 2011;121:3412–3424.

16  Tornblom H, Lindberg G, Nyberg B and Veress B. Full-thickness biopsy of the jejunum reveals inflammation and enteric neuropathy in irritable bowel syndrome. *Gastroenterology* 2002;123:1972–1979.

17  Yu S and Ouyang A. TRPA1 in Bradykinin-induced Mechano-hypersensitivity of Vagal C Fibers in Guinea Pig Esophagus. *Am J Physiol Gastrointest Liver Physiol* 2009;296(2): G255–G265.

18  Jones RC 3rd, Xu L and Gebhart GF. The mechanosensitivity of mouse colon afferent fibers and their sensitization by inflammatory mediators require transient receptor potential vanilloid 1 and acid-sensing ion channel 3. *J Neurosci* 2005;25:10981–10989.

19  Knowles CH and Aziz Q. Visceral hypersensitivity in non-erosive reflux disease. *Gut* 2008;57:674–683.

20  Winston J, Shenoy M, Medley D *et al*. The vanilloid receptor initiates and maintains colonic hypersensitivity induced by neonatal colon irritation in rats. *Gastroenterology* 2007;132:615–627.

21  Levine JD and Alessandri-Haber N. TRP channels: targets for the relief of pain. *Biochim Biophys Acta* 2007;1772:989–1003.

22  Caterina MJ, Schumacher MA, Tominaga M *et al*. The capsaicin receptor: a heat-activated ion channel in the pain pathway. *Nature* 1997;389:816–824.

23  Holzer P. TRPV1 and the gut: from a tasty receptor for a painful vanilloid to a key player in hyperalgesia. *Eur J Pharmacol* 2004;500:231–241.

24  Akbar A, Walters JR and Ghosh S. Review article: visceral hypersensitivity in irritable bowel syndrome: molecular mechanisms and therapeutic agents. *Aliment Pharmacol Ther* 2009;30:423–435.

25  Akbar A, Yiangou Y, Facer P *et al*. Increased capsaicin receptor TRPV1-expressing sensory fibres in irritable bowel syndrome and their correlation with abdominal pain. *Gut* 2008;57:923–929.

26  Gomes RB, Brodskyn C, de Oliveira CI *et al*. Seroconversion against Lutzomyia longipalpis saliva concurrent with the development of anti-Leishmania chagasi delayed-type hypersensitivity. *J Infect Dis* 2002;186:1530–1534.

27  Gunthorpe MJ, Szallasi A. Peripheral TRPV1 receptors as targets for drug development: new molecules and mechanisms. *Curr Pharm Des* 2008;14:32–41.

28  Broad LM, Keding SJ and Blanco MJ. Recent progress in the development of selective TRPV1 antagonists for pain. *Curr Top Med Chem* 2008;8:1431–1441.

29  Caterina MJ. On the thermoregulatory perils of TRPV1 antagonism. *Pain* 2008; 136:3–4.

30  Brierley SM, Page AJ, Hughes PA *et al*. Selective role for TRPV4 ion channels in visceral sensory pathways. *Gastroenterology* 2008;134:2059–2069.

31  Cenac N, Altier C, Chapman K *et al*. Transient receptor potential vanilloid-4 has a major role in visceral hypersensitivity symptoms. *Gastroenterology* 2008;135:937–946, 46 e1–2.

32  Vergnolle N. Modulation of visceral pain and inflammation by protease-activated receptors. *Br J Pharmacol* 2004;141:1264–1274.

33  Vergnolle N, Wallace JL, Bunnett NW and Hollenberg MD. Protease-activated receptors in inflammation, neuronal signaling and pain. *Trends Pharmacol Sci* 2001;22:146–1452.

34  Landis RC. Protease activated receptors: clinical relevance to hemostasis and inflammation. *Hematol Oncol Clin North Am* 2007;21:103–113.

35  Vergnolle N. Postinflammatory visceral sensitivity and pain mechanisms. *Neurogastroenterol Motil* 2008;20(Suppl 1):73–80.

36  Cenac N, Andrews CN, Holzhausen M *et al*. Role for protease activity in visceral pain in irritable bowel syndrome. *J Clin Invest* 2007;117:636–647.

37  Barbara G, Wang B, Stanghellini V *et al*. Mast cell-dependent excitation of visceral-nociceptive sensory neurons in irritable bowel syndrome. *Gastroenterology* 2007;132: 26–37.

38  Toda N, Kishioka S, Hatano Y and Toda H. Modulation of opioid actions by nitric oxide signaling. *Anesthesiology* 2009;110:166–181.

39  Takeuchi K, Yokota A, Tanaka A and Takahira Y. Factors involved in upregulation of inducible nitric oxide synthase in rat small intestine following administration of nonsteroidal anti-inflammatory drugs. *Dig Dis Sci* 2006;51:1250–1259.

40  Shamshiri H, Paragomi P, Paydar MJ *et al*. Antinociceptive effect of chronic lithium on visceral hypersensitivity in a rat model of diarrhea-predominant irritable bowel syndrome: The role of nitric oxide pathway. *J Gastroenterol Hepatol* 2009;24(4):672–680.

41  Coutinho SV, Urban MO, Gebhart GF. Role of glutamate receptors and nitric oxide in the rostral ventromedial medulla in visceral hyperalgesia. *Pain* 1998;78:59–69.

42  Tjong YW, Ip SP, Lao L *et al*. Role of neuronal nitric oxide synthase in colonic distension-induced hyperalgesia in distal colon of neonatal maternal separated male rats. *Neurogastroenterol Motil* 2011;23(7):666–e278.

43  Kuiken SD, Klooker TK, Tytgat GN *et al*. Possible role of nitric oxide in visceral hypersensitivity in patients with irritable bowel syndrome. *Neurogastroenterol Motil* 2006;18:115–122.

44  McKeown ES, Parry SD, Stansfield R *et al*. Postinfectious irritable bowel syndrome may occur after non-gastrointestinal and intestinal infection. *Neurogastroenterol Motil* 2006;18:839–843.

45  Lee KJ, Kim YB, Kim JH *et al*. The alteration of enterochromaffin cell, mast cell, and lamina propria T lymphocyte numbers in irritable bowel syndrome and its relationship with psychological factors. *J Gastroenterol Hepatol* 2008;23:1689–1694.

46  Piche T, Saint-Paul MC, Dainese R *et al*. Mast cells and cellularity of the colonic mucosa correlated with fatigue and depression in irritable bowel syndrome. *Gut* 2008;57:468–473.

47  Ohashi K, Sato Y, Kawai M and Kurebayashi Y. Abolishment of TNBS-induced visceral hypersensitivity in mast cell deficient rats. *Life Sci* 2008;82:419–423.

48  Ohashi K, Sato Y, Iwata H *et al*. Colonic mast cell infiltration in rats with TNBS-induced visceral hypersensitivity. *J Vet Med Sci* 2007;69:1223–1228.

49  Leri O, Tubili S, De Rosa FG *et al*. Management of diarrhoeic type of irritable bowel syndrome with exclusion diet and disodium cromoglycate. *Inflammopharmacology* 1997;5:153–158.

50  Klooker TK, Braak B, Koopman KE *et al*. The mast cell stabiliser ketotifen decreases visceral hypersensitivity and improves intestinal symptoms in patients with irritable bowel syndrome. *Gut*;59:1213–1221.

51  Grundy D. 5-HT system in the gut: roles in the regulation of visceral sensitivity and motor functions. *Eur Rev Med Pharmacol Sci* 2008;12(Suppl 1):63–67.

52  Fidelholtz J, Smith W, Rawls J *et al*. Safety and tolerability of tegaserod in patients with irritable bowel syndrome and diarrhea symptoms. *Am J Gastroenterol* 2002;97: 1176–1181.

53 Mayer EA and Bradesi S. Alosetron and irritable bowel syndrome. *Expert Opin Pharmacother* 2003;4:2089–2098.

54 Friedel D, Thomas R and Fisher RS. Ischemic colitis during treatment with alosetron. *Gastroenterology* 2001;120:557–560.

55 Schiller LR and Johnson DA. Balancing drug risk and benefit: toward refining the process of FDA decisions affecting patient care. *Am J Gastroenterol* 2008;103:815–819.

56 Drossman DA, Danilewitz M, Naesdal J *et al.* Randomized, double-blind, placebo-controlled trial of the 5-HT1A receptor antagonist AZD7371 tartrate monohydrate (robalzotan tartrate monohydrate) in patients with irritable bowel syndrome. *Am J Gastroenterol* 2008;103:2562–2569.

57 Storr M, Gaffal E, Saur D *et al.* Effect of cannabinoids on neural transmission in rat gastric fundus. *Can J Physiol Pharmacol* 2002;80:67–76.

58 Sanson M, Bueno L and Fioramonti J. Involvement of cannabinoid receptors in inflammatory hypersensitivity to colonic distension in rats. *Neurogastroenterol Motil* 2006;18:949–956.

59 Croci T, Manara L, Aureggi G *et al.* In vitro functional evidence of neuronal cannabinoid CB1 receptors in human ileum. *Br J Pharmacol* 1998;125:1393–1395.

60 Guagnini F, Cogliati P, Mukenge S *et al.* Tolerance to cannabinoid response on the myenteric plexus of guinea-pig ileum and human small intestinal strips. *Br J Pharmacol* 2006;148:1165–1173.

61 Klooker TK, Leliefeld KE, Van Den Wijngaard RM and Boeckxstaens GE. The cannabinoid receptor agonist delta-9-tetrahydrocannabinol does not affect visceral sensitivity to rectal distension in healthy volunteers and IBS patients. *Neurogastroenterol Motil*;23:30–35, e2.

62 D'Argenio G, Valenti M, Scaglione G *et al.* Up-regulation of anandamide levels as an endogenous mechanism and a pharmacological strategy to limit colon inflammation. *FASEB J* 2006;20:568–570.

63 Kimball ES, Schneider CR, Wallace NH and Hornby PJ. Agonists of cannabinoid receptor 1 and 2 inhibit experimental colitis induced by oil of mustard and by dextran sulfate sodium. *Am J Physiol Gastrointest Liver Physiol* 2006;291:G364–G371.

64 Breyer RM, Bagdassarian CK, Myers SA and Breyer MD. Prostanoid receptors: subtypes and signaling. *Annu Rev Pharmacol Toxicol* 2001;41:661–690.

65 Haupt W, Jiang W, Kreis ME and Grundy D. Prostaglandin EP receptor subtypes have distinctive effects on jejunal afferent sensitivity in the rat. *Gastroenterology* 2000;119: 1580–1589.

66 Maubach KA and Grundy D. The role of prostaglandins in the bradykinin-induced activation of serosal afferents of the rat jejunum in vitro. *J Physiol* 1999;515(Pt 1): 277–285.

67 Sarkar S, Hobson AR, Hughes A *et al.* The prostaglandin E2 receptor-1 (EP-1) mediates acid-induced visceral pain hypersensitivity in humans. *Gastroenterology* 2003;124: 18–25.

68 Cummins TR, Sheets PL and Waxman SG. The roles of sodium channels in nociception: Implications for mechanisms of pain. *Pain* 2007;131:243–257.

69 Sheets PL, Jackson JO 2nd, Waxman SG *et al.* A Nav1.7 channel mutation associated with hereditary erythromelalgia contributes to neuronal hyperexcitability and displays reduced lidocaine sensitivity. *J Physiol* 2007;581:1019–1031.

70 Cummins TR and Rush AM. Voltage-gated sodium channel blockers for the treatment of neuropathic pain. *Expert Rev Neurother* 2007;7:1597–1612.

71 Yiangou Y, Facer P, Chessell IP *et al.* Voltage-gated ion channel Nav1.7 innervation in patients with idiopathic rectal hypersensitivity and paroxysmal extreme pain disorder (familial rectal pain). *Neurosci Lett* 2007;427:77–82.

72 Verne GN, Sen A and Price DD. Intrarectal lidocaine is an effective treatment for abdominal pain associated with diarrhea-predominant irritable bowel syndrome. *J Pain* 2005;6:493–496.

73 Tarnawa I, Bolcskei H and Kocsis P. Blockers of voltage-gated sodium channels for the treatment of central nervous system diseases. *Recent patents on CNS drug discovery* 2007;2:57–78.

74 Waldmann R, Champigny G, Bassilana F *et al*. A proton-gated cation channel involved in acid-sensing. *Nature* 1997;386:173–177.

75 Page AJ, Brierley SM, Martin CM *et al*. Acid sensing ion channels 2 and 3 are required for inhibition of visceral nociceptors by benzamil. *Pain* 2007;133:150–160.

76 Jones RC 3rd, Otsuka E, Wagstrom E *et al*. Short-term sensitization of colon mecha-noreceptors is associated with long-term hypersensitivity to colon distention in the mouse. *Gastroenterology* 2007;133:184–194.

77 Aziz Q. Visceral hypersensitivity: fact or fiction. *Gastroenterology* 2006;131:661–664.

78 Amira S, Morrison JF and Rayfield KM. The distribution of substance P-containing nerves to the rat small intestine. *Exp Physiol* 1990;75:119–121.

79 Greenwood-Van Meerveld B, Gibson MS, Johnson AC *et al*. NK1 receptor-mediated mechanisms regulate colonic hypersensitivity in the guinea pig. *Pharmacol Biochem Behav* 2003;74:1005–1013.

80 Lee OY MJ, Naliboff BD, Chang L and Mayer EA. A double blind parallel group pilot study of the effects of CJ-11,974 and placebo on perceptual and emotional responses to rectosigmoid distension in IBS patients. *Gastroenterology* 2000;118:A846.

81 Julia V, Su X, Bueno L and Gebhart GF. Role of neurokinin 3 receptors on responses to colorectal distention in the rat: electrophysiological and behavioral studies. *Gastroenterology* 1999;116:1124–1131.

82 McLean PG, Picard C, Garcia-Villar R *et al*. Effects of nematode infection on sensitiv-ity to intestinal distension: role of tachykinin NK2 receptors. *Eur J Pharmacol* 1997;337:279–282.

83 Gaudreau GA, Plourde V. Role of tachykinin NK1, NK2 and NK3 receptors in the modulation of visceral hypersensitivity in the rat. *Neurosci Lett* 2003;351:59–62.

84 Houghton LA, Cremonini F, Camilleri M *et al*. Effect of the NK(3) receptor antagonist, talnetant, on rectal sensory function and compliance in healthy humans. *Neurogastroenterol Motil* 2007;19:732–743.

85 Rogers RC and Hermann GE. Mechanisms of action of CCK to activate central vagal afferent terminals. *Peptides* 2008;29:1716–1725.

86 Dockray GJ. Cholecystokinin and gut-brain signalling. *Regul Pept* 2009;155:6–10.

87 Dizdar V, Spiller R, Singh G *et al*. Relative importance of abnormalities of CCK (chol-ecystokinin) and 5-HT (serotonin) in Giardia-induced post-infectious irritable bowel syndrome and functional dyspepsia. *Aliment Pharmacol Ther* 2010;31(8):883–891.

88 Sabate JM, Gorbatchef C, Flourie B *et al*. Cholecystokinin octapeptide increases rectal sensitivity to pain in healthy subjects. *Neurogastroenterol Motil* 2002;14:689–695.

89 Cann PA, Rovati LC, Smart HL *et al*. Loxiglumide, a CCK-A antagonist, in irritable bowel syndrome. A pilot multicenter clinical study. *Ann N Y Acad Sci* 1994;713:449–450.

90 Cremonini F, Camilleri M, McKinzie S *et al*. Effect of CCK-1 antagonist, dexloxiglu-mide, in female patients with irritable bowel syndrome: a pharmacodynamic and pharmacogenomic study. *Am J Gastroenterol* 2005;100:652–663.

91 Bagnol D, Mansour A, Akil H and Watson SJ. Cellular localization and distribution of the cloned mu and kappa opioid receptors in rat gastrointestinal tract. *Neuroscience* 1997;81:579–591.

92 Coffin B, Bouhassira D, Chollet R *et al*. Effect of the kappa agonist fedotozine on perception of gastric distension in healthy humans. *Aliment Pharmacol Ther* 1996;10: 919–925.

93 Delvaux M, Louvel D, Lagier E *et al*. The kappa agonist fedotozine relieves hypersensitivity to colonic distention in patients with irritable bowel syndrome. *Gastroenterology* 1999;116:38–45.

94 Dapoigny M, Abitbol JL and Fraitag B. Efficacy of peripheral kappa agonist fedotozine versus placebo in treatment of irritable bowel syndrome. A multicenter dose-response study. *Dig Dis Sci* 1995;40:2244–2249.

95 Mangel AW, Bornstein JD, Hamm LR *et al*. Clinical trial: asimadoline in the treatment of patients with irritable bowel syndrome. *Aliment Pharmacol Ther* 2008;28(2): 239–249.

96 Anand P, Aziz Q, Willert R and van Oudenhove L. Peripheral and central mechanisms of visceral sensitization in man. *Neurogastroenterol Motil* 2007;19:29–46.

97 Sarkar S, Aziz Q, Woolf CJ *et al*. Contribution of central sensitisation to the development of non-cardiac chest pain. *Lancet* 2000;356:1154–1159.

98 Sarkar S, Hobson AR, Furlong PL *et al*. Central neural mechanisms mediating human visceral hypersensitivity. *Am J Physiol Gastrointest Liver Physiol* 2001;281: G1196–G1202.

99 Grundy D, Al-Chaer ED, Aziz Q *et al*. Fundamentals of neurogastroenterology: basic science. *Gastroenterology* 2006;130:1391–1411.

100 Willert RP, Woolf CJ, Hobson AR *et al*. The development and maintenance of human visceral pain hypersensitivity is dependent on the N-methyl-D-aspartate receptor. *Gastroenterology* 2004;126:683–692.

101 Hobson AR, Khan RW, Sarkar S *et al*. Development of esophageal hypersensitivity following experimental duodenal acidification. *Am J Gastroenterol* 2004;99:813–820.

102 Ness TJ, Metcalf AM and Gebhart GF. A psychophysiological study in humans using phasic colonic distension as a noxious visceral stimulus. *Pain* 1990;43:377–386.

103 Sach J, Bolus R, Fitzgerald L *et al*. Is there a difference between abdominal pain and discomfort in moderate to severe IBS patients? *Am J Gastroenterol* 2002;97:3131–3138.

104 Spiller R, Aziz Q, Creed F *et al*. Guidelines on the irritable bowel syndrome: mechanisms and practical management. *Gut* 2007;56:1770–1798.

105 Khan S and Chang L. Diagnosis and management of IBS. *Nat Rev Gastroenterol Hepatol*;7:565–581.

106 Moret C and Briley M. Antidepressants in the treatment of fibromyalgia. *Neuropsychiatr Dis Treat* 2006;2:537–548.

107 Morgan V, Pickens D, Gautam S *et al*. Amitriptyline reduces rectal pain related activation of the anterior cingulate cortex in patients with irritable bowel syndrome. *Gut* 2005;54:601–607.

108 Van Oudenhove L, Coen SJ and Aziz Q. Functional brain imaging of gastrointestinal sensation in health and disease. *World J Gastroenterol* 2007;13:3438–3445.

109 Gorelick AB, Koshy SS, Hooper FG *et al*. Differential effects of amitriptyline on perception of somatic and visceral stimulation in healthy humans. *Am J Physiol* 1998;275:G460–G466.

110 Thoua NM, Murray CD, Winchester WJ *et al*. Amitriptyline modifies the visceral hypersensitivity response to acute stress in Irritable Bowel Syndrome. *Aliment Pharmacol Ther* 2009;29(5):552–560.

111 Ford AC, Talley NJ, Schoenfeld PS *et al*. Efficacy of antidepressants and psychological therapies in irritable bowel syndrome: systematic review and meta-analysis. *Gut* 2009;58:367–378.

112 Rahimi R, Nikfar S, Rezaie A and Abdollahi M. Efficacy of tricyclic antidepressants in irritable bowel syndrome: a meta-analysis. *World J Gastroenterol* 2009;15:1548–1553.

113 Tack J, Broekaert D, Fischler B *et al*. A controlled crossover study of the selective serotonin reuptake inhibitor citalopram in irritable bowel syndrome. *Gut* 2006;55: 1095–1103.

114 Lyseng-Williamson KA and Siddiqui MA. Pregabalin: a review of its use in fibromyalgia. *Drugs* 2008;68:2205–2223.

115 Ravnefjord A, Brusberg M, Larsson H *et al*. Effects of pregabalin on visceral pain responses and colonic compliance in rats. *Br J Pharmacol* 2008;155:407–416.

116 Houghton LA, Fell C, Whorwell PJ *et al*. Effect of a second-generation alpha2delta ligand (pregabalin) on visceral sensation in hypersensitive patients with irritable bowel syndrome. *Gut* 2007;56:1218–1225.

117 Lackner JM, Jaccard J, Krasner SS *et al*. Self-administered cognitive behavior therapy for moderate to severe irritable bowel syndrome: clinical efficacy, tolerability, feasibility. *Clin Gastroenterol Hepatol* 2008;6:899–906.

118 Whorwell PJ, Prior A and Faragher EB. Controlled trial of hypnotherapy in the treatment of severe refractory irritable-bowel syndrome. *Lancet* 1984;2:1232–1234.

119 Webb AN, Kukuruzovic RH, Catto-Smith AG and Sawyer SM. Hypnotherapy for treatment of irritable bowel syndrome. Cochrane Database Syst Rev 2007:CD005110.

120 Spiller P. Review article: probiotics and prebiotics in irritable bowel syndrome (IBS). *Aliment Pharmacol Ther* 2008;28(4):385–396.

121 Brenner DM, Moeller MJ, Chey WD and Schoenfeld PS. The utility of probiotics in the treatment of irritable bowel syndrome: a systematic review. *Am J Gastroenterol* 2009;104:1033–1049; quiz 50.

122 Pimentel M, Lembo A, Chey WD *et al*. Rifaximin therapy for patients with irritable bowel syndrome without constipation. *N Engl J Med*;364:22–32.

# Multiple Choice Questions

1 Which of the following statements is false concerning visceral hypersensitivity?
   A Is always associated with IBS.
   B Can be caused by peripheral or central sensitization.
   C Can occur in the fore, mid and hindgut.
   D TRPV1 has been implicated in its aetiology.
   E Intra-rectal lignocaine can reduce visceral hypersensitivity.

Answer: A

2 Which of the following has not been associated with the development of peripheral sensitization?
   A Protease activated receptors.
   B Acid sensing ion channels.
   C Mast cells.
   D Transient vallinoid potential 6.
   E Cannabinoid receptor.

Answer: D

3 Which of the following forms of stimulation results in nociceptor activation?
   A Heat
   B Acid
   C Mechanical
   D Inflammation
   E All of the above

Answer: E

**4** Which of the following antispasmodics does not have proven efficacy for treating visceral pain associated with IBS?

**A** Cimetropium.

**B** Otilonium.

**C** Trimebutine.

**D** Mebeverine.

**E** Pinaverium.

Answer: D

**5** Which of the following has the least side effects in treating visceral pain associated with IBS?

**A** Mebeverine.

**B** Amitriptylline.

**C** Cognitive behavioural therapy.

**D** Fluoxetine.

**E** Bifidobacterium spp

Answer: C

# CHAPTER 13

# Abdominal Bloating

*Peter J. Whorwell*

Education and Research Centre, Wythenshawe Hospital and University Hospital of South Manchester, Manchester, UK

---

**Key points**

- Bloating and distension are common and often very intrusive features of irritable bowel syndrome and related functional gastrointestinal disorders.
- In approximately 50% of individuals reporting bloating this symptom is accompanied by an actual increase in girth (distension) which can be by as much as twelve centimetres.
- Bloating is associated with abnormal gas handling, hypersensitivity of the gastrointestinal tract, a loose bowel habit, fermentation and possibly an abnormal gut flora.
- Distension is associated with weak abdominal musculature, an abnormal accommodation reflex, slow gastrointestinal transit, constipation, fermentation and changes in bacterial flora.
- Treatment should take into account the possible underlying pathophysiology but often still has to involve a process of trial and error.

---

## Background

Most patients with irritable bowel syndrome complain of the symptom of abdominal bloating but it is now realized that there may be two components to this problem. Firstly, it may reflect a sensation of increased intra-abdominal pressure or, secondly, this feeling can be accompanied by an actual increase in girth, which should more appropriately be referred to as distension. However, it should be noted that most patients will refer to both features as bloating whereas for the physician it is important to know whether there is bloating on its own or co-existent distension, as treatment approaches may be different. Research in our laboratory has suggested that in approximately 50% of patients reporting bloating, the symptom is accompanied by actual distension [1]. A further complication is that the word bloating does not necessarily translate well into different languages

---

*Irritable Bowel Syndrome: Diagnosis and Clinical Management*, First Edition.
Edited by Anton Emmanuel and Eamonn M.M. Quigley.
© 2013 John Wiley & Sons, Ltd. Published 2013 by John Wiley & Sons, Ltd.

and in the literature, until relatively recently, the terms bloating and distension have been used synonymously.

Bloating and distension seem to be more common in females but this may be partly due to the fact that men often describe them differently using terms such as tightness or hardness of the abdomen. This could be because men tend to have stronger anterior abdominal musculature but other possibilities exist and these are described later. These symptoms tend to increase during the course of the day being at their worst in the evening and then the problem usually subsides overnight. This diurnal variation is absolutely characteristic of the bloating that accompanies functional gastrointestinal disorders and can almost be regarded as diagnostic of such a condition. In contrast, if distension does not wax and wane over a twenty four hour period this should be regarded as an alarm symptom which deserves further investigation as, among other things, ovarian cancer can lead to a progressive increase in girth. Other characteristics of bloating and distension include a tendency to be exacerbated by eating, to improve on lying down, to suddenly come on very quickly and to not necessarily be relieved by the passage of wind [2]. In addition, patients frequently say that this problem occurs very frequently, often on a daily basis, which can be in contrast to the other features of irritable bowel syndrome, such as pain and bowel dysfunction, which can be more intermittent in nature.

## Pathophysiology

The pathophysiology of bloating and distension is only just beginning to be understood as, until recently, there have been no reliable techniques for investigating this rather enigmatic problem. This has now changed with the advent of approaches such as the gas challenge technique [3, 4], abdominal inductance plethysmography [1], abdominal and diaphragmatic electromyography, CT scanning and magnetic resonance imaging. The principles behind the latter three do not need elaborating here but the other two are briefly described. The gas challenge test (Figure 13.1) involves the insufflation of a gas mixture of nitrogen, carbon dioxide and oxygen at the same partial pressures of venous blood, so that it remains within the lumen of the gut and therefore allows the study of the way the gut handles gas and how this might be influenced by physiological events, nutrients or pharmacological manipulation. Azpiroz's group in Barcelona have undertaken a series of elegant studies using this methodology some of which are described later. Abdominal inductance plethysmography (Figure 13.2) is a technique for recording change in girth over a period of up to 24 hours [5]. It is based on the principle that a loop of wire has a certain inductance which changes according to its shape and this can be

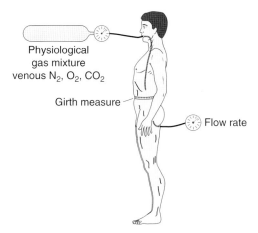

**Figure 13.1** The gas challenge technique: a mixture of nitrogen, carbon dioxide and oxygen at similar partial pressures to venous blood is infused into the jejunum allowing measurement of gas handling under a variety of different conditions.
(© Department of Medical Illustration, University Hospital of South Manchester.)

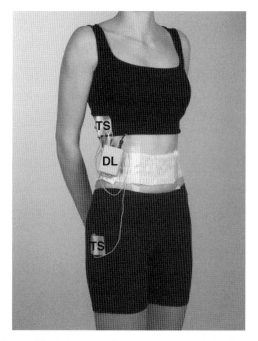

**Figure 13.2** Abdominal inductance plethysmography: the girth of a patient together with information on whether they are lying, sitting or standing can be recorded over a period of 24 hours.
(Reproduced from *Alimentary Pharmacology & Therapeutics*, A Agrawal, PJ Whorwell, 2007 with permission from John Wiley & Sons Ltd.)

captured and transposed into a measurement accurate down to 1 mm. The output from the loop, as well as of tilt switches for recording the position of the patient in terms of lying, sitting or standing, is captured by a data logger which can be subsequently interrogated by a computer and displayed graphically.

In the 1940s Alvarez suggested that abdominal distension was largely psychological in origin with an individual deliberately protruding their abdomen by increasing their lumbar lordosis and depressing their diaphragm [6]. This hypothesis was subsequently dismissed as unlikely but, as will be seen later, recent research has suggested that he was perhaps nearer the truth than he was given credit for, although the mechanism is likely to be a reflex rather than necessarily being a deliberate act on the part of the patient. Alvarez's work led to the concept that true distension does not exist, but with the advent of abdominal inductance plethysmography this question could be answered definitively and in a series of studies we have consistently found that in approximately half of those individuals reporting bloating there is also significant distension. Furthermore, the change in girth can be substantial and it is not necessarily unusual for some individuals to experience an increase of as much as twelve centimetres during the course of the day [1]. Having the ability to divide patients into those with bloating on its own and those in whom it is also accompanied by distension facilitates research into whether different mechanisms might be involved. As a consequence, we have been able to show that distension is more common in patients with constipation [1] and in those where gastrointestinal transit is delayed [7]. However, it does not seem to be related to body mass index, age, parity or psychological status [1].

It would seem reasonable to assume that bloating and distension may result from the accumulation of excessive amounts of gas within the gastrointestinal tract. However, there are no good data to support this view although there is a considerable body of evidence that the way the gut handles gas is important. The Barcelona group has shown that, compared to controls, patients with irritable bowel syndrome tend to retain more infused gas (Figure 13.3) and this is accompanied by a feeling of bloating as well as an increase in abdominal girth [8]. In subsequent studies, they have shown that this gas retention occurs more in the small bowel [9, 10], where it probably results in focal trapping, pooling and stretching of the mucosa, which it is thought could lead to symptoms. They have also shown that gas transit can be influenced by certain nutrients, such as fat, which obviously opens up the possibility of treatment by dietary advice [11].

There is still considerable debate about whether there is any specific abnormality of gut motor activity in patients with irritable bowel syndrome. However, the motor activity of the gut is reduced by sleep and, as bloating and distension improve overnight, it is possible to speculate that a reduc-

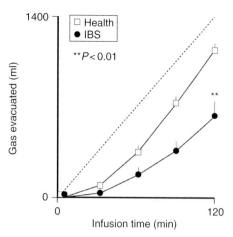

**Figure 13.3** Evacuation of intestinal gas in patients with irritable bowel syndrome
(n = 20) and healthy subjects (n = 20). Gas was infused into the intestine at a constant
rate (represented by the broken line) for two hours and collected via an anal cannula.
Note that IBS patients expelled a significantly lower volume of gas. Values are means
(SEM). **P<0.01.
(Reproduced from Impaired Transit and Tolerance of Intestinal Gas in the Irritable
Bowel Syndrome, J Serra, F Azpiroz, J-R Malagelada, 2001 with permission from BMJ
Publishing Group Ltd.)

tion in motility might be responsible. However, there has been relatively
little work to confirm this hypothesis but the observation that antispasmodics
appear to be relatively ineffective in relieving either bloating or distension suggests that at least phasic motor activity does not probably play an
important role. It has been suggested that tonic motor activity might be
important in gas transit [12] and, consequently, this concept deserves
further investigation. In contrast to the rather equivocal findings on motility in irritable bowel syndrome in general and bloating in particular, one
physiological finding that is relatively consistent in irritable bowel syndrome is that of excessive sensitivity to balloon distension of the gut which
is usually referred to as visceral hypersensitivity [13]. As a result of this
phenomenon patients seem more 'aware' of gastrointestinal events and we
hypothesized that this problem might contribute to the symptom of bloating in those subjects who do not experience distension. This notion was
confirmed in a study comparing sensory thresholds in bloating patients
with or without distension [14], where the latter proved to be more sensitive than the former (Figure 13.4).

   With respect to distension, it is entirely possible that there may be a component which is completely outside the gastrointestinal tract. One possibility
is weak abdominal musculature leading to protrusion of the abdominal
contents and this has been assessed by comparing the ability of patients
with irritable bowel syndrome and controls to do sit-ups [15]. IBS patients

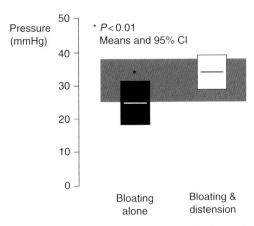

**Figure 13.4** Sensory thresholds to pain in patients with bloating without distension and bloating accompanied by distension. Sensory thresholds are significantly lower in those with bloating alone.
(© Department of Medical Illustration, University Hospital of South Manchester.)

did perform less well but the study was rather small and it is difficult to draw any firm conclusions. An alternative mechanism which could be related to anterior abdominal wall function is some form of abnormal accommodation reflex. It seems reasonable to assume that in order for the abdomen to accommodate an increase in the volume of its contents, such as that which occurs following a meal or during pregnancy, there must be some form of accommodation reflex to allow for the increase in volume. As the diaphragm and the anterior abdominal wall are the only structures surrounding the abdomen that are potentially 'elastic', such a reflex would have to involve either one or both of these structures and possibly be triggered by mechanoreceptors within the gut or abdominal cavity. There is now evidence, from a combination of electromyographic and CT studies, that such a reflex does exist and involves both the diaphragm and abdominal muscles [16–18]. Furthermore, it appears that this reflex is abnormal in patients with irritable bowel syndrome where, in response to a bloating stimulus, there is relaxation of the anterior abdominal musculature coupled with diaphragmatic descent, which is the opposite to what happens in normal individuals [16].

In addition to exhibiting visceral hypersensitivity, it appears that some patients with IBS have a tendency to have a more generalized distortion of perception that is not necessarily confined to the gut. For instance, they appear to rate the quality of their sleep as poor when, in fact, it is not necessarily any worse than that of controls [19] and they also appear to be hypersensitive to auditory [20–22] as well as visual stimuli [23]. This then raises the possibility that the symptom of bloating, as opposed to distension, could in some irritable bowel syndrome sufferers result from heightened perception of normal abdominal events rather than necessarily indicating an intrinsic abnormality within the abdomen.

Two relatively new concepts which are generating considerable interest in relation to the pathophysiology of irritable bowel syndrome are, firstly, that the microbiota of the gut may have a role to play [24] and, secondly, that low-grade inflammation could also be important [25]. In relation to bloating and distension, it is entirely conceivable that such factors could influence some of the mechanisms already thought to be involved, such as visceral sensitivity and abnormal handling of gas resulting from bacterial fermentation of nutrients in the gastrointestinal tract.

## Treatment

From what has been said already, the pathophysiological mechanisms involved in bloating and distension appear to be different but overlapping. It also seems likely that that these problems are multifactorial and vary in causality from individual to individual. However, as we begin to unravel this problem we can at least begin to offer treatment based on what we know although 'trial and error' will still have to be used.

### Lifestyle and diet

As abnormal gas handling is such a common phenomenon in these patients it seems reasonable to recommend the restriction of foods or drinks that can produce gas. Consequently, foods high in insoluble fibre should be eaten with caution and carbonated drinks are probably best avoided. There has also been an upsurge of interest in fermentable oligo- di- mono-saccharides and polyols (FODMAPs) with which our diets are becoming increasingly burdened. These carbohydrates occur in fruit and vegetables as well as being widely used in the food and drinks industry as artificial, low calorie, sweeteners. They are poorly absorbed, fermentable and appear to be particularly poorly tolerated by patients with irritable bowel syndrome [26, 27]. Although there are currently no data on whether FODMAP restriction might improve bloating or distension, this approach is worthy of a short therapeutic trial in a patient in whom symptoms are refractory. It has also been shown that the infusion of lipid into the duodenum can increase visceral hypersensitivity [28] and, therefore, it is not surprising that some patients find that the consumption of fatty foods can exacerbate their bloating.

Exercise is generally considered to be beneficial in terms of promoting good health although there is relatively sparse data on its effect on gastrointestinal physiology in relation to irritable bowel syndrome. However, there has been one recent study showing some improvement in symptoms, including bloating, with relatively modest amounts of exercise [29]. There have been no studies to assess whether strengthening the weak abdominal musculature, that has been previously reported, might be of any value.

## Medication

Simethicone is an old fashioned remedy for 'gaseousness' which is harmless, available in a variety of over-the-counter preparations and can sometimes prove to be useful. Based on the fact that constipation and slow transit are related to distension, it seems reasonable to assume that laxatives might help to relieve this symptom. However, there are no trial data to support this view although clinical experience suggests this strategy does sometimes lead to benefit. Another option worth considering is the use of a prokinetic medication. This approach is supported by the observation that the prokinetic drug neostigmine reduces the retention of infused gas in patients with irritable bowel syndrome and this is accompanied by a decrease in girth as well as symptoms [30]. Furthermore, in the clinical trial setting, prokinetics such as tegaserod [31] and possibly prucalopride [32] appear to help relieve the symptom of bloating which may be a reflection of a reduction in girth, although girth was not actually measured in these studies.

As visceral hypersensitivity is more closely related to bloating than distension, targeting this abnormality should have a positive effect on this symptom. There have been studies suggesting that both the tricyclic and the selective serotonin re-uptake inhibitors may modulate visceral sensation [33–35] and they are well known to be effective in the treatment of irritable bowel syndrome [36, 37]. Unfortunately, in none of the clinical trials of tricyclics has the symptom of bloating ever been recorded, although it has been assessed in four trials using selective serotonin re-uptake inhibitors, with two of the four studies showing a positive effect. Consequently, the use of antidepressants has currently to be on an empirical basis, although they are certainly worth trying.

With the increasing interest in disturbances of the gut microbiota in patients with irritable bowel syndrome, the therapeutic potential of modifying the bacterial contents of the gastrointestinal tract is being intensively investigated. One approach is to administer nonabsorbable antibiotics and following some initial reports suggesting benefit from neomycin [38], rifaximin has become the centre of most attention [39–41] with an apparent effect on bloating but there have, as yet, been no studies to ascertain whether this has been accompanied by a reduction in girth. Obviously, it would be inadvisable to administer an antibiotic on a continuous basis but some of the trial data suggest that short courses of up to two weeks may give benefit for a period of up to three months, making this a more viable proposition. However, the possible long-term consequences of repeated courses of antibiotics will need to be evaluated.

Probiotics provide another way of possibly altering the microbiota and there have been in excess of thirty trials of these products in irritable bowel syndrome to date, with at least two thirds being positive to some extent [42] and some, such as *Bifidobacterium infantis* 35624, actually showing a positive effect on bloating [43]. *Bifidobacterium lactis* DN-173-010 has previously been shown to accelerate gastrointestinal transit [44] and improve bloating in constipation-predominant IBS [45] and these are the very characteristics that should theoretically lead to an improvement in distension by reducing girth. Consequently, we have compared this organism with placebo in a study using abdominal inductance plethysmography and it showed that the active probiotic did significantly improve distension [46]. Thus, it seems that probiotics are worthy of trial for this indication although the availability of those that have a good evidence base is somewhat variable.

## Behavioural treatments

Hypnotherapy has been shown to improve the symptoms of irritable bowel syndrome [47] and this can be accompanied by a normalization of visceral hypersensitivity [48]. In addition, hypnosis has been shown to have an effect on other gastrointestinal physiological events as well as modulating the way the brain processes noxious stimuli [49]. Thus, it is perhaps not surprising that hypnosis has been shown to improve bloating, as it has the potential to modulate several of the mechanisms involved in its pathogenesis. However, to date there have been no studies assessing the effect of hypnosis on objectively measured distension. If, as seems likely in some cases, distension is the result of an abnormal accommodation reflex it seems reasonable to suppose it might also be amenable to modification by a behavioural technique such as biofeedback training and there are preliminary data to support this view [50]. It is also of interest that biofeedback for constipation has been reported to improve the symptom of bloating [51].

## Conclusion

Although closely related, there appear to be subtle but probably overlapping mechanisms involved in the pathophysiology of bloating and distension, and this probably explains why patients vary in their response to different therapeutic modalities. However, as we begin to identify these mechanisms and find clinically applicable ways of identifying them, more logical approaches to treatment should be forthcoming.

## CASE STUDY 13.1

A 23-year-old girl presented to her GP with gross distension of her abdomen which was leading to many comments about when she was expecting a baby. She also suffered from severe constipation and intermittent abdominal pain. Because of the extremely large size of her abdomen she was referred to a gastroenterologist who confirmed gross swelling although it was not quite so bad when she was in the recumbent position. Repetitive ultrasound examinations revealed no obvious abnormalities and, in particular, no evidence of an ascites or gynaecological pathology. Gastroscopy, colonoscopy as well as CT scanning provided no further useful information and all blood tests were normal.

### Comment
Distension of this degree clearly merits full investigation but once this has proved negative repetitive testing is completely unnecessary. On review in our Unit it was felt that her distension was part of irritable bowel syndrome and she was started on regular laxatives and a low fibre diet with some improvement. Distension of this extreme degree is likely to be associated with exaggerated reflex relaxation of the anterior abdominal wall and diaphragmatic contraction. Consequently, she was referred for 'retraining' using hypnotherapy; this led to further improvement in her symptoms.

## CASE STUDY 13.2

A 47-year-old women presented to her GP with a six month history of abdominal bloating but she denied any other gastric symptoms. She had read about ovarian cancer in a woman's magazine and was concerned about this possibility but an ultrasound examination and a CA125 blood test were both negative. A gastroenterological opinion was sought and on more detailed questioning it emerged that the bloating subsided at night and that her bowels were only opened twice a week but 'they have been like that for years'. She also added that her tummy was frequently uncomfortable although it didn't really amount to pain.

### Comment
Based on the detailed history that subsequently emerged this is unlikely to be anything sinister. The bloating exhibited diurnal fluctuation and she has clearly had other gastrointestinal symptoms for years which strongly suggests a functional problem. Patients often ignore mild functional symptoms until a particular feature rings an alarm bell for them, which then leads them to focus on that symptom without even mentioning other symptoms that would confirm the diagnosis because they class these other features as just normal for them.

# References

1 Houghton LA, Lea R, Agrawal A *et al.* Relationship of abdominal bloating to distention in irritable bowel syndrome and effect of bowel habit. *Gastroenterology* 2006;131(4): 1003–1010.
2 Maxton DG, Morris J and Whorwell PJ. Abdominal distension in irritable bowel syndrome: the patient's perception. *Eur J Gastroenterol Hepatol* 1992;4:241–243.

3  Galati JS, McKee DP and Quigley EM. Response to intraluminal gas in irritable bowel syndrome. Motility versus perception. *Dig Dis Sci* 1995;40(6):1381–1387.

4  Serra J, Azpiroz F and Malagelada JR. Intestinal gas dynamics and tolerance in humans. *Gastroenterology* 1998;115(3):542–550.

5  Reilly BP, Bolton MP, Lewis MJ *et al*. A device for 24 hour ambulatory monitoring of abdominal girth using inductive plethysmography. *Physiol Meas* 2002;23(4):661–670.

6  Alvarez WC. Hysterical type of nongaseous abdominal bloating. *Arch Intern Med (Chic)* 1949;84(2):217–245.

7  Agrawal A, Houghton LA, Reilly B *et al*. Bloating and distension in irritable bowel syndrome: the role of gastrointestinal transit. *Am J Gastroenterol* 2009;104(8):1998–2004.

8  Serra J, Azpiroz F and Malagelada JR. Impaired transit and tolerance of intestinal gas in the irritable bowel syndrome. *Gut* 2001;48(1):14–19.

9  Harder H, Serra J, Azpiroz F *et al*. Intestinal gas distribution determines abdominal symptoms. *Gut* 2003;52(12):1708–1713.

10  Salvioli B, Serra J, Azpiroz F *et al*. Origin of gas retention and symptoms in patients with bloating. *Gastroenterology* 2005;128(3):574–579.

11  Salvioli B, Serra J, Azpiroz F and Malagelada JR. Impaired small bowel gas propulsion in patients with bloating during intestinal lipid infusion. *Am J Gastroenterol* 2006;101(8):1853–1857.

12  Tremolaterra F, Villoria A, Serra J *et al*. Intestinal tone and gas motion. *Neurogastroenterol Motil* 2006;18(10):905–910.

13  Azpiroz F, Bouin M, Camilleri M *et al*. Mechanisms of hypersensitivity in IBS and functional disorders. *Neurogastroenterol Motil* 2007;19(1 Suppl):62–88.

14  Agrawal A, Houghton LA, Lea R *et al*. Bloating and distension in irritable bowel syndrome: the role of visceral sensation. *Gastroenterology* 2008;134(7):1882–1889.

15  Sullivan SN. A prospective study of unexplained visible abdominal bloating. *N Z Med J* 1994;107(988):428–430.

16  Tremolaterra F, Villoria A, Azpiroz F *et al*. Impaired viscerosomatic reflexes and abdominal-wall dystony associated with bloating. *Gastroenterology* 2006;130(4):1062–1068.

17  Villoria A, Azpiroz F, Soldevilla A *et al*. Abdominal accommodation: a coordinated adaptation of the abdominal wall to its content. *Am J Gastroenterol* 2008;103(11):2807–2815.

18  Accarino A, Perez F, Azpiroz F *et al*. Abdominal distention results from caudo-ventral redistribution of contents. *Gastroenterology* 2009;136(5):1544–1551.

19  Elsenbruch S, Harnish MJ and Orr WC. Subjective and objective sleep quality in irritable bowel syndrome. *Am J Gastroenterol* 1999;94(9):2447–2452.

20  Blomhoff S, Jacobsen MB, Spetalen S *et al*. Perceptual hyperreactivity to auditory stimuli in patients with irritable bowel syndrome. *Scand J Gastroenterol* 2000;35(6):583–589.

21  Berman SM, Naliboff BD, Chang L *et al*. Enhanced preattentive central nervous system reactivity in irritable bowel syndrome. *Am J Gastroenterol* 2002;97(11):2791–2797.

22  Andresen V, Bach DR, Poellinger A *et al*. Brain activation responses to subliminal or supraliminal rectal stimuli and to auditory stimuli in irritable bowel syndrome. *Neurogastroenterol Motil* 2005;17(6):827–837.

23  Carruthers HR, Morris J, Tarrier N and Whorwell PJ. Reactivity to images in health and irritable bowel syndrome. *Aliment Pharmacol Ther* 2010;31(1):131–142.

24  Collins SM, Denou E, Verdu EF and Bercik P. The putative role of the intestinal microbiota in the irritable bowel syndrome. *Dig Liver Dis* 2009;41(12):850–853.

25  Ohman L and Simren M. Pathogenesis of IBS: role of inflammation, immunity and neuroimmune interactions. *Nat Rev Gastroenterol Hepatol* 2010;7(3):163–173.

26 Staudacher HM, Whelan K, Irving PM and Lomer MC. Comparison of symptom response following advice for a diet low in fermentable carbohydrates (FODMAPs) versus standard dietary advice in patients with irritable bowel syndrome. *J Hum Nutr Diet* 2011;24(5):487–495.

27 Gibson PR and Shepherd SJ. Evidence-based dietary management of functional gastrointestinal symptoms: The FODMAP approach. *J Gastroenterol Hepatol* 2010;25(2):252–258.

28 Caldarella MP, Milano A, Laterza F *et al.* Visceral sensitivity and symptoms in patients with constipation- or diarrhea-predominant irritable bowel syndrome (IBS): effect of a low-fat intraduodenal infusion. *Am J Gastroenterol* 2005;100(2):383–389.

29 Johannesson E, Simren M, Strid H *et al.* Physical activity improves symptoms in irritable bowel syndrome: a randomized controlled trial. *Am J Gastroenterol* 2011;106(5):915–922.

30 Caldarella MP, Serra J, Azpiroz F and Malagelada JR. Prokinetic effects in patients with intestinal gas retention. *Gastroenterology* 2002;122(7):1748–1755.

31 Tack J, Muller-Lissner S, Bytzer P *et al.* A randomised controlled trial assessing the efficacy and safety of repeated tegaserod therapy in women with irritable bowel syndrome with constipation. *Gut* 2005;54(12):1707–1713.

32 Emmanuel AV, Kamm MA, Roy AJ *et al.* Randomised clinical trial: the efficacy of prucalopride in patients with chronic intestinal pseudo-obstruction – a double-blind, placebo-controlled, cross-over, multiple n = 1 study. *Aliment Pharmacol Ther* 2012;35(1):48–55.

33 Morgan V, Pickens D, Gautam S *et al.* Amitriptyline reduces rectal pain related activation of the anterior cingulate cortex in patients with irritable bowel syndrome. *Gut* 2005;54(5):601–607.

34 Broekaert D, Fischler B, Sifrim D *et al.* Influence of citalopram, a selective serotonin reuptake inhibitor, on oesophageal hypersensitivity: a double-blind, placebo-controlled study. *Aliment Pharmacol Ther* 2006;23(3):365–370.

35 Thoua NM, Murray CD, Winchester WJ *et al.* Amitriptyline modifies the visceral hypersensitivity response to acute stress in the irritable bowel syndrome. *Aliment Pharmacol Ther* 2009;29(5):552–560.

36 Jackson JL, O'Malley PG, Tomkins G *et al.* Treatment of functional gastrointestinal disorders with antidepressant medications: a meta-analysis. *Am J Med* 2000;108(1):65–72.

37 Ford AC, Talley NJ, Schoenfeld PS *et al.* Efficacy of antidepressants and psychological therapies in irritable bowel syndrome: systematic review and meta-analysis. *Gut* 2009;58(3):367–378.

38 Pimentel M, Chow EJ and Lin HC. Normalization of lactulose breath testing correlates with symptom improvement in irritable bowel syndrome. a double-blind, randomized, placebo-controlled study. *Am J Gastroenterol* 2003;98(2):412–419.

39 Pimentel M, Lembo A, Chey WD *et al.* Rifaximin therapy for patients with irritable bowel syndrome without constipation. *N Engl J Med* 2011;364(1):22–32.

40 Sharara AI, Aoun E, Abdul-Baki H *et al.* A randomized double-blind placebo-controlled trial of rifaximin in patients with abdominal bloating and flatulence. *Am J Gastroenterol* 2006;101(2):326–333.

41 Pimentel M, Park S, Mirocha J *et al.* The effect of a nonabsorbed oral antibiotic (rifaximin) on the symptoms of the irritable bowel syndrome: a randomized trial. *Ann Intern Med* 2006;145(8):557–563.

42 Whorwell PJ. Do probiotics improve symptoms in patients with irritable bowel syndrome? *Therap Adv Gastroenterol* 2009;2(4):37–44.

43 Whorwell PJ, Altringer L, Morel J *et al.* Efficacy of an encapsulated probiotic Bifidobacterium infantis 35624 in women with irritable bowel syndrome. *Am J Gastroenterol* 2006;101(7):1581–1590.

44 Marteau P, Cuillerier E, Meance S *et al*. Bifidobacterium animalis strain DN-173 010 shortens the colonic transit time in healthy women: a double-blind, randomized, controlled study. *Aliment Pharmacol Ther* 2002;16(3):587–593.

45 Guyonnet D, Chassany O, Ducrotte P *et al*. Effect of a fermented milk containing Bifidobacterium animalis DN-173 010 on the health-related quality of life and symptoms in irritable bowel syndrome in adults in primary care: a multicentre, randomized, double-blind, controlled trial. *Aliment Pharmacol Ther* 2007;26(3):475–486.

46 Agrawal A, Houghton LA, Morris J *et al*. Clinical trial: the effects of a fermented milk product containing Bifidobacterium lactis DN-173-010 on abdominal distension and gastrointestinal transit in irritable bowel syndrome with constipation. *Aliment Pharmacol Ther* 2008;29:104–114.

47 Whorwell PJ. Review article: The history of hypnotherapy and its role in the irritable bowel syndrome. *Aliment Pharmacol Ther* 2005;22(11–12):1061–1067.

48 Lea R, Houghton LA, Calvert EL et al. Gut-focused hypnotherapy normalizes disordered rectal sensitivity in patients with irritable bowel syndrome. *Aliment Pharmacol Ther* 2003;17(5):635–642.

49 Miller V and Whorwell PJ. Hypnotherapy for functional gastrointestinal disorders: a review. *Int J Clin Exp Hypn* 2009;57(3):279–292.

50 Burri E, Azpiroz A, Hernandez C *et al*. Biofeedback treatment of abdominal distension: proof of concept (Abstract). *Gut* 2010;59:A137.

51 Chiotakakou-Faliakou E, Kamm MA, Roy AJ *et al*. Biofeedback provides long-term benefit for patients with intractable, slow and normal transit constipation. *Gut* 1998;42(4):517–521.

# Multiple Choice Questions

1 Bloating and distension are:
  **A** Most commonly experienced in the morning and improve during the course of the day.
  **B** Usually improve with eating.
  **C** Usually improve if the bowels are opened.
  **D** Should be further investigated if there is no fluctuation over 24 hours.
  **E** Have somewhat different underlying mechanisms.

Answer: D and E are correct.

2 Distension:
  **A** Is associated with visceral hypersensitivity.
  **B** May respond to treatment with laxatives.
  **C** Is associated with abnormal relaxation of the anterior abdominal musculature.
  **D** The change in girth does not usually exceed 5 cm during the course of the day.
  **E** Is associated with depression of the diaphragm.

Answer: B, C and E are correct.

3 Bloating:
  **A** Is associated with abnormal gas handling.
  **B** Is associated with constipation rather than diarrhoea.
  **C** Occurs in 50% of patients complaining of distension.
  **D** Is associated with visceral hyposensitivity.
  **E** Often responds to a low fibre diet.

Answer: A and E are correct.

# CHAPTER 14

# Sequencing the Treatments: The Book in One Chapter!

*Hans Törnblom and Magnus Simrén*
Department of Internal Medicine, Institute of Medicine, Sahlgrenska Academy, University of Gothenburg, Gothenburg, Sweden

---

**Key points**

- Making and explaining the diagnosis and its benign nature are the first treatment actions.
- Symptom assessment can be difficult. Use of validated questionnaires may be helpful.
- Psychosocial factors should be addressed.
- All IBS patients should be given basic dietary advice.
- If pharmcological treatments are given, they should be directed at the predominant symptom and given one at the time.
- Patients with the most severe symptom load, often including extra-intestinal components and psychiatric comorbidity, can benefit from a multidisciplinary approach.

---

## Introduction

Irritable bowel syndrome (IBS) is a benign and highly prevalent disease, which inevitably means that a structured approach to the existing treatment options is crucial in order to use available resources properly. The majority of patients are managed adequately in primary care and only a minority need to be seen by hospital specialists. Both doctor and patient preferences are factors of importance in selection of treatment, where irrational grounds for decision making may result if a good therapeutic relationship is not been developed early on. A confident and experienced doctor seems to increase the chances of improvement, even if the clinical efficacy of available treatment methods is limited [1, 2]. This is exemplified by the high placebo response to treatment interventions in IBS [3], which can be good as a short-term success but, on the other hand, may increase

---

*Irritable Bowel Syndrome: Diagnosis and Clinical Management*, First Edition.
Edited by Anton Emmanuel and Eamonn M.M. Quigley.
© 2013 John Wiley & Sons, Ltd. Published 2013 by John Wiley & Sons, Ltd.

the risk of continued use of ineffective drugs and repeated and unnecessary diagnostic investigations by multiple physicians if a follow-up is not performed.

Communicating symptoms is notoriously difficult. In IBS, assessment of the symptom pattern is the basis both for the diagnosis *per se* [4] and for decision making regarding diagnostic tests and symptom-guided treatment. To take a careful patient history during the visit, focusing on symptoms, is therefore of paramount importance for the continued clinical management of the patient. To combine this with the clinical use of validated questionnaires in a prospective manner is potentially helpful in the clinical decision making. For instance, characterization of the bowel habits with the Bristol Stool Form (BSF) scale [5] is the basis for the current definition of IBS subgroups (constipation (C), diarrhoea (D), mixed (M) or un-subtyped (U)) and may serve as a guide when choosing therapies aimed at improving altered bowel habits in IBS patients. From clinical experience it is often evident that the information about bowel habits, that is stool frequency and consistency, differs between retrospectively recalled information (i.e. taking patient history during a visit) and prospectively collected diary data. Moreover, predominantly ($\geq25\%$) hard (BSF 1–2) or loose (BSF 6–7) stools is a reasonably good predictor for defining patients with slow or fast colonic transit, which can be helpful in choosing the optimal therapy for the patients [6].

The severity of IBS symptoms and the influence of IBS-related and extra-intestinal symptoms on daily life is also of importance when determining the optimal therapeutic approach; this can be assessed with the IBS symptom severity score (IBS-SSS) [7] or the Gastrointestinal Symptom Rating Scale (GSRS)-IBS (only GI symptoms) [8]. Psychosocial factors that may influence illness perception and illness behaviour may also help to guide treatment options, not necessarily directed at IBS symptoms but rather towards comorbidity affecting the way IBS can be coped with. In this respect, the Hospital Anxiety and Depression (HAD) scale [9] is an easy to use, 14-item questionnaire that may identify patients that need psychiatric counselling/therapy. The Patient Health Questionnaire-15 (PHQ-15) [10] is a good predictor for somatization and can help the doctor to identify if there are multiple somatic symptoms, which predicts low quality of life and is a general risk factor for treatment dissatisfaction.

The suggestions regarding the sequencing of the treatment options that are presented here are based on a confident diagnosis of IBS. If so, it is also important that the initial reason for seeking health care brought forward by the patient is adequately addressed, even if it was not related to the IBS diagnosis *per se*. There is probably less hope for improvement of IBS symptoms by any treatment option if the patient still fears a life-threatening disease being the cause of the symptoms. We have divided the treatment options into three levels and the recommendations are partly evidence-based and partly based on clinical experience. All IBS patients are assumed to benefit from the treatment options in level 1, regardless of symptom severity and psychological comorbidity. The recommendations in treatment level 2 are probably useful mainly for patients with moderate symptom severity, for example with an IBS-SSS score >175 [11], or with frequent counselling despite seemingly mild symptoms. Treatment level 3 is intended foremost for IBS patients with abdominal pain predominance, severe IBS symptoms in general (IBS-SSS >300) [11], a complex situation with several extra-intestinal complaints or a difficult psychosocial situation that may include psychiatric illness or drug dependence.

As stated, it is not possible to put forward the suggested sequencing on an evidence-based approach, rather it is mainly based on clinical experience, where safety, availability and costs are important factors to take into account. It must also be remembered that most treatment options will be of benefit in only a minority of the IBS patients, and if we are unable to help, we must not harm our IBS patients by potentially dangerous or ill-defined treatment options.

## Treatment level 1

### Reassurance and explanation

The first and probably most important therapeutic intervention is to make sure that the patient is confident with the IBS diagnosis and has a basic understanding of IBS. Even if the information regarding IBS is steadily increasing in widely available media, it is difficult for the individual to assess its reliability. Therefore, education and information from the healthcare provider is important as a complement to the publicly available information. Local education resources will determine what is feasible in this respect. In most instances an interactive and open discussion during the outpatient visit, where the patient is encouraged to put forward fears and troubles, is sufficient, possibly combined with a written information pamphlet or a repeat consultation with a trained nurse. If available, a structured patient group education, an 'IBS school', has been found to be superior to written information to enhance knowledge of IBS and improve GI symptoms and GI-specific anxiety in IBS patients, even though the cost effectiveness of this kind of education remains to be investigated [12].

The healthcare provider should convey a realistic message regarding the prognosis, where it should be pointed out that IBS is not associated with the development of any medically serious disease, and that the life expectancy is the same as in the general population [13, 14]. Symptom severity fluctuates over time in the majority of IBS patients and some

**Physician–patient interaction**
- Concerns adequately addressed
- Psychosocial factors assessed
- Evaluation of factors that precipitated health care seeking
- Patient involved in the clinical work-up
- Continuity offered
- Realistic goals
- Cost-effective evaluation
- Reassurance of the diagnosis

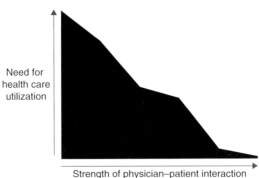

**Figure 14.1**  A good physician–patient interaction decreases the need for multiple consultations. (Modified from Owens *et al.* [2].)

patients improve dramatically, while others continue to have severe symptoms from time to time. Few prognostic risk factors determining the course of IBS are known but a sudden onset of symptoms after an infection (post-infectious IBS) means a better chance for improvement over a period of six years [15]. On the other hand, chronic continuing life stress is a risk factor for not improving, regardless of type of onset [15, 16]. A discussion about the role of food intake in symptom generation and the possible underlying pathophysiologic mechanisms, such as visceral hypersensitivity, gastrointestinal dysmotility and brain–gut interactions, as well as elements of psychosocial nature is to be encouraged as soon as an IBS diagnosis is made or if it is the most probable outcome of a diagnostic work-up.

At the initial stage, good interaction between the patient and all the healthcare professionals involved is key to the subsequent outcome (Figure 14.1). By adequately addressing the concerns of the patient, assessing relevant psychosocial factors and evaluating factors that precipitated health care seeking, the basis for a continuous good relationship is founded. Treatment goals should be realistic. No single therapy has been shown to change the long-term course in IBS and an explanation that treatment is intended to decrease specific symptoms rather than curing the disease is important. Expecting a cure compatible with a course of antibiotics in bacterial infection will inevitably create patient disbelief in the skills of the caregiver. Moreover, involving the patient in the clinical work-up, offering continuity, performing a cost-effective evaluation and reassuring the patient about the diagnosis will diminish the need for continuous healthcare treatment [2].

## Dietary factors
Approximately two out of three patients with IBS experience worsening of gastrointestinal symptom related to food intake [17, 18]. However, today

there is no convincing evidence that food allergy is the mechanism underlying symptom deterioration. It should be kept in mind that perceived food intolerance is not a phenomenon unique to IBS but is very common in the general population as well [19]. Even though the mechanisms underlying adverse food reactions in IBS are incompletely understood, and the evidence supporting the effectiveness of dietary interventions is weak, dietary advice has the highest treatment priority among the patients [20] and should be approached in a serious way by the doctor. If needed, the expertise of a dietician may be added. The latter intervention is especially important for patients who tend to exclude a large number of food items and reduce food intake because of a fear of food allergies or in order to decrease postprandial symptoms with a long-term risk of weight loss and malnutrition. In general, regular meals should be encouraged, even if it provokes symptoms, and advice to eat smaller and more frequent meals and to eat in a nonstressful manner is often of help for the patient.

Traditionally, IBS patients have been advised to increase their fibre intake. This is still useful as long as the goal is to improve stool consistency and frequency; increasing the daily fibre intake seems to be most efficient in IBS-C. The drawback of increasing fibre intake is the risk of worsening other IBS symptoms, such as flatulence, bloating and visible abdominal distension, due to colonic fermentation. Worsening of these symptoms may overshadow a positive effect on bowel habits, leading to a global impression that the advice is negative. In a recent meta-analysis of existing studies, fibre supplementation was modestly effective in relieving global IBS symptoms, but the effect was limited to isphagula, whereas bran was not effective [21]. Water-soluble fibre such as psyllium hydrophilic mucilloid seems to be superior to non-soluble fibre like wheat bran and to produce less side effects [22–24].

Unfortunately, the link between the patient's own experience of food items that trigger IBS symptoms and the outcome of excluding these foods from the diet is lacking. Despite that, many IBS patients use exclusion of foods they find symptom provoking from their diet [17] and often ask for tests to exclude allergies. At this moment, there is no evidence to support a widespread use of food allergy test-panels of any kind in adults with IBS, except for transglutaminase antibodies to exclude coeliac disease. In the same manner, lactose intolerance and the relationship with IBS symptoms is also controversial. In a double-blind, placebo-controlled provocation study in IBS patients, including both lactose tolerant and intolerant patients, there was no difference in symptoms after drinking lactose-containing milk or a lactose-free product [25]. In the clinical situation, a reduction in intake of dairy products is reasonable advice to give, without the necessity to do further diagnostic testing, if milk provokes diarrhoea and gas production. However, a critical evaluation of the symptomatic response to this dietary intervention is necessary. Knowledge of regional and ethnic differences in the prevalence of lactase deficiency may help the physician to selectively give this advice, so that a good source of nutrients is not withheld from large groups of adults. In the western world, the intake of artificial sweeteners like mannitol and sorbitol in chewing gums, soft drinks and candy may also be of importance for gas-related symptoms in IBS and should be taken into account when taking a dietary history. Moreover, emerging evidence suggests that reduced intake of fermentable carbohydrates (FODMAPs – fermentable oligosaccharides, disaccharides, monosaccharides and polyols) might be helpful for subgroups of IBS patients [26].

Furthermore, based on physiological and pathophysiological knowledge, reduced intake of fat may be indicated in IBS patients with food-related symptoms, especially abdominal pain, gas and bloating, as well as urgency and diarrhoea. No formal trials to test this advice have been published, but fat increases colorectal sensitivity [27, 28] and gas retention [29] in IBS patients, so a diet low in fat is theoretically compelling, and based on clinical experience many patients find this advice to be useful.

## Probiotics

The use of probiotics in IBS appears to be safe and may be of benefit in some individuals. Their modes of action are to a large extent unknown, but underlying mechanisms involving inhibition of pathogen binding, immunomodulation and enhancement of mucosal barrier function have been postulated [30]. A major problem is the abundance of probiotic products claiming effectiveness, and our current knowledge is limited by the variety of species, strains and doses of probiotics used in studies published so far. Many of these are small and of low quality, and few formal comparisons between different probiotic products exist. Recent meta-analyses suggest that the majority of probiotic therapies tested show a trend to be effective in IBS, but this finding in part can be questioned because of suspected publication bias, with an over-representation of small, positive studies [31, 32]. Of the individual IBS symptoms reported as an outcome, the effects on abdominal pain and bloating after probiotic treatment are most convincing, and, of the individual bacteria, *Bifidobacterium infantis* 35624 has demonstrated efficacy in two well-designed clinical trials [33, 34], but positive effects with other probiotic products have also been demonstrated [35]. However, in general, it is still too early to give specific strain recommendations, based on the lack of comparative trials, and there are insufficient data to recommend certain probiotics to different patient groups. Long-term data of the efficacy and safety of probiotic treatment in IBS are largely lacking, but results of a six-months trial have been published [35].

## Treatment level 2

At this level of treatment, pharmacotherapy directed towards specific IBS symptoms (summarized in Figure 14.2) may be initiated by the doctor in close collaboration with the patient. It is good advice to test one drug or make one treatment adjustment at a time, with a predefined time point for evaluation. One must not prescribe drugs in an attempt to 'get rid' of the patient without follow-up. Instead, a state of mutual understanding that the pharmacological agent may help for the specific symptom should be reached but, if it does not, it should be stopped. It is also important from time to time to give advice to temporarily stop a treatment in order to evaluate if it is still needed. An effective pharmacotherapy should be able to regain its positive effects if symptoms recur during a 'drug holiday'. When there are no more pharmacological treatment options to try, this should be clearly stated, but together with the message that the patient–doctor relationship continues, and that nonpharmacological treatment options, self-management strategies (Chapter 7) and general support measures are still available to reduce the symptom burden.

### Treatment directed towards specific IBS symptoms

As a general rule, based on the shortcomings with alosetron and tegaserod, where unexpected side effects appeared in the early phase of clinical use, new IBS drugs should probably be used mainly in specialist gastroenterology outpatient clinics in order to optimize their use and to have tight control of side effects. A repeat analysis of the symptom pattern, especially if not done during the initial work-up, may also need to be performed where treatment fails. In selected cases where difficult rectal passage of stool is the predominant symptom, assessment of pelvic floor function can be done to evaluate if biofeedback training is indicated.

### Constipation

Most patients with IBS who fulfil criteria for constipation predominance have a normal transit time [36]. With this in mind, fibre supplementation and bulking agents like psyllium, methylcellulose and calcium poly-carbophil, rather than stimulant laxatives or prokinetics, are used as first-line treatment options for patients with IBS-C, but the evidence supporting the use of bulking agents and fibre supplementation is relatively weak [21, 37]. To avoid common side effects like bloating, flatulence and intensified abdominal discomfort and pain [22, 38], a gradual dose-titration is recommended on an empirical basis. As during the initial evaluation of symptoms, a symptom diary may help to evaluate effects and side effects of the treatment regimen. If this measure fails, a trial with osmotic laxatives like polyethylene glycol (PEG) or lactulose is indicated to ease passage of stool, even if formal trials in IBS are largely lacking except for a small study that included PEG in one of the treatment arms (27 patients). After four weeks of treatment, a significant improvement in stool frequency was seen, but with no effect on the intensity of abdominal pain [39]. From a clinical point of view, it is reasonable that PEG will affect bowel habits in IBS-C in a similar way as in patients with chronic idiopathic constipation as shown in a recent meta-analysis [40]. The treatment effect should be evaluated during a follow-up period of at least 4–12 weeks.

In the USA and Switzerland, where lubiprostone, a chloride channel activator, is available for women with IBS-C, this drug can be prescribed to patients who have failed fibre, bulking agents and laxatives. The recommended dose in IBS-C is 8 μg twice daily; this has shown significant benefit compared to placebo [41], also for IBS symptoms other than constipation. Increasing the dose is not recommended because of a parallel increase in side effects like nausea, diarrhoea and abdominal pain [42].

$5HT_4$ antagonists have been developed for treatment of IBS-C and chronic idiopathic constipation. Tegaserod, a partial $5-HT_4$ receptor agonist intended for women with IBS-C, has been withdrawn because of increased risk for cardiovascular events. It can still be prescribed under restricted license, also with an age restriction (<55 years). Prucalopride is a selective, high-affinity $5HT_4$ agonist authorized by the European Medicines Agency for symptomatic treatment of females with chronic constipation in whom laxatives fail to provide adequate relief; this is based upon the results from three big trials [43–45] and has shown good long-term effects [46]. However, although no formal trials in IBS-C exist so far, it can be expected that prucalopride can be useful also in subsets of IBS-C patients, as the overlap between IBS-C, functional constipation and chronic idiopathic constipation is substantial [47].

Linaclotide represent a new type of intestinal secretagogue that acts by binding to the guanylate cyclase C receptor on the intestinal epitheium without any systemic effects. A series of intracellular events involving cGMP formation ends up with the opening of CFTR channels resulting in chloride secretion. Linaclotide was during the autumn 2012 approved for use in moderate to severe IBS-C by US Food and Drug Administration and received a a positive opinion recommending marketing approval by the European Committee for Medicinal Products for Human Use (CHMP), and is expected to be available for use in 2013. Two large phase-III trials [48, 49] showed positive effects on stool frequency and stool form and decreased abdominal pain and discomfort, in a similar way as in chronic constipation, where a number of studies exist. Interestingly, beside the effect on secretion, linaclotide also has antinociceptive effects with improvement of abdominal pain, discomfort and bloating, which of course is favourable for IBS patients.

### Diarrhoea

Loperamide is the first choice for intermittent or chronic use in IBS patients with predominant diarrhoea; the dose range is 2–16 mg/day. There is good evidence that loperamide reduces stool frequency and improves stool consistency [20, 50–53], but it should not be expected to decrease other IBS symptoms such as abdominal pain or bloating. There is no evidence that the positive effects, which are mediated by binding to the $\mu$-receptor in the myenteric plexus and thereby decreasing gut motility and secretion, has any tendency to decrease over time or carry any risk for drug dependency. Most patients need it on an intermittent basis in situations where they need to be confident with their bowel habits, but, for those with severe diarrhoea, chronic and regular use can be encouraged. Most doctors will also meet patients that report severe constipation already after a single pill. If anything, that probably provides evidence that the diarrhoea is not due to an accelerated intestinal transit and should not be treated with loperamide.

Whether or not bile-acid malabsorption is a common underlying reason for diarrhoea in IBS is not clear. However, there are studies suggesting that approximately one out of three patients with diarrhoea who do not respond to loperamide treatment has bile acid malabsorption and that their symptoms are more responsive to the bile-acid binding agent cholestyramine than to loperamide [54]. Especially in IBS patients with nocturnal diarrhoea and in those with an acute onset of their IBS symptoms after a gastroenteritis (post-infectious IBS) [55, 56], a trial period with a bile-acid binding agent is indicated, as it as well as in patients with more severe diarrhoeal symptoms that do not respond to loperamide. If this treatment option is used, it is important to keep the nonspecific binding properties to other medications in mind, which potentially may decrease their bioavailability.

5-HT$_3$ receptor antagonists have shown efficacy in IBS-D patients [57]. Unfortunately, side effects, mainly ischemic colitis, have stopped further development of drugs from this class or have led to withdrawal. Alosetron, intended for women with IBS-D, is available in the United States under restricted license, but will not appear in Europe.

### Abdominal pain

Antispasmodics seem to be helpful in IBS in patients where the abdominal pain attacks are more or less predictable and episodic with symptom free intervals in between. A common way of using these pharmacological agents is by trying to prevent postprandial symptoms. The majority of these drugs have an antimuscarinic effect, which is proposed to relieve smooth muscle spasm; these drugs include hyoscine, mebeverine, otilonium bromide, pinaverium bromide and cimetropium bromide. The clinical trials evaluating antispasmodics are quite old with suboptimal quality. Moreover, the availabilities of the different drugs are limited, since several of the drugs from the clinical trials are not available in all countries and, therefore, there are problems in finding an equivalent dose for the available antispasmodics. However, repeated meta-analyses supports their efficacy in IBS compared to placebo treatment [21, 37, 58–62], but the small sample size in many studies together with a potential publication bias make this finding weak. The commonly reported side effects are related to the antimuscarinic action of the drugs, such as dry mouth, constipation, blurred vision and palpitations.

Peppermint oil is an over-the-counter drug alternative belonging to the group of antispasmodics, but it does not act via an antimuscarinic effect, rather as a nonspecific smooth muscle relaxant. Studies with peppermint oil are scarce, but when combining the four randomized trials, the drug is superior to placebo, and it seems to be a safe and cheap alternative to the more traditional antispasmodics, and perhaps just as effective [21].

Antidepressants are useful in patients with more or less daily abdominal pain of troublesome character [63]. The older tricyclic antidepressants (TCAs) are still considered as first choice, but with new data appearing the more modern selective serotonin reuptake inhibitors (SSRIs) seem to be effective as well; these drugs probably act more on symptoms in general, including depression and anxiety, rather than specifically on pain. In most IBS patients, there is a need to explain the rationale for using antidepressants and quite often to downplay the antidepressive effect. Most patients find it easier to accept and understand the possibility of TCAs modulating the central pain experience and reducing primary afferent nerve firing. The recommended low starting dose also underscores and reassures that the doctor does not believe that 'it is all in the head' of the patient, because these doses do not affect depressive symptoms. For those patients not responding to a dose equivalent to 10–25 mg/day of, for example, amitriptyline within a month, the dose can gradually be increased to levels used in psychiatry if tolerated by the patients. Common side effects like sedation, constipation, dry mouth and palpitations often limit the use of higher doses. Nocturnal pain may be particularly suitable to treat with TCAs since the sedative effect may be of additional help. TCAs can also be worth a trial in the patient situation mentioned above, where an IBS-D situation may be related to a pronounced rectal hypersensitivity.

### Abdominal gas and bloating

For the moment, dietary advice, as stated under treatment level 1, is probably the most effective recommendation for these symptoms. Some probiotics may also have a positive effect. Since visceral sensory function may be involved as a pathophysiologic mechanism, a trial with a TCA may be initiated without any good formal evidence.

## Other pharmacological agents

The nonabsorbable antibiotic rifaximin has received a lot of interest as an IBS treatment based on the assumption that some patients have their symptoms because of a small intestinal bacterial overgrowth (SIBO). An early trial showed promising results in reducing IBS symptoms, and among the symptoms bloating was the one that responded most favourably [64]. However, already at the level of the putative pathogenetic mechanism lies a problem in definitions, leading to prevalence figures for SIBO in IBS to vary from 78 [65] to 4% [66]. Recently, two multicentre trials combined were published showing that a two-week course of rifaximin, 550 mg three times daily in nonconstipated IBS patients, gave a small but statistically significant improvement compared to placebo regarding global relief of symptoms (9% better than placebo) and bloating (10% better than placebo). Given the relative small effect and lack of data from other parts of the world, this type of antibiotic treatment cannot be recommended for use in IBS patients outside controlled clinical trials. More information about predictors of treatment responsiveness, the risk of development of antibiotic resistance, the efficacy and safety of re-treatment schedules and the optimal dosing regimen is needed before further recommendations can be made.

Herbal medicines have been tested in IBS and other functional GI disorders and demonstrated efficacy [67, 68]. Iberogast is one example, but the clinical studies focus mainly on functional dyspepsia. Pregabalin, an $\alpha_2\delta$ ligand, is sometimes used for patients with severe therapy refractory abdominal pain and anxiety: The scientific evidence supporting its use is still very weak, but from clinical experience some patients fare well with this therapy [69].

## Psychological treatment

For patients with more severe GI symptoms with or without comorbid psychological symptoms, a range of psychological treatment alternatives has been investigated [70]. The psychological therapies that have been evaluated in IBS are mainly cognitive behavioural therapy (CBT), dynamic psychotherapy, hypnotherapy and relaxation therapy. Except for relaxation therapy, pooling of data suggests that psychological treatment options are more effective than usual care to improve global symptom severity [31, 63]. This kind of intervention can be used at treatment level 2, but in clinical practice the main problem with this type of treatment is availability, and partly, therefore, it is mainly used for patients who are refractory to other types of treatments, that is at level 3. Based on the fact that there is no clear evidence suggesting clinically important differences in effectiveness between CBT, dynamic psychotherapy or hypnotherapy, the recommendation can be to choose the type of treatment that is available at the local level. To have good access to these therapies and to

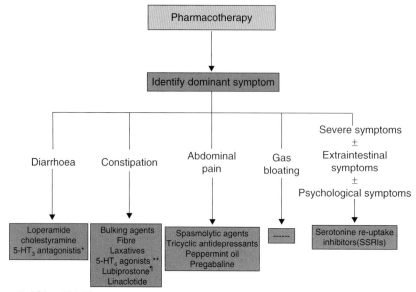

\*   USA, restricted licence
\*\*  Restricted licence (tegaserod) or limited C-IBS evidence (prucalopride)
¶   Available in USA and Switzerland for women

**Figure 14.2** Pharmacologic treatment options directed towards dominant IBS symptom.

obtain good clinical results, regular and good communication between the referring physicians and the therapists is very important. Moreover, motivating the patient for this kind of treatment probably also affects the clinical outcome, and explaining that this is a way to manage the severe IBS symptoms and not just a way to treat depression or anxiety is helpful. An innovative approach to increase the availability of these treatment options is to use the Internet and promising results exist for the effectiveness of Internet-based CBT in patients with IBS [71]. Moreover, treating patients in groups instead of individually is another option to increase the availability (For summary, see Figure 14.3).

## CASE STUDY

### Clinical Case Scenarios
A 34-year-old female patient seeks advice regarding her severely troublesome bowel habits at a GP's office. She is an otherwise healthy, nonsmoking, low-alcohol consuming individual working full time as a high-school teacher. Her mother had problems of the same kind, but less severe.

A GP colleague at another clinic investigated her two years ago including blood-chemistry, serology to rule out coeliac disease and stool samples for culture. She was told the diagnosis was IBS after a brief telephone call follow-up. Her main problem at that time point was her irregular bowel habits, ranging from constipation to a severe rush to the toilet with mushy stool, and also the abdominal cramps preceding a bowel movement. Her impression of the information given was that her problems were more or less stress-related and would go away if she 'relaxed a bit'. At the same consultation, tramadol was prescribed for a headache problem that she complained about for which paracetamol did not suffice. This prescription has been repeated without further consultation since then, even if she for now takes it on a daily basis to relieve her abdominal pain and distension that is associated with her current bowel problem, constipation. The reason for consulting another GP is because she has problems in getting a face-to-face appointment with her first doctor.

A physical examination reveals nothing abnormal.

You confirm the initial diagnosis of IBS without any further investigations. A full 20 minutes is spent to get a more extensive history from the patient and also to explain the nature of IBS. Since it turns out that she has a fear that her bowel problems might develop into cancer, its benign nature is stressed. Questioning her about food habits reveal that the lunch meal is nonexistent during workdays in order to reduce the risk of unacceptable bloating in the afternoon and that her fibre intake is exceptionally high in an attempt to relieve her constipation.

You present her with the following suggestion:

1.  Stop tramadol in order to get rid of its probable side effects, which could be a big part of her current symptoms.

2.  Reduction in fibre intake to decrease bloating.

3.  Start having a regular lunch meal of medium size and a complementary snack like a piece of fruit in the morning and afternoon.

4.  Repeat consultation in 6–8 weeks as follow up.

### Scenario 1

A much improved and somewhat surprised patient comes to your office six weeks later. She managed to stop tramadol after three weeks of tapering the dose and has once more the well-known irregular bowel-habits from before. Bloating is less prominent and pain attacks less frequent and of lower intensity. Most of all, she dares to have lunch during workdays.

This time, the only suggestion is to further reduce the type of cereal fibre she is adding and exchange it for ispaghula husk 3.5 g OD or b.d. A phone-call in another six weeks reveals more regular bowel habits without any worsening of bloating and abdominal pain.

The plan from now on is to have an on-demand appointment.

### Scenario 2

A disappointed patient comes to your office. None of your suggestions have been possible to achieve. The dose of tramadol is unchanged. When lowering it, she cannot sleep. Her constipation is so far unaffected or worsened when trying to decrease fibre intake a bit.

You tell her about a probable physical addiction to tramadol and the importance of getting rid of it. Her answer to this is disbelief, since she experienced that a dose reduction also unveils a tendency of arthralgias that she has not been aware of before. She suspects an arthrosis, definitely no tendency of addiction. After further discussion of the nature of problems, a week of filling in a stool diary is decided and yet another appointment after that.

A week later, she turns up with a diary where there have been three bowel movements with the shape of Bristol Stool Form (BSF) scale 2 for all of them. You are even more strengthened in your conviction that tramadol needs to be stopped, and after having the patient to fill out a HAD questionnaire with a high score for anxiety [17] and a borderline score for depression [11], you suggest to her that she has a psychiatric consultation as well. A bit hesitantly, she accepts it and at an appointment 12 weeks later returns in a much more satisfied mood. She is now on regular dose SSRI-therapy and has more or less managed to get rid of tramadol. Bloating is less prominent, constipation reasonable and pain attacks less frequent and of lower intensity. Ispaghula husk 3.5 g OD is added and she will continue to have a psychiatric contact for another three-month period and an on-demand contact with you.

## Treatment level 3

A proportion of patients have severe symptoms that do not respond to any of the treatment options in level 1 and 2 (Figure 14.3). Some of these also have psychiatric comorbidities and numerous extra-intestinal symptoms, as well as severe GI symptoms. In some of these patients, use of multiple drugs may have become a part of the problem, especially the use of analgesics and excessive laxative use.

In these patients with severe IBS, most often including extra-intestinal symptoms and related diagnoses such as fibromyalgia, chronic headache, insomnia, anxiety and mood disorders, a multidisciplinary approach is indicated. It is important to define if IBS is the sole problem or if there are parallel problems like a primary psychiatric disease, psychosocial problems, drug dependency or use of opioid analgesics, which will need specific interventions besides the regular IBS treatment. As previously mentioned, somatization is more common in this group of IBS patients than in the general population. A substantial proportion of these patients benefits from psychotropic drugs, and SSRIs are often beneficial, both for GI and psychiatric symptoms.

The multidisciplinary approach used in this patient group should use patient-centred care, and the key to success is to have different healthcare providers take part in the management. The healthcare provider leading the management can differ based on the clinical presentation; for some patients it can be a gastroenterologist, whereas others are better off with a psychiatrist, psychologist or a behavioural therapist. Some of these patients need combinations of pharmacological treatment alternatives in order to control the severe symptoms, but one of the main goals for this patient group is to avoid opioid analgesics, since these may worsen the situation [72]. Even though a multidisciplinary approach is advocated, for some patients the main focus may still be on specific problems, such as on treating psychiatric comorbidity when this dominates the clinical picture

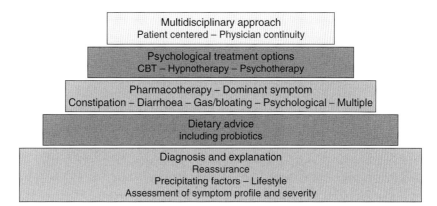

**Figure 14.3** Sequencing of treatments where the IBS diagnosis is the first and fundamental treatment step.

or to focus on pain management when this is the predominant feature. Regardless of how the multidisciplinary approach for these patients is organized, health care continuity is of great importance for this group of patients in order to avoid 'doctor shopping'. (Figure 14.3)

## Summary

A graduated treatment approach is recommended for IBS patients. For patients with mild symptoms reassurance, education and lifestyle and dietary changes, when appropriate, are sufficient. Patients with moderately severe symptoms can often be managed successfully with symptom modifying drugs. Psychological treatment alternatives, such as CBT, hypnotherapy and dynamic psychotherapy can, from a theoretical point of view, also be offered at this stage, but limited availability limits the use of these treatment options widely in clinical practice, and is therefore often reserved for patients with more severe and intrusive symptoms. Furthermore, for the small group with severe and incapacitating symptoms, a multidisciplinary approach is recommended and psychotropic drugs are often used in the management of these patients. Opioid analgesics should be avoided as far as possible.

## References

1 Kaptchuk TJ, Kelley JM, Conboy LA *et al.* Components of placebo effect: randomised controlled trial in patients with irritable bowel syndrome. *BMJ* 2008;336(7651):999–1003.
2 Owens DM, Nelson DK and Talley NJ. The irritable bowel syndrome: long-term prognosis and the physician-patient interaction. *Ann Intern Med* 1995;122(2):107–112.

3 Patel SM, Stason WB, Legedza A *et al*. The placebo effect in irritable bowel syndrome trials: a meta-analysis. *Neurogastroenterol Motil* 2005;17(3):332–340.

4 Longstreth GF, Thompson WG, Chey WD *et al*. Functional bowel disorders. *Gastroenterology* 2006;130(5):1480–1491.

5 O'Donnell LJ, Virjee J and Heaton KW. Detection of pseudodiarrhoea by simple clinical assessment of intestinal transit rate. *BMJ* 1990;300(6722):439–440.

6 Sadik R, Bjornsson E and Simren M. The relationship between symptoms, body mass index, gastrointestinal transit and stool frequency in patients with irritable bowel syndrome. *Eur J Gastroenterol Hepatol* 2010;22(1):102–108.

7 Francis CY, Morris J and Whorwell PJ. The irritable bowel severity scoring system: a simple method of monitoring irritable bowel syndrome and its progress. *Aliment Pharmacol Ther* 1997;11(2):395–402.

8 Wiklund IK, Fullerton S, Hawkey CJ *et al*. An irritable bowel syndrome-specific symptom questionnaire: development and validation. *Scand J Gastroenterol* 2003;38(9):947–954.

9 Zigmond AS and Snaith RP. The hospital anxiety and depression scale. *Acta Psychiatr Scand* 1983;67(6):361–370.

10 Spitzer RL, Williams JB, Kroenke K *et al*. Utility of a new procedure for diagnosing mental disorders in primary care. The PRIME-MD 1000 study. *JAMA* 1994; 272(22):1749–1756.

11 Francis CY, Morris J and Whorwell PJ. The irritable bowel severity scoring system: a simple method of monitoring irritable bowel syndrome and its progress. *Aliment Pharmacol Ther* 1997;11(2):395–402.

12 Ringstrom G, Storsrud S, Posserud I *et al*. Structured patient education is superior to written information in the management of patients with irritable bowel syndrome: a randomized controlled study. *Eur J Gastroenterol Hepatol* 2010;22(4):420–428.

13 Harvey RF, Mauad EC and Brown AM. Prognosis in the irritable bowel syndrome: a 5-year prospective study. *Lancet* 1987;1(8539):963–965.

14 Sloth H and Jorgensen LS. Chronic non-organic upper abdominal pain: diagnostic safety and prognosis of gastrointestinal and non-intestinal symptoms. A 5- to 7-year follow-up study. *Scand J Gastroenterol* 1988;23(10):1275–1280.

15 Neal KR, Barker L and Spiller RC. Prognosis in post-infective irritable bowel syndrome: a six year follow up study. *Gut* 2002;51(3):410–413.

16 Bennett EJ, Tennant CC, Piesse C *et al*. Level of chronic life stress predicts clinical outcome in irritable bowel syndrome. *Gut* 1998;43(2):256–261.

17 Simren M, Mansson A and Langkilde AM *et al*. Food-related gastrointestinal symptoms in the irritable bowel syndrome. *Digestion* 2001;63(2):108–115.

18 Park MI and Camilleri M. Is there a role of food allergy in irritable bowel syndrome and functional dyspepsia? A systematic review. *Neurogastroenterol Motil* 2006;18(8): 595–607.

19 Young E, Stoneham MD, Petruckevitch A *et al*. A population study of food intolerance. *Lancet* 1994;343(8906):1127–1130.

20 Halpert A, Dalton CB, Palsson O *et al*.. What patients know about irritable bowel syndrome (IBS) and what they would like to know. National Survey on Patient Educational Needs in IBS and development and validation of the Patient Educational Needs Questionnaire (PEQ). *Am J Gastroenterol* 2007;102(9):1972–1982.

21 Ford AC, Talley NJ, Spiegel BM *et al*. Effect of fibre, antispasmodics, and peppermint oil in the treatment of irritable bowel syndrome: systematic review and meta-analysis. *BMJ* 2008;337:a2313.

22 Francis CY and Whorwell PJ. Bran and irritable bowel syndrome: time for reappraisal. *Lancet* 1994;344(8914):39–40.

23 Rees G, Davies J, Thompson R *et al*. Randomised-controlled trial of a fibre supplement on the symptoms of irritable bowel syndrome. *J R Soc Health* 2005; 125(1):30–34.

24 Bijkerk CJ, de Wit NJ, Muris JW *et al*. Soluble or insoluble fibre in irritable bowel syndrome in primary care? Randomised placebo controlled trial. *BMJ* 2009;339:b3154.

25 Savaiano DA, Boushey CJ and McCabe GP. Lactose intolerance symptoms assessed by meta-analysis: a grain of truth that leads to exaggeration. *J Nutr* 2006;136(4): 1107–1113.

26 Gibson PR and Shepherd SJ. Evidence-based dietary management of functional gastrointestinal symptoms: The FODMAP approach. *J Gastroenterol Hepatol* 2010; 25(2):252–258.

27 Caldarella MP, Milano A, Laterza F *et al*. Visceral sensitivity and symptoms in patients with constipation- or diarrhea-predominant irritable bowel syndrome (IBS): effect of a low-fat intraduodenal infusion. *Am J Gastroenterol* 2005;100(2):383–389.

28 Simren M, Abrahamsson H and Bjornsson ES. An exaggerated sensory component of the gastrocolonic response in patients with irritable bowel syndrome. *Gut* 2001; 48(1):20–27.

29 Serra J, Salvioli B, Azpiroz F and Malagelada JR. Lipid-induced intestinal gas retention in irritable bowel syndrome. *Gastroenterology* 2002;123(3):700–706.

30 Spiller R. Review article: probiotics and prebiotics in irritable bowel syndrome. *Aliment Pharmacol Ther* 2008;28(4):385–396.

31 Brandt LJ, Chey WD, Foxx-Orenstein AE *et al*. An evidence-based position statement on the management of irritable bowel syndrome. *Am J Gastroenterol* 2009;104 (Suppl 1):S1–35.

32 Moayyedi P, Ford AC, Talley NJ *et al*. The efficacy of probiotics in the therapy of irritable bowel syndrome: a systematic review. *Gut* 2010;59(3):325–332.

33 O'Mahony L, McCarthy J, Kelly P *et al*. Lactobacillus and bifidobacterium in irritable bowel syndrome: symptom responses and relationship to cytokine profiles. *Gastroenterology* 2005;128(3):541–551.

34 Whorwell PJ, Altringer L, Morel J *et al*. Efficacy of an encapsulated probiotic Bifidobacterium infantis 35624 in women with irritable bowel syndrome. *Am J Gastroenterol* 2006;101(7):1581–1590.

35 Kajander K, Hatakka K, Poussa T *et al*. A probiotic mixture alleviates symptoms in irritable bowel syndrome patients: a controlled 6-month intervention. *Aliment Pharmacol Ther* 2005;22(5):387–394.

36 Tornblom H, Van Oudenhove L, Sadik R *et al*. Colonic transit time and IBS symptoms: what's the link? *Am J Gastroenterol* 2012;107(5):754–60.

37 Jailwala J, Imperiale TF and Kroenke K. Pharmacologic treatment of the irritable bowel syndrome: a systematic review of randomized, controlled trials. *Ann Intern Med* 2000;133(2):136–147.

38 Snook J and Shepherd HA. Bran supplementation in the treatment of irritable bowel syndrome. *Aliment Pharmacol Ther* 1994;8(5):511–514.

39 Khoshoo V, Armstead C and Landry L. Effect of a laxative with and without tegaserod in adolescents with constipation predominant irritable bowel syndrome. *Aliment Pharmacol Ther* 2006;23(1):191–196.

40 Ford AC, Suares NC. Effect of laxatives and pharmacological therapies in chronic idiopathic constipation: systematic review and meta-analysis. *Gut* 2011;60(2):209–218.

41 Drossman DA, Chey WD, Johanson JF *et al*. Clinical trial: lubiprostone in patients with constipation-associated irritable bowel syndrome–results of two randomized, placebo-controlled studies. *Aliment Pharmacol Ther* 2009;29(3):329–341.

42 Johanson JF, Drossman DA, Panas R *et al*. Clinical trial: phase 2 study of lubiprostone for irritable bowel syndrome with constipation. *Aliment Pharmacol Ther* 2008; 27(8):685–696.

43 Camilleri M, Kerstens R, Rykx A and Vandeplassche L. A placebo-controlled trial of prucalopride for severe chronic constipation. *N Engl J Med* 2008;358(22):2344–2354.

44 Quigley EM, Vandeplassche L, Kerstens R and Ausma J. Clinical trial: the efficacy, impact on quality of life, and safety and tolerability of prucalopride in severe chronic constipation – a 12-week, randomized, double-blind, placebo-controlled study. *Aliment Pharmacol Ther* 2009;29(3):315–328.

45 Tack J, van Outryve M, Beyens G *et al*. Prucalopride (Resolor) in the treatment of severe chronic constipation in patients dissatisfied with laxatives. *Gut* 2009;58(3):357–365.

46 Camilleri M, Van Outryve MJ, Beyens G *et al*. Clinical trial: the efficacy of open-label prucalopride treatment in patients with chronic constipation - follow-up of patients from the pivotal studies. *Aliment Pharmacol Ther* 2010;32(9):1113–1123.

47 Wong RK, Palsson OS, Turner MJ *et al*. Inability of the Rome III criteria to distinguish functional constipation from constipation-subtype irritable bowel syndrome. *Am J Gastroenterol* 2010;105(10):2228–2234.

48 Rao S, Lembo AJ, Shiff SJ, Lavins BJ, Currie MG, Jia XD, *et al*. A 12-Week, Randomized, Controlled Trial with a 4-Week Randomized Withdrawal Period to Evaluate the Efficacy and Safety of Linaclotide in Irritable Bowel Syndrome with Constipation. *Am J Gastroenterol* 2012 Sep 18.

49 Chey WD, Lembo AJ, Lavins BJ, Shiff SJ, Kurtz CB, Currie MG, *et al*. Linaclotide for Irritable Bowel Syndrome with Constipation: A 26-to Evaluate Efficacy and Safety. *Am J Gastroenterol* 2012 Sep 18.

50 Cann PA, Read NW, Holdsworth CD and Barends D. Role of loperamide and placebo in management of irritable bowel syndrome (IBS). *Dig Dis Sci* 1984;29(3):239–247.

51 Efskind PS, Bernklev T, Vatn MH. A double-blind placebo-controlled trial with loperamide in irritable bowel syndrome. *Scand J Gastroenterol* 1996;31(5):463–468.

52 Hovdenak N. Loperamide treatment of the irritable bowel syndrome. *Scand J Gastroenterol* (Suppl) 1987;130:81–84.

53 Lavo B, Stenstam M and Nielsen AL. Loperamide in treatment of irritable bowel syndrome – a double-blind placebo controlled study. *Scand J Gastroenterol* (Suppl) 1987;130:77–80.

54 Smith MJ, Cherian P, Raju GS *et al*. Bile acid malabsorption in persistent diarrhoea. *J R Coll Physicians Lond* 2000;34(5):448–451.

55 Niaz SK, Sandrasegaran K, Renny FH and Jones BJ. Postinfective diarrhoea and bile acid malabsorption. *J R Coll Physicians Lond* 1997;31(1):53–56.

56 Sinha L, Liston R, Testa HJ and Moriarty KJ. Idiopathic bile acid malabsorption: qualitative and quantitative clinical features and response to cholestyramine. *Aliment Pharmacol Ther* 1998;12(9):839–844.

57 Camilleri M, Northcutt AR, Kong S *et al*. Efficacy and safety of alosetron in women with irritable bowel syndrome: a randomised, placebo-controlled trial. *Lancet* 2000;355(9209):1035–1040.

58 Systematic review on the management of irritable bowel syndrome in the European Union. *Eur J Gastroenterol Hepatol* 2007;19(Suppl 1):S11–S37.

59 Akehurst R and Kaltenthaler E. Treatment of irritable bowel syndrome: a review of randomised controlled trials. *Gut* 2001;48(2):272–282.

60 Brandt LJ, Bjorkman D, Fennerty MB *et al*. Systematic review on the management of irritable bowel syndrome in North America. *Am J Gastroenterol* 2002;97(11 Suppl):S7–S26.

61 Poynard T, Naveau S, Mory B and Chaput JC. Meta-analysis of smooth muscle relaxants in the treatment of irritable bowel syndrome. *Aliment Pharmacol Ther* 1994;8(5):499–510.

62 Quartero AO, Meineche-Schmidt V, Muris J *et al.* Bulking agents, antispasmodic and antidepressant medication for the treatment of irritable bowel syndrome. *Cochrane Database Syst Rev* 2005(2):CD003460.

63 Ford AC, Talley NJ, Schoenfeld PS *et al.* Efficacy of antidepressants and psychological therapies in irritable bowel syndrome: systematic review and meta-analysis. *Gut* 2009 Mar;58(3):367–378.

64 Pimentel M, Park S, Mirocha J *et al.* The effect of a nonabsorbed oral antibiotic (rifaximin) on the symptoms of the irritable bowel syndrome: a randomized trial. *Ann Intern Med* 2006 Oct 17;145(8):557–563.

65 Pimentel M, Chow EJ and Lin HC. Eradication of small intestinal bacterial overgrowth reduces symptoms of irritable bowel syndrome. *Am J Gastroenterol* 2000;95(12):3503–3506.

66 Posserud I, Stotzer PO, Bjornsson ES *et al.* Small intestinal bacterial overgrowth in patients with irritable bowel syndrome. *Gut* 2007;56(6):802–808.

67 Bensoussan A, Talley NJ, Hing M *et al.* Treatment of irritable bowel syndrome with Chinese herbal medicine: a randomized controlled trial. *JAMA* 1998; 280(18):1585–1589.

68 Rosch W, Liebregts T, Gundermann KJ *et al.* Phytotherapy for functional dyspepsia: a review of the clinical evidence for the herbal preparation STW 5. *Phytomedicine* 2006;13(Suppl 5):114–121.

69 Gale JD and Houghton LA. Alpha 2 Delta (alpha(2)delta) Ligands, Gabapentin and Pregabalin: What is the Evidence for Potential Use of These Ligands in Irritable Bowel Syndrome. *Front Pharmacol* 2011;2:28.

70 Lackner JM, Mesmer C, Morley S *et al.* Psychological treatments for irritable bowel syndrome: a systematic review and meta-analysis. *J Consult Clin Psychol* 2004;72(6):1100–1113.

71 Ljotsson B, Hedman E, Andersson E *et al.* Internet-delivered exposure-based treatment vs. stress management for irritable bowel syndrome: a randomized trial. *Am J Gastroenterol* 2011;106(8):1481–1491.

72 Grunkemeier DM, Cassara JE, Dalton CB and Drossman DA. The narcotic bowel syndrome: clinical features, pathophysiology, and management. *Clin Gastroenterol Hepatol* 2007;5(10):1126–39; quiz 1–2.

# Multiple Choice Questions

## Choose the best answer

1  A 35-year-old female with an IBS diagnosis for 10 years is seeking your advice regarding her problems with intermittent tendency for diarrhoea. She had an appointment at your office three weeks ago for the same problem and you prescribed loperamide PRN. After trying 4 mg on two separate occasions which resulted in constipation for two days at each time she is convinced about her being extremely sensitive to medications in general. She still wants help for the diarrhoea. What do you do next?

   **A** Order a SeHCAT test.

   **B** Recommend she tries an eight-week trial with a probiotic preparation.

   **C** Ask her to fill in a stool diary and have a repeat consultation.

   **D** Give loperamide another try but with 2 mg as the preferred dose.

Answer: C

Communicating stool habits is difficult. This particular patient returned a stool diary with frequent passage of stool two mornings in one week, both mornings identified as stressful because her children where extremely slow to get ready for school, almost making her late for work. The first faecal passage those mornings had BSF scale 3, thereafter 3–4 times within 30 min with small amounts of faecal matter with BSF scale 6–7. The other days she had one or two bowel movements during the day with formed stool. Completing the diary and reflecting about it made the patient realize the psychological component involved and she no longer wanted any medications.

2  A 21-year-old male patient originating from Bosnia but living in Sweden for 13 years had a diagnosis of IBS with mixed bowel habits (IBS-M) two years ago. Among the investigations done, coeliac disease was ruled out. He is very troubled by increasing problems with flatulence and abdominal distension that is socially disturbing,

particularly when dining with friends. He is otherwise healthy and does not use any pharmacological agents. What is your next step?

**A**  Recommend the patient tries a period without dairy products.

**B**  Order a blood test for lactase-DNA.

**C**  Send the patient to a dietician for food advice.

**D**  Recommend he tries a probiotic product.

Answer: A

Since the patient is from a geographic region where adult lactose intolerance is common, a formal testing may not be needed if the clinical result is positive and coeliac disease already has been ruled out, which minimizes the risk of treating lactose intolerance secondary to other conditions.

**3**  One of your regular IBS patients is seeking advice for increasing problems with abdominal pain related to her constipation-predominant IBS that has been a more or less lifelong companion to her. She is now 62 years old and has mild diabetes that has responded well to dietary intervention and hypertension treated with a beta-blocker. The last year has been terrible for her after her husband died in a car accident. A physical examination reveals nothing alarming and routine laboratory tests are normal with her usual haemoglobin level (134 g/l) and a sedimentation rate of 5 mm/h. She normally takes a bulking agent on a regular basis and an osmotic laxative PRN to have a daily bowel movement and thereby decreased abdominal pain for the most part of the day, a strategy that is now failing. She has read about a new drug intended for her symptom profile, prucalopride, and would like to try it. A bit ashamed, she also asks for a sleeping pill, since her normal good nights sleep still has not returned to normal after the death of her husband. What will your recommendation to her be?

**A**  Order a colonoscopy before deciding further.

**B**  Recommend a trial period with a SSRI.

**C**  Recommend a trial period with a tricyclic antidepressant (TCA).

**D**  Prescribe prucalopride as requested.

Answer: B

The combination of increased IBS-symptoms and a possibility of a sleep-disorder related to a depression after the death of her husband make a trial period with a SSRI reasonable. This may have dual positive effects, both for her IBS-related abdominal pain and a parallel psychiatric problem. A TCA could be an alternative but the dosage intended for IBS may not suffice for her possible depressive problem. Prucalopride still does not have enough evidence for this clinical situation, but is intended for females with functional constipation where treatment with standard laxatives has failed. A colonoscopy in a patient without any alarm symptoms or findings is not likely to lead to significant findings.

4 A 40-year-old female patient with IBS diagnosed in a city nearby, from where she has just moved to live in your catchment area, has an appointment in your primary care outpatient clinic. The main problem for years is terrible abdominal pain. Because of the associated constipation she takes a random mixture of bulking agents, osmotic and irritant laxatives. After opening her bowels, there is an hour of slight abdominal pain relief and, because of that, her treatment goal is to have a bowel movement at least twice daily. She also has a diagnosis of fibromyalgia and suffers from frequent attacks of migraine headache, the latter as often as every second day and for which she justifies the use of codeine analgesics. Since she has been told that every patient has the right to receive a good analgesic treatment, she now wants you to prescribe a better painkiller. A friend of hers with rheumatoid arthritis has oxycodone that seems very effective. Which treatment approach may help this patient?

A Tell the patient you cannot help her and end the consultation.

B A two-week trial period with oxycodone bid.

C Suggest a consultation with a gastroenterologist aiming at a multi-disciplinary approach to her complex pain and GI problem where there seems to be a risk for her to develop drug addiction.

D Suggest a consultation with a psychiatrist aiming at an evaluation of psychiatric comorbidity and risk for drug addiction.

Answer: C or D

If the local resources allow for a multidisciplinary approach guided by a gastroenterologist this is probably the preferred option for a patient who does not recognize the impact of psychosocial factors on her symptom burden. If agreed upon, a primary psychiatric counselling is an option as good as (c), as long as the referring doctor continues to take care of her IBS-problem. Opioid analgesics must not be used for IBS-related abdominal pain.

5 A woman, 23 years of age, attending your primary care office for long-standing diarrhoea-predominant IBS, has found out that a FODMAP diet approach is helping her quite a lot. She has fewer problems with intestinal gas and bloating and fewer bowel movements per day.

After a 10-day Penicillin V treatment for streptococcal tonsillitis she experienced a definite improvement of the gas-related symptoms. After studying information on the Internet she now would like to try rifaximin. What do you do?

**A** Tell her that, for the moment, our knowledge is not sufficient to recommend this treatment outside clinical trials, and that the best option for her is to continue with her dietary modification.

**B** Prescribes rifaximin 550 mg tid for two weeks.

**C** Tell her that this is a treatment option she will not get and that gut bacteria has nothing to do with IBS.

**D** Send her to the gastroenterologist to see if they can check for SIBO by the use of small bowel aspirate culture.

Answer: A

Antibiotic treatment in IBS cannot be recommended at this time and the clinical use of small bowel culture in a patient without risk factors for small intestinal bacterial overgrowth has low diagnostic value. Even so, an open-minded approach to continuing research regarding the potential role of gut microbiota in IBS should be discussed.

# PART 4

# What's next in Irritable Bowel Syndrome

# CHAPTER 15

# Diagnostic and Therapeutic Horizons for Irritable Bowel Syndrome

*Jan Tack*

Translational Research Center for Gastrointestinal Disorders (TARGID), University of Leuven, Leuven, Belgium

---

**Key points**

***Diagnostic horizons for IBS***

- Physician awareness and application of a positive diagnosis of IBS needs to be increased.
- Tools to facilitate positive diagnosis are needed.
- The search for reliable biomarkers is continuing.
- The role of gluten sensitivity and other food factors in IBS deserves further studies.

***Therapeutic horizons for IBS***

- Drug development has been hampered by the heterogeneous nature of IBS.
- The 'zero tolerance' for adverse events for IBS drugs needs to be overcome.
- Titrating therapeutic approaches to severity levels of IBS may help to overcome some of the current regulatory biases in this condition.
- Current focus is on luminally acting agents, but there is a clear need for novel centrally acting agents.
- Improved physician communication skills may improve satisfaction in management of IBS patients.
- Patient education, using group sessions or digital media, may contribute to symptom improvement.

---

## Introduction

Irritable bowel syndrome (IBS) is one of the most common disorders seen by physicians, not only at the internist or gastroenterologist level, but also at the primary care level [1, 2]. In spite of its high prevalence, physicians often consider the diagnosis and, especially, the management of IBS

---

*Irritable Bowel Syndrome: Diagnosis and Clinical Management*, First Edition.
Edited by Anton Emmanuel and Eamonn M.M. Quigley.
© 2013 John Wiley & Sons, Ltd. Published 2013 by John Wiley & Sons, Ltd.

patients challenging, or even frustrating in some of the more difficult cases [3–5]. This chapter reviews some of the challenges with IBS management and provides an outlook of approaches that may help to overcome them in the near future.

## Challenges in managing IBS in clinical practice

Several factors contribute to the unease of physicians towards the management of IBS patients, including a sense of diagnostic uncertainty and the perceived lack of effective therapeutic interventions. Moreover, a large proportion of physicians consider IBS not so much a currently poorly explained gastrointestinal disorder but rather a psychosomatic condition and, therefore, outside of the usual (organic) scope of medicine [6]. IBS patients, and especially those with more severe symptoms, are characterized by higher levels of anxiety, neuroticism and a tendency towards pain catastrophizing [7, 8], and physicians may experience more difficulty interacting with patients with these personality traits.

'Refractory' IBS patients, who respond poorly to several pharmacotherapeutic interventions, who continue to seek medical aid or further diagnostic procedures, or those who are incapacitated by their symptoms, are especially difficult to manage. These patients may experience reluctance of physicians to treat them or even clear rejection, which may lead them to 'doctor shopping' with health care overuse, or to seeking relief in alternative and complementary medicine [9].

## IBS diagnosis and diagnostic uncertainties

### Historical perspective

For a long time, a diagnosis of IBS has been considered a diagnosis of exclusion and many physicians currently in clinical practice were taught to exclude organic disease in case of presumed IBS. This approach suggests extensive diagnostic evaluation before a diagnosis of IBS can be made, and this may lead to excessive use of technical examinations with low relevant yield, especially in the patient with refractory symptoms. In addition, inherently this principle is associated with persisting diagnostic uncertainty, as an exhaustive work-up to exclude all possible underlying organic disease is not feasible in practice. International consensus and guidelines have abandoned the concept of diagnosis of exclusion for IBS and clinicians are consistently encouraged to make a positive diagnosis of IBS using the Rome criteria [1, 10–14].

## Positive diagnosis of IBS

Evidence from population surveys and cross-sectional patient studies shows that the majority of IBS patients undergo technical examinations which are unlikely to be necessary [15–20]. These observations may reflect either inadequate knowledge of symptom-based criteria or persisting diagnostic uncertainty when physicians are dealing with IBS patients.

There is strong evidence from the literature that primary care physicians, internists and even gastroenterologists are unaware of the Rome criteria, or do not use them in clinical practice [20–22]. These observations suggest that a major educational effort is needed to increase the awareness of the existence of these criteria by practicing physicians and how to use them to avoid unnecessary diagnostic investigations. On the other hand, Rome diagnostic criteria have been criticized as being too complex or too restrictive or not in line with clinical practice reality [23, 24]. An easier-to-use form or version of the diagnostic IBS criteria is therefore desirable, for example using screening questionnaires (in paper or electronic application form) that the patient can fill out, or through an easier-to-understand phrasing of symptom and duration criteria. Moreover, strong evidence that Rome and other diagnostic criteria for IBS are accurate is still lacking, and the best available data used Rome I criteria [25]. Indeed, in a cohort of patients with IBS according to Rome I criteria, Vanner *et al.* showed that symptom criteria and the absence of alarm features had a positive predictive value of 98% for IBS. Similar data are currently lacking for the more recent Rome II and III iterations. Hence, in addition to improving awareness and applicability of diagnostic criteria, further validation of the diagnostic accuracy of the Rome criteria and their ability to avoid diagnostic additional investigations is mandatory to increase their appeal.

## Diagnostic uncertainty

Diagnosing IBS based on symptom pattern alone remains challenging, even to experienced clinicians, because the symptoms are not truly specific, symptoms may vary over time and a multitude of organic diseases may mimic IBS [12]. In the absence of a reliable biomarker, and with a lack of therapeutic interventions whose success may confirm a tentative diagnosis, diagnostic uncertainty is most likely to linger in the physician who is confronted with a patient who responds poorly to traditional management. It is conceivable that such uncertainties contribute to the high number of technical examinations that IBS patients are exposed to, and to the increased likelihood for IBS patients to undergo abdominal surgical interventions, whose necessity can also be questioned [15–19, 26–28].

## Stool markers

A number of faecal biomarkers, mainly protease resistant neutrophil derived proteins, have been evaluated for their potential to noninvasively detect mucosal inflammation in the gastrointestinal tract. Calprotectin is present in the cytoplasm of neutrophils, it resists metabolic degradation by intestinal bacteria and is stable for up to one week at room temperature. Therefore, it has the potential to provide an attractive screening tool for intestinal inflammation. Several studies have evaluated the ability of faecal calprotectin measurement by enzyme-linked immunosorbent assay (ELISA) to distinguish IBS from inflammatory bowel disease, and most of these find diagnostic accuracies of 80% or higher [29]. In contrast, the accuracy of faecal calprotectin testing to screen for colorectal neoplasia is insufficient. Lactoferrin is another marked derived from neutrophils which is resistant to proteolysis in the faeces and can be measured in stool by ELISA to screen for organic disease. Several studies have evaluated the accuracy of this test to identify organic disease with sensitivities of 78% and higher and specificities of 67% and higher [30]. The numbers of subjects in these studies are relatively limited and large-scale studies assessing the clinical application of faecal inflammatory marker testing in patients suspected to have IBS, to select those undergoing further work-up, including colonoscopy, are still needed before these tests can be added to routine clinical work-up. A number of other markers, including faecal myeloperoxidase, lysozyme and polymorphonuclear-elastase for the detection of intestinal inflammation, and assays for tryptase and eosinophil cationic protein for the detection of food hypersensitivity and are still under evaluation [31, 32].

## Serum markers

More recently, based on analysis of serum markers that differentiated subjects with IBS from those without IBS, a 10-biomarker algorithm was proposed, which could serve as an aid in the diagnosis of IBS [33]. The panel consists mainly of markers linked to (intestinal) inflammatory processes, and placebo therapeutic response in IBS was shown to be associated with baseline levels or evolution over time of some of the markers [34], suggesting that some of them may be relevant to IBS symptom generation. However, current diagnostic accuracy (70%) and positive and negative predictive values (respectively 81 and 64%) seem below a clinically useful level, and clearly further studies are needed before this panel can be implement in diagnostic management, especially for difficult patients.

## Gluten sensitivity

Coeliac disease is one of the few organic conditions which guidelines recommend to exclude in IBS patients with diarrhoea, especially in areas with an increased background prevalence of coeliac disease [35, 36].

Recently, gluten sensitivity has emerged as a condition separate from coeliac disease, and related to IBS. Patients with gluten sensitivity present with IBS-like symptoms, do not have classical serological markers for coeliac disease such as immunoglobulin A tissue transglutaminase antibodies, but respond to exclusion of gluten from the diet [37]. At present, it is unclear whether gluten sensitivity is a specific mechanism, related to immune activation and antigliadin antibodies, or whether this is nonspecific, related to a broader context of increased mucosal permeability and low-grade intestinal inflammation in response to a number of food allergens, of which gluten is only one [38]. Continuing and future studies will be needed to determine the role of gluten, and other food hypersensitivities, in triggering IBS symptoms [39].

## Treatment of IBS patients

### General considerations

The management of IBS patients is challenging and, to general practitioners, IBS is amongst the conditions where patient satisfaction is most difficult to achieve [40]. Besides diagnostic uncertainty and difficulties related to psychosocial comorbidities and personally traits in IBS, the lack of effective therapeutic modalities has been a major factor. From a pharmacotherapeutic point of view, the unmet need in IBS remains major [41]. A number of behavioural and psychotherapeutic treatments have shown efficacy in IBS, but to the average physician they are outside of the usual therapeutic approaches and they are difficult to organize in everyday practice [42].

### Drug development in IBS

Drug development for IBS has been hampered by the heterogeneous nature of the condition, both in underlying pathophysiological mechanisms and in comorbidities and overlap with other functional gastrointestinal disorders. Traditionally, altered intestinal motility has been considered the primary target in IBS; this has led to the development of antispasmodics and antidiarrhoeals, with demonstrable efficacy, but small margins over placebo and highly variable availability in different countries [41]. During the last decade, visceral hypersensitivity has been the main target for new drug development but this approach has suffered from poor translation from animal models to clinical reality, and from inadequate methodologies to assess colorectal sensitivity in humans [43, 44]. Hence, in spite of a research focus on visceral sensitivity modulation, new drugs with demonstrable efficacy in IBS, such as tegaserod, alosetron and cilansetron, mainly altered intestinal motility, and hence were targeted towards stool-pattern-specific subtypes of IBS [45]. However, the efficacy over placebo for these drugs was considered low by some authors and the drugs are no longer widely available due to concerns over associated adverse events.

## Risk–benefit and severity issues in IBS

A major problem with IBS is the broad symptom profile description and low frequency threshold of the symptom-based definitions for diagnosing IBS [1, 46]. Population surveys based on Rome and other criteria generate impressively high prevalence numbers, reaching approximately 10% or more of the adult population [15, 47]. The assumption that a condition with such high prevalence can hardly be considered a true or major disease has had major implications for the approval and risk–benefit appraisal of newly developed drugs. Alosetron, with established efficacy in diarrhoea-predominant IBS, was withdrawn from the market because of the occurrence of severe constipation and, especially, because of an associated low-prevalence risk of ischemic colitis; cilansetron was not approved for the same reason [45, 48]. Use of alosetron in a restricted access risk management plan in the United States revealed acceptable tolerability (low incidence of ischemic colitis and constipation without major consequences) and good safety in 29 072 treated patients [49]. Tegaserod, with established efficacy in constipation-predominant IBS, was withdrawn worldwide because of an imbalance in pooled 'cardiovascular events' that was observed in an update of the trial database [45, 50]. Subsequent larger studies have questioned this signal [51, 52].

The regulatory decisions in these cases reveal a tendency for 'zero tolerance' for any perceived risk with a drug for a non-life-threatening condition like IBS. The efficacy of benefit for symptoms and quality of life improvement with these drugs was clearly considered of secondary importance compared to the safety profile. Considerations of safety (including development of bacterial antibiotic resistance) over efficacy are also likely to have played a role in the US Food and Drug Administration's decision not to approve rifaximin for IBS after two positive phase 3 studies [53, 54].

The high epidemiology numbers suggest that IBS is a common disorder, and part of daily life, and this may play a role in some of the regulatory decisions regarding drugs for IBS. However, the majority of subjects with IBS symptoms in the community will never consult a physician for their symptoms, and in clinical practice IBS patients also display a broad range of symptom severity and impact. A subset of IBS patients has symptoms with important severity (e.g. abdominal pain) and with major impact on daily life. In these patients, the tolerance of (mild to moderate) adverse events for a drug with demonstrable efficacy could arguably be considered to be higher, and this is in fact supported by surveys of risk acceptance and therapeutic efficacy balance in IBS patients [55, 56]. A well-accepted and validated severity scale for IBS should be introduced in future clinical trials and decisions whether or not to approve a drug should consider different severity levels of the disease. This should include the ability to use drugs of proven efficacy that have a potential for mild to moderate adverse events, but to restrict their use to more severely affected patient subgroups.

## Current therapeutic developments for IBS

In response to the perceived 'zero tolerance' for adverse effects with IBS drugs at the regulatory level, drug development has switched to locally acting agents. Lubiprostone and linaclotide act from the lumen to promote secretion and alleviate IBS with constipation symptoms [57, 58]. Probiotics and prebiotics are an area of intense research for the treatment of IBS [59]. Other novel approaches with a potentially attractive safety profile are under evaluation. These include the spherical carbon absorbent AST-120 (Zysa®), which has shown potential benefit for the treatment of nonconstipating IBS [60]. These effects may be related to this carbon compound's ability to adsorb a number of irritant substances in the lumen, such as bile acids, bacterial products, histamines, serotonin and others. Another approach is the use of exogenously administered bile acids or the use of an ileal bile acid transporter to improve constipation [61, 62].

Treatment approaches such as these, restricted to actions in the gut lumen and on the mucosa, are likely to have a very reassuring safety profile, but will not address the central components, such as dysfunction of the brain–gut axis and psychosocial comorbidities that are an important part of IBS presentation in a large group of patients [63]. For these patients, centrally acting agents (antidepressants) can be used but their efficacy throughout different studies, many of them of small size, has been inconsistent [42]. Unfortunately, there is a lack of novel centrally acting agents being developed for IBS at the present time.

## Non-pharmacological management options in IBS

Patients expect adequate information, willingness to listen and support from their treating physician [64]. Physicians, especially in primary care, have difficulty providing satisfactory management of patients with IBS [40]. Specialists also feel less comfortable, and may even develop a sense of frustration, when dealing with patients with more resistant IBS symptoms [3–6, 65]. Enhancement of physicians' communication skills is likely to improve physicians' attitude towards these and other patients, and is not necessarily difficult to organize. There is evidence that a brief, physician-directed educational class may improve some of these uncertainties and attitudes [40, 65].

Patients with refractory IBS symptoms may experience lack of symptom relief, lack of empathy and even stigmatization and rejection in their contacts with the medical community [4]. Some of these experiences are likely to contribute to the high prevalence of alternative and complementary medicine use in IBS patients [9]. Emerging evidence shows that one or more education sessions, delivered either in group therapy or through an Internet-based care network, is able to generate significant symptom improvement in the short and long term [66, 67]. These measures may promote self-management by patients, as part of or complementary too pharmacotherapy. Organizing these types of sessions should be considered for centres with an interest in IBS and other functional gastrointestinal disorders. Organizing and implementing such sessions may benefit from involvement of dedicated 'practice nurses' devoted to interacting with and counselling IBS patients [68]. Dedicated nurses are likely to maintain a longer-lasting dialogue with the patients, allowing them to evaluate responses to previous therapeutic interventions, to identify triggering factors and participate in the management approach, thereby improving overall treatment outcomes in IBS patients.

# References

1 Longstreth GF, Thompson WG, Chey WD *et al*. Functional bowel disorders. *Gastroenterology* 2006;130:1480–1491.

2 Hungin AP, Whorwell PJ, Tack J and Mearin F. The prevalence, patterns and impact of irritable bowel syndrome: an international survey of 40000 subjects. *Aliment Pharmacol Ther* 2003;17: 643–650.

3 Blankenfeld H, Mehring M and Schneider A. Diagnostic uncertainty: irritable bowel syndrome in general practice. *MMW Fortschr Med* 2011;153(32–34):27–29.

4 Dixon-Woods M and Critchley S. Medical and lay views of irritable bowel syndrome. *Fam Pract* 2000;17(2):108–113.

5 Olden KW and Brown AR. Treatment of the severe refractory irritable bowel patient. *Curr Treat Options Gastroenterol* 2006;9(4):324–330.

6 Gladman LM and Gorard DA.General practitioner and hospital specialist attitudes to functional gastrointestinal disorders. *Aliment Pharmacol Ther*. 20031;17(5):651–654.

7 Tkalćić M, Hauser G and Stimac D. Differences in the health-related quality of life, affective status, and personality between irritable bowel syndrome and inflammatory bowel disease patients. *Eur J Gastroenterol Hepatol* 2010;22(7):862–867.

8 Lackner JM and Quigley BM. Pain catastrophizing mediates the relationship between worry and pain suffering in patients with irritable bowel syndrome. *Behav Res Ther* 2005;43(7):943–957.

9 Kong SC, Hurlstone DP, Pocock CY *et al*. The incidence of self-prescribed oral complementary and alternative medicine use by patients with gastrointestinal diseases. *J Clin Gastroenterol* 2005;39(2):138–141.

10 Thompson WG, Longsteth GF, Drossman DA *et al*. Functional bowel disorders and functional abdominal pain. *Gut* 1999;45(suppl. 2):43–47.

11 Vanner SJ, Depew WT, Paterson WG *et al*. Predictive value of the Rome criteria for diagnosing the irritable bowel syndrome. *Am J Gastroenterol* 1999;94(10):2912–2917.

12 Spiller RC and Thompson WG. Bowel disorders. *Am J Gastroenterol* 2010;105(4): 775–785.

13 Spiller R, Aziz Q, Creed F *et al*. (Clinical Services Committee of The British Society of Gastroenterology). Guidelines on the irritable bowel syndrome: mechanisms and practical management. *Gut* 2007;56(12):1770–1798.

14 Furman DL and Cash BD. The role of diagnostic testing in irritable bowel syndrome. *Gastroenterol Clin North Am* 2011;40(1):105–119.

15 Piessevaux H, Fischler B, and Tack J. Prevalence and impact of irritable bowel symptoms in the Belgian general population. *Gastroenterology* 134;4:A422.

16 Dapoigny M, Bellanger J, Bonaz B *et al*. Irritable bowel syndrome in France: a common, debilitating and costly disorder. *Eur J Gastroenterol Hepatol* 2004;16(10):995–1001.

17 Bellini M, Tosetti C, Costa F *et al*. The general practitioner's approach to irritable bowel syndrome: from intention to practice. *Dig Liver Dis* 2005;37(12):934–939.

18 Brun-Strang C, Dapoigny M, Lafuma A *et al*. Irritable bowel syndrome in France: quality of life, medical management, and costs: the Encoli study. *Eur J Gastroenterol Hepatol* 2007;19(12):1097–1103.

19 Nyrop KA, Palsson OS, Levy RL *et al*. Costs of health care for irritable bowel syndrome, chronic constipation, functional diarrhoea and functional abdominal pain. *Aliment Pharmacol Ther* 2007;26(2):237–248.

20 Lea R, Hopkins V, Hastleton J *et al*. Diagnostic criteria for irritable bowel syndrome: utility and applicability in clinical practice. *Digestion* 2004;70(4):210–213.

21 Corsetti M, Tack J. Are symptom-based diagnostic criteria for irritable bowel syndrome useful in clinical practice? *Digestion* 2004;70(4):207–209.

22 Charapata C and Mertz H. Physician knowledge of Rome symptom criteria for irritable bowel syndrome is poor among non-gastroenterologists. *Neurogastroenterol Motil* 2006;18:211–216.

23 Quigley EM. The 'con' case. The Rome process and functional gastrointestinal disorders: the barbarians are at the gate! *Neurogastroenterol Motil* 2007;19(10):793–797.

24 Camilleri M. Do the symptom-based, Rome criteria of irritable bowel syndrome lead to better diagnosis and treatment outcomes? The con argument. *Clin Gastroenterol Hepatol* 2009;8(2):129.

25 Ford AC, Talley NJ, Veldhuyzen van Zanten SJ *et al*. Will the history and physical examination help establish that irritable bowel syndrome is causing this patient's lower gastrointestinal tract symptoms? *JAMA* 2008;300(15):1793–1805.

26 Cole JA, Yeaw JM, Cutone JA *et al*. The incidence of abdominal and pelvic surgery among patients with irritable bowel syndrome. *Dig Dis Sci* 2005;50(12):2268–2275.

27 Lu CL, Liu CC, Fuh JL *et al*. Irritable bowel syndrome and negative appendectomy: a prospective multivariable investigation. *Gut* 2007 May;56(5):655–660.

28 Minocha A, Johnson WD and Wigington WC. Prevalence of abdominal and pelvic surgeries in patients with irritable bowel syndrome: comparison between Caucasian and African Americans. *Am J Med Sci* 2008;335(2):82–88.

29 Von Roon AC, Karamountzos L, Purkayastha S *et al*. Diagnostic prescision of fecal calprotectin for inflammatory bowel disease and colorectal malignancy. *Am J Gastroenterol* 2007;102:803–813.

30 Gisbert JP, McNicholl AG and Gomollon F. Questions and answers on the role of fecal lactoferrin as a biologiclal marker in inflammatory bowel disease. *Inflamm Bowel Dis* 2009;15:1746–1754.

31 Turkay C and Kasapoglu B. Noninvasive methods in evaluation of inflammatory bowel diseqse: where do we stand now? *Clinics* 2010; 65:221–231.

32 Caroccio A, Crusca I, Mansueto P *et al*. Fecal assays detect hypersensitivity to cow's milk protein and gluten in adults with irritable bowel syndrome. *Clin Gastroenterol Hepatol* 2011;9:956–971.

33  Lembo AJ, Neri B, Tolley J *et al*. Use of serum biomarkers in a diagnostic test for irritable bowel syndrome. *Aliment Pharmacol Ther* 2009;29(8):834–842.

34  Kokkotou E, Conboy LA, Ziogas DC *et al*. Serum correlates of the placebo effect in irritable bowel syndrome. *Neurogastroenterol Motil* 2010;22(3):285–e81.

35  Spiegel BM, DeRosa VP, Gralnek IM *et al*. Testing for celiac sprue in irritable bowel syndrome with predominant diarrhea: a cost-effectiveness analysis. *Gastroenterology* 2004;126(7):1721–1732.

36  National Institute for Health and Clinical Excellence. Irritable bowel syndrome in adults: diagnosis and management of irritable bowel syndrome in primary care. NICE clinical guideline 61, 2008. http://www.nice.org.uk/nicemedia/pdf/CG061NICEGuideline.pdf (accessed 18 October 2012).

37  Biesiekierski JR, Newnham ED, Irving PM *et al*. Gluten causes gastrointestinal symptoms in subjects without celiac disease: a double-blind randomized placebo-controlled trial. *Am J Gastroenterol* 2011;106(3):508–514

38  Verdu EF, Armstrong D and Murray JA. Between celiac disease and irritable bowel syndrome: the "no man's land" of gluten sensitivity. *Am J Gastroenterol* 2009; 104(6):1587–1594.

39  Eswaran S, Tack J and Chey WD. Food: the forgotten factor in the irritable bowel syndrome. *Gastroenterol Clin North Am* 2011;40(1):141–162.

40  Longstreth GF and Burchette RJ. Family practitioners' attitudes and knowledge about irritable bowel syndrome: effect of a trial of physician education. *Fam Pract* 2003;20(6):670–674.

41  Tack J, Fried M, Houghton LA *et al*. Systematic review: the efficacy of treatments for irritable bowel syndrome – a European perspective. *Aliment Pharmacol Ther* 2006;24(2):183–205.

42  Ford AC, Talley NJ, Schoenfeld PS *et al*. Efficacy of antidepressants and psychological therapies in irritable bowel syndrome: systematic review and meta-analysis. *Gut* 2009;58(3):367–378.

43  Camilleri M, Coulie B and Tack JF. Visceral hypersensitivity: facts, speculations, and challenges. *Gut* 2001;48(1):125–131.

44  Van Oudenhove L, Geeraerts B and Tack J. Limitations of current paradigms for visceral sensitivity testing. *Neurogastroenterol Motil* 2008;20(2):95–98.

45  Ford AC, Brandt LJ, Young C *et al*. Efficacy of 5-HT3 antagonists and 5-HT4 agonists in irritable bowel syndrome: systematic review and meta-analysis. *Am J Gastroenterol* 2009;104(7):1831–1843.

46  Kamm MA. Review article: the complexity of drug development for irritable bowel syndrome. *Aliment Pharmacol Ther* 2002;16(3):343–351.

47  Choung RS and Locke GR 3rd. Epidemiology of IBS. *Gastroenterol Clin North Am* 2011;40(1):1–10.

48  Chang L, Chey WD, Harris L *et al*. Incidence of ischemic colitis and serious complications of constipation among patients using alosetron: systematic review of clinical trials and post-marketing surveillance data. *Am J Gastroenterol* 2006;101(5): 1069–1079.

49  Chang L, Tong K and Ameen V. Ischemic colitis and complications of constipation associated with the use of alosetron under a risk management plan: clinical characteristics, outcomes, and incidences. *Am J Gastroenterol* 2010;105(4):866–875.

50  Pasricha PJ. Desperately seeking serotonin… A commentary on the withdrawal of tegaserod and the state of drug development for functional and motility disorders. *Gastroenterology* 2007;132(7):2287–2290.

51 Anderson JL, May HT, Bair TL *et al*. Lack of association of tegaserod with adverse cardiovascular outcomes in a matched case-control study. *J Cardiovasc Pharmacol Ther* 2009;14(3):170–175.

52 Loughlin J, Quinn S, Rivero E *et al*. Tegaserod and the risk of cardiovascular ischemic events: an observational cohort study. *J Cardiovasc Pharmacol Ther* 2010;15(2): 151–157.

53 Pimentel M, Lembo A, Chey WD *et al*. (TARGET Study Group). Rifaximin therapy for patients with irritable bowel syndrome without constipation. *N Engl J Med* 2011;364(1):22–32.

54 Tack J. Antibiotic therapy for the irritable bowel syndrome. *N Engl J Med* 2011; 364(1):81–82.

55 Drossman DA, Morris CB, Schneck S *et al*. International survey of patients with IBS: symptom features and their severity, health status, treatments, and risk taking to achieve clinical benefit. *J Clin Gastroenterol* 2009;43(6):541–550.

56 Drossman DA, Chang L, Bellamy N *et al*. Severity in irritable bowel syndrome: a Rome Foundation Working Team report. *Am J Gastroenterol* 2011;106(10): 1749–1759.

57 Schey R and Rao SS. Lubiprostone for the treatment of adults with constipation and irritable bowel syndrome. *Dig Dis Sci* 2011;56(6):1619–1625.

58 Johnston JM, Kurtz CB, Macdougall JE *et al*. Linaclotide improves abdominal pain and bowel habits in a phase IIb study of patients with irritable bowel syndrome with constipation. *Gastroenterology* 2010;139(6):1877–1886.e2.

59 Moayyedi P, Ford AC, Talley NJ *et al*. The efficacy of probiotics in the treatment of irritable bowel syndrome: a systematic review. *Gut* 2010;59(3):325–332.

60 Tack JF, Miner PB Jr, Fischer L and Harris MS. Randomised clinical trial: the safety and efficacy of AST-120 in non-constipating irritable bowel syndrome – a double-blind, placebo-controlled study. *Aliment Pharmacol Ther* 2011;34(8):868–877.

61 Rao AS, Wong BS, Camilleri M *et al*. Chenodeoxycholate in females with irritable bowel syndrome-constipation: a pharmacodynamic and pharmacogenetic analysis. *Gastroenterology* 2010;139(5):1549–1558.

62 Chey WD, Camilleri M, Chang L *et al*. A randomized placebo-controlled phase IIb trial of a3309, a bile acid transporter inhibitor, for chronic idiopathic constipation. *Am J Gastroenterol* 2011;106(10):1803–1812

63 Halpert A, Drossman D. Biopsychosocial issues in irritable bowel syndrome. *J Clin Gastroenterol* 2005;39(8):665–669.

64 Halpert A, Dalton CB, Palsson O *et al*. Irritable bowel syndrome patients' ideal expectations and recent experiences with healthcare providers: a national survey. *Dig Dis Sci* 2010;55(2):375–383.

65 Tuinman PR, Oberink HH, Wieringa-de Waard M and Hoekstra JB. Difficult consultations rather than difficult patients. *Ned Tijdschr Geneeskd* 2011;155: A2821.

66 Saito YA, Prather CM, Van Dyke CT *et al*. Effects of multidisciplinary education on outcomes in patients with irritable bowel syndrome. *Clin Gastroenterol Hepatol* 2004;2(7):576–584.

67 Ljótsson B, Hedman E, Lindfors P *et al*. Long-term follow-up of internet-delivered exposure and mindfulness based treatment for irritable bowel syndrome. *Behav Res Ther* 2011;49(1):58–61.

68 Harris LA and Heitkemper MM. Practical considerations for recognizing and managing severe irritable bowel syndrome. *Gastroenterol Nurs* 2012;35(1):12–21.

# Multiple Choice Questions

1 A diagnosis of IBS should be based on:
   **A** Typical symptoms and the exclusion of organic disease.
   **B** The presence of typical symptoms.
   **C** The absence of alarm symptoms.
   **D** Typical symptoms in the absence of alarm symptoms.
   **E** Typical symptoms with a normal colonoscopy.

Answer: D

2 Drug development for IBS is hampered by:
   **A** The absence of a biomarker.
   **B** The heterogeneous nature of the condition.
   **C** The instability of symptoms over time.
   **D** The need for absolute absence of adverse events.
   **E** All of the above.

Answer: E

# Index

Note: Page numbers in *italics* refer to Figures; those in **bold** to Tables.